BOUND
FOR
BROADMOOR

BOUND FOR BROADMOOR

by
Peter Thompson

HODDER AND STOUGHTON
LONDON SYDNEY AUCKLAND TORONTO

To all my friends in Broadmoor
and particularly Charlie, Don,
Dick and Fred.

 First printed 1972. Second impression 1972. ISBN 0 340 14787 3. *Printed in Great Britain for Hodder and Stoughton Limited, St. Paul's House, Warwick Lane, London, EC4P 4AH, by Compton Printing Ltd, London and Aylesbury.*

Introduction

by Lord Longford

No-one, surely, can read Peter Thompson's manuscript without recognising the idealism and the courage that lie behind it. The public spirit is evident throughout, but what gives the book a special, perhaps a unique poignancy and an extra dimension is the tension between his indomitable concern for his fellow human beings and his own psychological afflictions which he describes here without self-glorification or self-pity.

Through all his tribulations in recent years he has struggled nobly to maintain his religious faith and has, in fact, been much sustained by it.

Peter Thompson erupted quite unexpectedly into my own life in 1958 when he called on me out of the blue and insisted that I should play my part in an enquiry into the after-care of ex-prisoners which he was about to initiate. Soon this young and at that time totally unknown Public Relations Officer had collected a group of experts and other representative people all strangers to him hitherto. Without false modesty I can say that the Pakenham-Thompson Committee which followed would be better called the Thompson-Donaldson Committee from its founder and driving force, Peter Thompson, and its amazingly energetic secretary, the present Lord Donaldson. Be that as it may it must be held to have played no inconsiderable part in the substantial improvement in our after-care arrangements since that time. They are anything but satisfactory yet today are perhaps less inadequate that what is done or rather what is not done for ex-patients of mental hospitals of one kind or another. To this latter cause Peter Thompson is now devoting himself ardently and in so far as his fund-raising work for charity permits.

No-one but Peter could probably have secured following his discharge from Broadmoor an interview with Sir Keith Joseph, Secretary of State for Health and Social Security, which is not to diminish the credit due to Sir Keith, who greeted his nervous visitor with the words "How are you Peter? Sit down and have a cup of tea." In a moment Peter found himself reclining on the most agreeable of couches. Against that background the exchange between Sir Keith and Mrs Shirley Williams, M.P. on February 2nd 1971 in the House of Commons is noteworthy. Mrs Shirley Williams asked the Secretary of State for Social Services what proposals he has received for an after-care service for long-stay patients discharged from mental hospitals, and for long-stay patients discharged from special hospitals; and what reply he has sent. Sir Keith Joseph: "I have received suggestions from a former patient at one of the special hospitals that a national after-care service should be provided for patients discharged from psychiatric hospitals, including the special hospitals.

"I am studying the availability and adequacy of the existing after-care services and their need for development." (This exchange followed a meeting Peter had with Mrs Shirley Williams at the House of Commons.)

Peter Thompson recalls that the idea of this book was discussed at a lunch we took part in soon after he emerged from Broadmoor. Certainly the idea began to take shape on that occasion. I am proud to accept any responsibility that

Prologue

The massive gates closed behind me, and I stood there in my ill-fitting suit, various bags, boxes and cases all around me, and more scared than I would have admitted by the sheer spaciousness of the outside world. I felt my inside pocket. The wallet was there, containing ten one pound notes provided by a thoughtful charity – my total financial resources. After four years in Broadmoor I was free at last. I had fought and fought for my discharge, but now that it had actually happened I could hardly resist the urge to turn round and hammer on the gates to be let back in again.

I had relied heavily on that strange institution that loomed behind me, and now, with what seemed almost indecent haste, the prop was about to disappear. Through years of mental strain and breakdown this community of the confused had shielded me from the harsh realities of a world which had broken me – or, perhaps, on which I had broken myself. Now that world lay before me again, and I was going to face the same sort of pressures and strains that had wrecked me before.

Indeed, there would be one extra pressure: the popular idea of Broadmoor as a 'criminal lunatic asylum', and all the associated ideas of violence, horror and madness that people associate with it. I would have to face people who would know how for years I had lived a double life in a kind of mental twilight zone: by day an ardent and well-known penal reformer, friend of peers and politicians; by night a man gripped by dark fears and fantasies, which finally led to a violent outburst, a trial at the Old Bailey, and detention in Broadmoor. My heart sank even lower at the mere thought of it. The mentally ill always carry this extra burden, that sympathy for them is tinged with suspicion. Obviously a patient discharged from Broadmoor would find things even worse.

It was possibly at that very moment that the idea of this book began to germinate. The ordinary person, no matter how sympathetic or 'liberal', cannot be expected to visualise the circumstances of a mentally ill offender. The media concentrate, for the most part, on the more horrific cases ('Mad Axeman at Large', and so on), which attaches all kinds of emotional over-tones to the names of the Special Hospitals, as they are now called: Rampton, Moss-Side and Broadmoor. Obviously people find it very hard to think of the inmates as *people,* or their disorders as very often caused, or at least aggravated, by contemporary public and social attitudes towards the mentally ill.

So I decided to tell my 'story' – not because it is unique, or sensational, or scandalous (though some will inevitably see it that way), but because it is more typical than most people would admit of a whole group of sufferers. In a sense, perhaps I can speak for hundreds of patients in Broadmoor who for various reasons can never hope to speak for themselves. I think I can speak, too, for many others who are aware of emotional problems in their lives which threaten to destroy them, and cannot find the help or the understanding that they need.

I have tried to write without self-pity, or at least with no more of it than is unavoidable in an account of this nature. I am only too aware how much I have disappointed and hurt people I respect and love. And I am not trying to evade responsibility for the things I have done, at any rate where I knew what I was doing at the time. The events I recount reflect very little credit on me, as a person. I know that. But I also feel that they reflect very little credit on the society of which we are all members. That is why I have set them down.

In relating this story I suppose I might fairly be accused of exhibitionism. All I can say is that simply to recall, let alone record, these events has been a costly and painful experience. I would never have attempted it had I not believed that somehow, in some way, this book may contribute something to a change of attitude towards those of us who, almost from our cradles, are 'bound for Broadmoor'.

Chapter I

I WAS BORN on October 15, 1933, at St Thomas's Hospital London. We lived in Golders Green at the time. It was not a happy home. My parents fought endlessly. My father was a professional singer, coming from a working class background, but my mother had a genteel middle class upbringing of a totally different kind, which even poverty could not eradicate. My father beat me, despite my mother's objections, and the inevitable soon happened – they separated. At the age of three I was sent with my sister – who was only a year old – to live with foster-parents, as my mother was working.

All I can remember about this period of my life is that we were beaten badly for stealing food, and once locked in a pitch black rat-infested cellar for twenty-four hours. It is hard to credit, looking back, but it is a fact. My mother knew these things were happening, but could not persuade my father to have us moved. I was always stealing Energen rolls, simply because I was so hungry, and had sores on my body caused by malnutrition. I still bear the marks to this day.

My father was having an affair with the foster-mother, so that whenever I complained to him about our conditions I got another beating for telling lies. However, eventually we were taken away – but by that time I was six and my sister was four.

Father took us back with him to a house in Finsbury Park, in North London. By now the war was on. I vividly recall an incident in the blitz when there was a direct hit on a house three doors away. My sister and I awoke with the explosion to find the windows shattered. I ran downstairs screaming to tell my father and he simply smacked my face, bundled me back upstairs and locked us both in our first floor bedroom.

When my mother heard about this she insisted on taking us away. In fact, father would not let my sister go with me to Swanage, in Dorset, but sent her instead to Gillingham. So I travelled alone to Swanage, at the age of seven, where I was to live with my mother throughout the war.

For a year or two I went to a Roman Catholic convent school, where I got frequently caned for stealing apples from the orchard, but I was very much the boy without friends. I was persistently bullied by a boy who was really quite brutal in his attentions. I eventually persuaded my mother to change my school, and I was transferred to the Swanage Elementary School, where I stayed until I left at fifteen. Unhappily, the beastly boy dogged my steps and followed me there, so that I was under this boy's thumb right up to the day I finally left school.

Mother and I lived in a single room all this time. A man called George Johnson shared the house in which we were tenants, and I really think he was the kindest and gentlest man I have ever met. Kindness and gentleness, as may be gathered, were rather lacking in my childhood. Several traumatic emotional events only served to heighten my sense of inadequacy and isolation. One involved my best friend, John, who was run over by an R.A.F. truck and died soon afterwards in hospital. I can still see his head lolling backwards as they lifted him into the ambulance. He was my age – nine – and his death hit me in a way nothing had done before.

I suppose this was the contrast of my childhood: a great fear of communicating myself to people in friendship (John was a rare exception, which explains my grief when he died), harsh and even deprived circumstances, and a broken home; and on the other side a growing sense of a need to find another world of acceptance and achievement: a private world, at times even a fantasy world. At ordinary 'bread and butter' lessons I was hopeless, unable to concentrate; and I was no good at all at sports. I was even described as a 'backward' child, but I could read and write fluently. I failed entrance exams to three grammar schools, and ended up leaving school at fifteen, as my mother was quite unable to support me any longer.

I went along to the employment exchange to look for a job. The manager offered me two – one as an apprentice to a dental technician, the other as apprentice to a plumber. Not surprisingly, I chose the former, and my adult life had begun.

My mother was unable to get work in Swanage, and so went away to London when I was fifteen. I moved into digs. As an apprentice, during my first two years with the dentist I was earning only fifteen shillings a week, and my board cost ten shillings a week – which meant money for clothes and so on was pretty scarce. After a year or so of this I reckoned I needed more, so to supplement my income, I took on a paper round. This meant that from 6.30 a.m. to 8.30 a.m. I did my paper round, and then from nine to six I did my day's work in the laboratory.

When I reached seventeen another section of my time was mortgaged. I was living at the time in the home of a solicitor, and he suggested that I ought to do evening classes. To do this I needed to travel into Bournemouth, to the Municipal College, as it was called in those days, where I began to study for eight 'O' level G.C.E. subjects, including maths and physics. I needed to do the paper round to pay for the courses.

I had a motor bike, bought out of my precious 'savings', and this was my means of transport. So from the age of seventeen my routine on many days began at 6 a.m., when I got up, and ended at three in the morning when I would finish my revision and 'homework', having driven the twenty-five miles home from Bournemouth, getting in about eleven-thirty. This was my programme for about two and a half years. It was a great strain, but I was conscious – probably too conscious – of the weaknesses in my formal education, and was rather desperate to make amends. In any case, I had few friends, and a schedule like this gave me less time to feel lonely.

I was lonely, very lonely: not that I was lacking social activities during my mid and late teens. I was secretary of the local Toc H, a Sunday school teacher at the Congregational Church, a keen Scout (a troop leader and holder of the Scout cord), a chess club member, an occasional yachtsman and lobster fisher, a squash player, a news delivery boy and a very diligent evening class student. And yet the inescapable fact remains that I was an essentially lonely and isolated person. All this time-consuming activity separated me from people, rather than bring me closer to them.

Where religion was concerned, I had a strangely ambivalent attitude. From the time when I 'moved over' to the Congregationalists – at about fifteen – I had phases of quite strong piety. I 'said my prayers' at night, and was regular at church services and (later) as a Sunday school teacher. I had a strong conviction that God existed, but an equally strong suspicion that He was ineffective: I felt He was 'there' to be worshipped, but could not bring myself to believe that He would actually help me in my life and problems.

I suppose at heart I rejected the idea of a personal God,

and of God 'almighty'. At any rate, while my religion satisfied some aesthetic impulses, it really did nothing to counter my sense of loneliness and isolation. If God was 'there' at all, it was a very long way off; and this remote Being was quite incapable of affecting my rather strange, distorted life in any significant way. Actually, at nineteen I went through a period when I felt drawn to train for and enter the Congregational ministry, but this phase in fact led on into the first major emotional crisis of my life.

Possibly the thought of becoming a Minister, or at least starting theological training, aroused some hitherto dormant anxieties about my own emotional problems. Certainly over the months following my nineteenth birthday I became more and more oppressed by the thought of my moral and spiritual failures. Like many boys, I suppose, I became quite obsessively worried over the practice of masturbation, and this and other anxieties built up, over against my sincere longings to be 'holy', until, at the end of six months or so, I found myself suffering from a severe and worsening depression.

This built up to an intolerable level, and finally brought me to a point of desperation. On an afternoon when the dental surgeon was out, I took what I believed to be a tray of carbon dioxide gas from his surgery, got a dental gas mask and dosed myself with the gas.

I was found collapsed on the laboratory floor by the surgeon's wife, who heard me groaning. I was in fact delirious – the gas I had taken was not the lethal carbon dioxide but nitrous oxide, commonly known as 'laughing gas'. I made a swift recovery. Nevertheless, it was a serious suicide attempt, and goes some way to revealing my state of mind at the time.

Not long after this the dental surgeon broke my apprenticeship and dismissed me – and I only had six months to go as an apprentice. It also meant that my deferment from National Service lapsed, and I was liable to be called up at any time.

A couple of very contrasted jobs filled in the intervening months. First I worked as a trainee manager in a high class hotel, which gave me both a taste for good living and also some social polish and expertise that stood me in good stead later. The second was as a housemaster at a Barnardo's Children's Village.

All I got for my pains, financially, was my keep, but I felt that as a job it was consistent with my hopes of entering the Christian ministry, and tackled the task with a fair degree of fervour. At the age of nineteen, then, I found myself in charge of a 'cottage' with twenty children aged three to fifteen, a matron, two nurses, cleaners and cooks all under my 'control'. My experience at the hotel proved invaluable, but it is typical of a developing pattern in my life that I should find myself in this precocious position.

I was distressed in many ways by what I saw at Barnardo's. On the whole the children – who mostly came from very unsatisfactory homes, many of them broken – resented authority, which represented to them, I suppose, the society which had dealt them such a loaded hand. However, my own background, including a broken home, at least gave me an ability to share in this, and to use my own experience to help them. I took simple Bible study and prayers in the dormitories, and managed to establish a pretty good relationship with the children.

National Service now lay across my path. I was called up in November 1953, and after the usual 'trade tests' was solemnly told that I was to train as a dental technician, which was fairly predictable. For that training I was posted to R.A.F. Halton, near Aylesbury, in Buckinghamshire, where the principal R.A.F. hospital and many associated medical schools were situated.

Within a day or two of getting there, and before being

formally 'signed up', I was taken ill. A doctor diagnosed what he called 'twenty-four-hour flu', and sent me home for a few days to recover. On the train journey I fainted twice, and had to take a taxi from Paddington to my mother's flat in Fulham. I felt really grim, and was not very surprised when it was discovered that I was running a temperature of 104·5°. A friend of my mother's fetched a doctor, who diagnosed not 'twenty-four-hour flu' but acute double pneumonia. In fact I was seriously ill for six weeks, and for a few days there was even some question as to whether I was likely to recover at all.

Eventually I returned to Halton, to be much more sympathetically handled, I must say – perhaps because of the pneumonia incident. I was sent to Bridgnorth, in Shropshire, early in 1954 to do my 'square bashing' – initial recruit training. Almost at once I got myself across some of the minor functionaries of the camp.

As any National Serviceman from that period will recall, the Drill Instructors were petty tyrants of the worst sort, foulmouthed, thick and vindictive. Cheap and vulgar humour was heaped upon any recruit who had a slight abnormality or any degree of sensitivity, and this brutalising behaviour was ignored, if not condoned, by the senior officers.

An additional burden was my continuing inability to achieve satisfactory relationships with those around me. I had no real friends in my flight, although the fellows were pleasant enough, and felt desperately lonely and isolated again. Depression began to return, darker and more oppressive than ever. All of this came to a head with a nightmare experience towards the end of my time at Bridgnorth.

In our billet there were a number of lads from the Durham mines. They regarded me as a bit odd – Southern accent, and a few social 'graces', I suppose – and on this particular night they set on me. They probably meant no more than to have a bit of horseplay, but for me it quickly turned into an affair of horror. They pulled off my pyjama trousers and 'blackened' me – covered my genitals with boot polish. I was sickened and appalled, and a great wave of depression and despair swept over me. I ran to the end of the billet, grabbed a bayonet – we had spent the day bayonetting dummies on a gantry – and cut myself on the chest. Then I pulled a jersey on over my pyjamas, picked up my '1250' (identity card) – an oddly rational action in the circumstances – and ran out of the billet.

It was raining outside, and the camp, a huge one with several square miles of hutted accommodation in neat squares around parade grounds, was lit only by the occasional lights outside billets. I ran along the concrete camp roads, not sure what I intended to do but desperate to get away.

Suddenly, there ahead of me was the guard room, an oasis of light in the darkness, and the two armed guards at the main gates. I hesitated, and then ran full pelt towards the gates. The sentries crossed their rifles to stop me, but I pushed them aside and ran out into the road, across it, over a gate and into a field on the other side. I ran for perhaps a mile, soaked to the skin, my pyjamas muddied and blood-stained, until I came to some cover where I collapsed exhausted and lay on the wet ground sobbing.

Soon all the sounds of the inevitable man-hunt reached my ears – shouts, whistles and the barking of dogs. It took them about an hour and a half to find me, and when they did they dragged me to my feet and frog-marched me back to the guard room. Clearly, so far as the military police were concerned, it was a simple case of an attempt at absconding.

The duty officer was sent for. I was rather incoherent, and must have looked a strange sight in my blood and mud-stained clothes. He got out of me that I had cut myself with a bayonet, but seemed to think that the explanation for my blackened crutch was that I had not been washing myself properly. Then, however, a flight sergeant took a closer look at me.

'Oh, my poor boy!' he said, and explained to the duty officer that I had been blackened. The atmosphere changed from that moment, and the flight sergeant in particular was very thoughtful and kind. An 'SP' (R.A.F. policeman) went with me back to the billet, and in fact slept in that billet each night of my remaining fortnight in Bridgnorth, to see that I was not attacked again.

I was not sorry to leave the place and return to Halton, I must say, though since my original trade test the authorities had changed their minds about my R.A.F. career and had now decided that I should train not as a dental technician but as a dental hygienist. In civilian life this is roughly equivalent to a dentist's nurse/receptionist.

It was at this moment that another turning point arose, and, as it is a very decisive and formative one in my life, I think it is worth recording in some detail.

I was quite friendly with another fellow on the dental course, Gordon. He was a very devout Christian of a kind I had hardly come across before, an evangelical and a great supporter of Billy Graham. This was the spring of 1954, the year of Graham's first big 'crusade' in Britain, in Harringay arena, London, and the papers were full of it.

Now, as I have indicated, I have always considered myself to be a Christian, and for several years had quite seriously been considering training for ordination. So when Gordon suggested I went along with him to Harringay I gladly agreed. It would be interesting, I felt, to see whether this man Graham was, in fact, a prophet for our day, calling people back to God.

In the event, any such detached, objective analysis proved impossible. I was hit, and hit hard, by what Billy Graham had to say and 'went forward' as an enquirer at the end of the meeting. I was given various little booklets by my

'Counsellor', but came away with the overwhelming impression that I had 'surrendered my life' to Jesus Christ and would from now on be living on a different plane altogether.

As it turned out, this experience only heightened and intensified my inner problems. Now I not only had my inability to relate to other people, and also various other not very remarkable personality problems (masturbation among them), but saw these as directly contradictory to my new standing as a man who had given himself to Christ. The contradiction was unbearable. It was like being compelled to watch my own humiliation. Billy Graham had said that conversion would put a 'smile on my face and a spring in my step'. It may have done that for others, but for me, twisted up inside with my tendency to depression and snared by my fantasies, it was a recipe for black despiair.

Within just three weeks of my visit to Harringay things had come to a head. One Sunday, unable to face myself any longer, I went into the 'ablutions' – washroom to the civilised world – with a leather stirrup strap of my mother's which I used on my suitcase. There was a water pipe about seven feet up the wall. I hung the strap around this, and then stood on a table and tied the strap round my neck.

At this point I more or less decided not to do what I had intended – jump off the table and strangle myself. Perhaps, indeed, I had never seriously intended things to go that far. But fate intervened. I slipped off the table and found myself clinging for my life to the water pipe, desperately trying to prevent the strap from tightening round my neck and asphyxiating me. But I simply could not support my own weight and lost consciousness.

Fortunately for me, I was found only seconds later by a medical corporal, my face distorted and on the verge of asphyxiation. He got me down, undid the strap, carried me to my bed – he was from my billet – and massaged my neck.

Slowly I came round, and as I did the horror of what had happened returned . . . the table slipping, the clutching fingers and the moment of bursting pressure as I had fallen.

Being a Sunday, there was no one around, and as soon as I could speak I began pleading with my rescuer not to tell anyone what had happened. I knew him fairly well – he was a very likeable man, a devout Roman Catholic – and I begged him to forget the whole incident, assuring him that in the end it was all an accident. Rather reluctantly, I felt, he agreed, and put me to bed. By morning I was little the worse for my ordeal and tried to put it all behind me. However, that was not to be.

Three weeks later I was sitting in my class in the hygiene school. A jeep drew up outside and four R.A.F. policemen walked into the classroom. One of them spoke to the instructor.

'Thompson.'

As he said my name I guessed what had happened. My corporal friend had not kept his word, and now the whole horrible incident was going to be dragged up again. Actually, it was worse than that. I was taken away by the R.A.F. police and driven, not to the CO's office as I expected, to explain my actions, but straight to the 'mental' block of the hospital, where I was to stay for thirteen weeks.

Looking back, I can quite understand the corporal's action. He told me later that he felt, on reflection, that he just could not accept the responsibility of keeping my suicidal inclinations to himself. He had been worried that it might happen again – and then, how would he feel?

The period in mental hospital was an interesting and perhaps helpful experience. I got psycho-therapy once a week, but probably more helpful, and certainly more pleasant, were the friendships I made there. A shared plight is a great solvent for social barriers.

At the end of the thirteen weeks I appeared before a senior

medical officer, Wing Commander O'Connor. He asked me whether I had at any stage *intended* to commit suicide. I admitted that at one point I had. He then explained that in those circumstances he had no alternative but to discharge me from the R.A.F. on medical grounds.

I pleaded with him, because at last I was finding my feet and settling down in service life, and I also wanted the chance to go abroad. But he was adamant, and so, barely six months after my call-up, there I was on a Metropolitan line train one August afternoon, travelling back to London, a civilian again. My career in the Air Force had not been a happy one, it is true, though recently I had had genuine hopes of 'winning through', so I suppose I should have been pleased. But I was not. And I think if I had had the remotest idea what lay ahead I would have thrown myself out of the carriage.

For the next three years or so I worked for several different Direct Mail firms, first as a telephone salesman, and then gradually inching my way up the ladder to quite a good job as general manager of a small business. However, an unpleasant incident led to my leaving that job.

The owner had brought in a 'partner', an experienced business man from the City, and a few months later he insisted that I offered a 'commission' (which means, in effect, a bribe) to a man who was responsible for placing a large contract which we hoped to get. I refused, for reasons I shall discuss later, saying that I would rather we got the contract simply on merit. He replied, not unreasonably, that it was 'not that sort of a world'. I suppose it could be said that his point was made when we failed to get the contract, and I was dismissed. Still, I took away two new assets: very good references and a driving licence – they had arranged lessons for me, as a senior employee.

The reasons for my strong stand over the 'bribery' issue

are highly relevant to the story of my life and reflected the growing importance of religion in my thinking.

After the Billy Graham experience, I had reacted to some degree, as I have explained: but following my discharge from the Air Force I took up evangelical Christianity again with rare zeal. I began preaching in a Congregational church, but eventually gravitated to that hot-bed of Anglican evangelicalism, All Souls, Langham Place. Here I found many kindred spirits – young business people and students mostly, whose enthusiasm for God and Christ was highly infectious. My association there lasted for several years.

It was a kind of love-hate relationship. On the one hand I loved and admired the fervour and zeal of these Christians, and tried to emulate them. On the other hand I was only too conscious that, in my case at least, the standards were simply too high. Later I came to discover they were too high for just about everybody else as well. From adolescence I had had strong Christian longings. If ever a young man *wanted* to be holy it was me. But, because of my increasingly complicated mental state, I was quite unable to accept myself *as I was,* and felt the need to assume a role which would be accepted in the community of which I wished to be a member. So I tried as hard as I could to act like a fervent evangelical Christian, attending Bible studies, prayer meetings and training courses, being commissioned as a parish worker, and doing Sunday school teaching and house visiting in my spare time. Only years later did I begin to see that, although I could not accept myself as I was, *God* could: indeed, that is what the 'gospel' of Christianity is all about. Whether other Christians could or would accept me was, in comparison, an irrelevance.

In fact, however, as with the 'Billy Graham' experience, a strong dose of religion only served to heighten, rather than solve, my tensions. I was well aware at that time that I was on the brink of further serious mental trouble. Indeed, I even had a private consultation with a West End doctor, who told me that he felt I should be in hospital. But I ignored his advice and continued to mount my tortured treadwheel of social and business success, bearing the lonely burden of my private failings and fears on my own shoulders.

So, for all this mingled uplift and despair, I was out of work; and out of work, as I saw it, for obeying God and my conscience rather than my employer. The whole incident led to a bad spell for me, covering some months. Its outward sympton was unemployment, but its inward cause was the build-up of depression, partly through circumstances, but mostly through my own inner contradictions.

I worked for two weeks at Fortnum & Mason's store, as a telephone enquiry clerk. This involved chasing goods and orders that had gone astray and dealing with customers' complaints. It would have been hard to find a job more calculated to disturb a person in my state. With all the anxieties and tensions I already had, the often trivial complaints and worries of the store's wealthy customers were the last straw.

On one occasion a wealthy Scottish lady phoned with some typically petty enquiry. Just about at the end of my tether, I sat listening to her heavily accented voice and finally interrupted the eloquent flow. 'It would be a great help if you could speak English,' I said.

The poor soul had probably never been addressed so rudely in her life. It takes little imagination to multiply a few similar incidents and deduce why my employment with the firm ended after only a fortnight. This incident was sadly typical of my behaviour at that stage of my life, when the main symptom of my mental illness (an illness which I largely refused to recognise) was the occasional act of almost total irresponsibility, as though I had no personal responsibility for my actions or the course my life was taking. My association with evangelical Christianity served only to heighten, or perhaps rationalise, this irresponsibility, in so far as I believed that every incident in life, however trivial, was planned for me by God, who would always 'see me through'. At times I felt like a spectator of my own life.

I got a temporary job in the Chelsea post office delivering Christmas parcels, and this led to one of the most important developments in my life. Again, I suppose, this belief in a providential ordering of life (a belief which, in a modified form, I still profoundly accept) played a significant role in events.

Among the students working in the post office over the pre-Christmas period was a girl I admired very much. I was delighted to notice that she, like me, was wearing a 'Scripture Union' badge – a sign at that time which performed roughly the same role for evangelicals as the cult handshake for freemasons. We got acquainted, at least to the level of familiarity that was more or less obligatory amongst evangelicals, but without getting to know very much about each other. I did discover, though, that she lived near me in Chelsea – I was staying near Sloane Square at that time with a member of All Souls who had taken pity on me.

Shortly after Christmas I went to a party in Paddington given by one of the curates of All Souls, and there, to our surprise, we met again. This time, fortified not only by our common faith but by the obviously providential ordering of events to bring us together, we became much more friendly. Janet was a qualified nurse and midwife, who was at that stage training at a ladies' Bible college for missionary service in the Congo. She was of average height, slightly plump, with a strikingly good complexion and a very placid temperament, it seemed. I admired her mature faith, her infectious sense of humour and her dedication.

I am less sure why she was attracted to me, though I think probably it was mostly that I needed her, and Janet needed to be needed. I was, after all, a bit of a liability: obviously unstable, unemployed, given to bouts of depression. But in between, and overlaying that, too, I was a talkative, socially alert sort of person, and I shared many of her interests in music and the theatre. Just before meeting her I had finally ended a long-drawn-out engagement with a Dutch girl, to our mutual relief, I believe; so I felt there was no serious barrier to prevent my courtship of Janet.

However, there was one big practical problem. I was broke. Worse than that, I was in debt. Early in 1958 I had moved into digs in Ealing, and by the spring I was in arrears with my rent, owed money to various firms for unpaid bills and altogether was in the red to the tune of fifty pounds or so. That may not seem a vast sum, but to a man on unemployment benefit, with holes in his shoes and no savings at all, it was an enormous amount of money.

A friend suggested that I went to see Sir Kenneth Grubb. He was, they told me, the sort of man who 'helped people in trouble'. Well, I was in trouble, so I pocketed my pride and asked if I could see him. It transpired that he was a former Public Relations advisor to the Rank Organisation, as well as being president of the Church Missionary Society.

He was very understanding and helpful: the sort of man one 'took to' immediately. He wrote a great number of letters about me, though without landing me a job, and then – because he was going out of the country for a while – 'passed me on' to another influential Christian business man, George Goyder, who was to keep an eye on my welfare in Sir Kenneth's absence.

I met Mr Goyder in an office in Whitehall, where he introduced me to yet another churchman, Nevill, who had an influential position in the City. Together they tackled my problem. They paid off my debts, and then Nevill got me a job in the City with an insurance firm. On the strength of this change in my fortunes I got engaged to Janet.

So, with my debts paid off, my engagement announced, and regular work, I had some reason to celebrate at last. For a time, indeed, the cloud over my life lifted. All along my most fundamental problem had been insecurity, stemming from my childhood. Now Janet was there, to provide security and love, and behind me there were two splendid 'father figures' as an apparent guarantee against isolation and social failure in the future. For the first time in my life, I knew something of what happiness means. For a year and more this state continued and, blissfully unaware of what lay ahead, I made the most of it.

Chapter 2

It was Guy Fawkes night, 1958. While the suburbs rattled to the noise of fireworks, the devoted younger Christians of All Souls Church gathered as usual for their 'Wednesday Club', held in the church's hall in Duke Street, near Selfridge's. Here each week over a hundred young men and women, mostly between twenty and thirty-five years old, I suppose, met for a buffet supper and then some sober diversion by an invited speaker. He or she might talk about some aspect of Christian belief, or about missionary work, or a current social problem. It was all very earnest and sincere, and supported by a well-defined social group of youngish business people, students and nurses. Of this club I was treasurer, and, as befitted such an appointment, I took the job very seriously.

On this particular night I had been handing over certain sums to various officials of the club and had about £100 in cash left in my briefcase, which I placed on a window sill in the upper hall.

Later in the evening I was introduced to a man called John Fitzgibbon, who told me he had been sent round to the club by the Rev. David Steele, a curate at St Paul's, Portman Square. Fitzgibbon had been discharged from prison, having served several years preventive detention, and David Steele thought the Wednesday Club might be able to help him. He was a man of about fifty, I suppose. We gave him some supper and talked. Later – and I can only describe it this way – both he and my briefcase, with the cash in it, disappeared.

I rang David Steele, who sounded worried and asked me what I intended to do. I said that it was obviously a matter for the police, as it was not my money. He asked me not to prosecute Fitzgibbon, as he would certainly be sent straight back to gaol, which Steele felt would destroy him completely. I was impressed by this, and agreed only to report the loss of the briefcase to the police, and not to press charges if Fitzgibbon were found. So I reported the matter to the local police.

Three days later I had a phone call at work from the Cardiff City police. They had got both Fitzgibbon and the briefcase, but no money. My address and phone number were in the case, which was why they had rung me.

Did I wish to prefer charges? No, I explained, I didn't. Was I Fitzgibbon's employer? No. Then in that case it was a public offence and the police would prosecute. All right, I said, but I shall refuse to give evidence. If you do, they told me, we shall simply *subpoena* you. The case, they added, would be heard in London the next Wednesday.

Very disturbed by all this, and confirmed in my determination that a Christian club should not be an indirect cause of a man's self-destruction, I rang a Christian lawyer whom I knew, and he agreed to represent Fitzgibbon.

The case created something of a stir. Our solicitor explained to the court that the man from whom Fitzgibbon had stolen this money was in fact paying for his defence. The magistrate was so impressed by this, apparently, that instead of the lengthy spell in prison which everyone expected, Fitzgibbon got off with a short, sharp six months in Pentonville.

It is very hard to explain why I went to such lengths for a

man I barely knew at all. He was not a personable character, but I think it was much more that I could not bear to see anyone crushed beyond endurance. Being so near annihilation myself, I was sensitive about people who were one step lower on the rung of self-destruction than I was. Fitzgibbon was a battered, defeated sort of man, who had had everything thrown at him. Perhaps it was self-identification, but I could not stand by and watch him finished off.

I visited him in prison, too, several times, and when he was discharged we arranged a job for him and a home with David Steele. More than that, Desmond Wilcox, who was a reporter on the *Daily Mirror,* gave a breakfast for him – the whole thing to be covered, of course, extensively in his paper. This gave birth to a new concern in me, which was gradually to assume a major role in my life: the plight of the discharged prisoner. I had seen it at first hand, and also had a glimpse of the enormous power of publicity, properly handled. I decided to do something, somehow, about it.

However, for the present I had other things on my mind. My engagement to Janet had run into all kinds of opposition, which caused us both a great deal of distress. Various people at All Souls had tried to persuade Janet to call the marriage off. This so incensed me that we both left All Souls and began to attend St Paul's Church in Kensington, near the place where we proposed to live after the wedding. In fact, Janet and I were married in that church on February 14, 1959.

Our wedding was, truthfully, a bit of a farce. The break with All Souls had dealt a shattering blow to my fervent evangelicalism. To be treated like this by people I had considered to be brothers and sisters in Christ, and with whom I had prayed and worked, was quite devastating. I took it out on God by refusing to pray any more or read the Bible. So I went into Christian marriage without Christian beliefs, or at least without Christian *feelings*.

I nearly went into it without a best man, too, because

Julian Inglis-Jones, a stockbroker friend I had invited, who knew rather more about my state of mind and health than most people, declined to take part. In fact he had tried to persuade Janet to call it off a fortnight before the wedding, and would have succeeded but for my going to her in a desperate and emotional state and pleading with her not to destroy me.

All of these events were nagging reminders that my psychological problems had not gone away for good. They had flared up in a severe depression during the previous winter, when I was unemployed, and were, I knew, only lying doggo, waiting for a suitable moment to pounce.

That moment was not long delayed. We had only been married a few months when some of my old problems began to arise again, but in even more insidious ways. It seemed as though the more I took external steps to counter them, the more deviously they worked away at the subconscious level. I began to cross the threshold of a double life, a life that became more and more of a waking nightmare as time went on: a nightmare that was all the more hideous because I could not share it with nor even explain it to those who were closest to me.

A part, or a symptom, of my problem was a state of acute depression, accompanied by irrational fears and fantasies. Some of these arose out of circumstances, but most were the product of my own disordered mind. I was terrified of ceasing to be, of self-destruction; and at times aware of malign forces driving me to that very thing. I had occasionally in the past tried to contain or control these feelings by getting into a car and driving it off on my own. Now I returned to this practice, hiring a car from time to time for a night, and driving for mile after mile quite aimlessly, under a compulsion to isolate myself from my problems. There is, I suppose, a strange isolation about being alone in a moving car, cut off by a metal box from the external world, constantly transient to every external situation. The driver, too, is in control totally, through steering wheel, brakes and accelerator, of all that happens – something I longed to be in my own life. So driving a car was a wonderful release from torment. It was to create a little world in which I was alive and yet isolated from life's cruelties, and in charge of my circumstances.

Not surprisingly, Janet could not understand this compulsion. Once a week or so I would hire a car and drive away, often staying out until the early hours of the morning. Once she pursued me to our front door, pleading with me in tears not to go out. I wanted to please her, but I could not break the compulsion, and I left her weeping on the pavement. The image of that moment has literally haunted me ever since.

Some of my fantasies concerned violence, but most at that time were concerned with the need to establish my own identity as against evil and destructive forces. I longed for people to need me and depend on me.

Perhaps it was this which, at about the same time as the car driving compulsion returned, also compelled me to take up the cause of some of our society's under-dogs. I had always had an acute sense of justice, and any unfairness or disparity of treatment angered and disturbed me – even more than when it happened to me. That, perhaps, lay behind my concern for John Fitzgibbon. It certainly lay behind my mounting involvement in the after-care of prisoners, which escalated after his release from prison in March 1959, despite my private troubles.

The Press had given the Fitzgibbon case enormous publicity, both at the time of his trial and now, on his release. I wanted to use this to get something done about the problems of ex-prisoners – though at that stage I was not sure what it ought to be. I got the services of a part-time secretary and began to try to gain influential support for at least a committee of enquiry into the whole subject. My own M.P., Mr

William Roots, Q.C., put the idea to Lord Butler, the then Home Secretary, but he felt such an enquiry was neither 'necessary nor timely'. He felt I should 'canalise my interest' towards publicising the difficulties of ex-prisoners in finding work, and the role voluntary agencies could play in this field.

However, with support promised from several national papers for a committee of enquiry, I was not inclined to be put off that easily. The Press are notorious for blowing hot and cold, and there was no guarantee at all that they would be so well disposed even in a few months' time. But I needed the support of influential men – men whose names and opinions counted for something in the affairs of the nation.

I worked on the basis of 'nothing venture, nothing gain'. My 'private' secretary – a delightful and lively woman of fifty, an ex-opera singer and still a lady pilot despite the loss of an eye – aided and abetted my plans, and Janet – who backed me wholeheartedly – helped to provide some of the financial support needed to get the project launched. We drew up a list of 'top men', and I began to approach them systematically.

First I got an interview with the chairman of Lloyd's who was sympathetic but could offer no practical help. The chairman of the Stock Exchange, however – Lord Ritchie of Dundee – proved very helpful, saying that I could use his name as a supporter of my cause, and also giving me an introduction to the influential chairman of the House of Lords' Lords Committees, Lord Merthyr. This proved to be a major step forward.

Lord Merthyr could not act as chairman in view of his official position, but suggested that I approach Lord Pakenham (now Lord Longford). That was, I suppose, the turning point in the whole enterprise. Lord Pakenham, unlike so many others, combined interest with a willingness to commit himself. He obviously cared a great deal about the problems of ex-prisoners, and said he was willing to get involved in their cause.

There followed a period of intense activity as I sought to get this committee formed. I had very little money – we were drawing on Janet's capital to keep our heads above water – and no 'professional' expertise, but the timing was right and things began to move.

The next major step was a reception at the St Ermine's Hotel, Victoria – paid for, incidentally, out of my own depleted pocket! But only such an occasion could validate the launching of a genuinely influential committee, even if it was organised by a £10-a-week insurance clerk.

Printed invitation cards went out to trades union leaders, employers, officials of the relevant Government ministries, and so on. Lord Pakenham agreed to chair the gathering, and in the event about eighty people turned up, including most of the men we had hoped would attend. It was a great success, and when the question was put whether the time had not come to set up a major committee to investigate the whole question of the after-care of prisoners, the meeting backed the idea wholeheartedly.* I there and then asked Lord Pakenham to serve as its chairman, members were appointed to the committee, and it was duly named the Pakenham-Thompson committee, with myself as its co-sponsor.

Two days before I had had the temerity to try to phone the Director-General of the B.B.C., Sir Ian Jacob, and to my surprise got put through to him. I explained our hopes for the committee and asked for the B.B.C.'s support through their news department. He promised me nothing, but said he would see what could be done. In the event, and all unknown to me, both B.B.C. and I.T.N. cameras were waiting in an adjoining room during the meeting, and excellent

* The exact terms of reference were: 'To examine the present methods of assisting discharged prisoners to find and keep employment with particular reference to the reasons for the difficulties experienced. To publish a report on these with suggested means of avoiding or overcoming them'.

coverage of its decisions was given in the networked news bulletins of both channels that evening.

On the other hand, Press coverage of the actual gathering at St Ermine's was inexplicably poor. Only the *Guardian,* through Antony Howard, who attended the meeting, carried a story, but once the decision to go ahead with the committee was taken the other papers fell in line and gave it good support.

So the Pakenham-Thompson Committee was formed, and at once received a substantial financial grant from the Leverhulme Trust. It was, I suppose, an ambition achieved. I had proved to myself that I could take on a major task and carry it through, despite apathy and opposition. I don't know how consciously that was a motive in my action at the time. I certainly had a genuine and quite intense concern for the ex-prisoner in the face of society's hypocritical approach to his problems. After-care and rehabilitation, I felt, should begin the moment a man is sentenced, rather than the day he is discharged from prison. But even that would achieve little unless public apathy and prejudice were overcome. I suppose I identified with the ex-prisoner. I saw myself in his loneliness, his sense of rejection, his inability to relate to the society around him. I became very angry when society rebuffed him, and very sensitive to his inclination to withdraw and opt out.

My concern for the ex-prisoner was 'sincere'. That is to say, I was not (so far as I can judge) doing this in order to advance myself socially, or work out my own inner problems: at least, not consciously. But the fact is that at that time I was also deeply ill mentally. The Peter Thompson who mixed with the chief men in the Establishment and made use of the mass communications media to advance the cause of the under-dog, was a very far cry from the other Peter Thompson whom even his own wife barely knew, who drove off on dark, lonely journeys at night, terrified of evil spirits and forces and swamped by a fantasy world too horrible to describe.

Indeed, during this period – the time when the Pakenham-Thompson Committee was being set up – my illness took another sinister turn. On my nocturnal travels I began to take knives, guns and other weapons with me. The reason for this was that I felt sure horrible forces of evil were out to attack me, and the protection of the metal shell of my hired car no longer seemed adequate to keep them out. In my confused state I believed that guns and knives might frighten them away.

I also developed a disturbing desire to pry into the private lives and thoughts of my acquaintances, possibly to deck out my own fantasy world with the realities of 'normal' lives. I even took away private diaries, in order to get some kind of 'power' over their owners, though in the event I threw them away unread. All of this, at least, will show the extent of my illness and its seriousness: an illness, of course, which was unknown to most of those associated with my humanitarian work.

Unknown to me, at about this time Janet approached the National Association for Mental Health, asking them to put her in touch with a psychiatrist on my behalf. As a result of this I went to see the Superintendent of Belmont Hospital, who urged me to become a voluntary in-patient for at least six months. My confused mind saw the whole thing as a plot to get me out of the way, and I refused. However, finally I did agree to become an out-patient of a consultant psychiatrist at a London hospital, and remained a patient of his for many years. He was rather more encouraging than most of the doctors I had seen. He hoped that I would get better with treatment, and put me on a course of drugs. In fact, for the present, I very rapidly deteriorated. My night driving got worse. Not only was I carrying knives and guns on these drives to protect myself from evil powers, but I now took to firing the guns at the windows of houses out in the country. I cannot explain why I did this, because until then all my 'violence' had been of a defensive nature – rather a pathetic protection against the imagined evils that hemmed in and threatened to destroy me. But now aggression was bursting out in these gun attacks.

My morals also disintegrated, and I became quite irresponsible, though in fact I got little pleasure out of odd incidents. I hardly need to add that this part of my disintegration had a disastrous effect on what was left of my Christian faith, and also, of course, on my relationship with Janet, although she was (so far as I could tell) unware of the details of my behaviour.

I was leading a double life. During the daytime I was doing complicated re-insurance in a City office, an active and increasingly well known worker in the cause of the ex-prisoner, a friend and associate of public figures and completely respectable. At night I was another man, gripped by depressive fantasies, driving off into the darkness in hired cars, armed with knives and guns to fight off the demons and firing shots into the homes of innocent people. Many people – journalists, statesmen, lawyers, businessmen – knew the first Peter Thompson. Only my psychiatrist (with whom I was totally frank) and – to a lesser extent – Janet, knew the second one.

Actually, early in 1960 my daytime routine changed too – but this had little to do with my illness. My voluntary work for ex-prisoners was increasingly invading the insurance offices. Phone calls from the Press, lunch-time committees, parcels being delivered – obviously sooner or later there would be complaints. At last the deputy chairman of the firm saw me and gave me an ultimatum: either I gave up my ex-prisoners' work, or I left the company. I took the latter course, and – doubtless to the firm's embarrassment – the *Daily Mirror* ran a story about Peter Thompson losing his job because of his work for ex-prisoners. However, this was not altogether a bad thing for me. As a result of the *Mirror's* story, I had a letter from the chairman of a Public Relations firm, offering me a job as a P.R. executive at twice my previous salary. I was very pleased, as I had for some time felt that I had some flair for P.R., and had hoped for an opportunity to develop it.

I enjoyed my new work, which both extended and satisfied me. Perhaps that was why my night driving diminished a bit and I was not so much on edge. However, after a time my illness began to take on new forms, coming back after a period of quiet with ominous inevitability.

One of these new aspects led to an event which almost wrecked my career in P.R. for good. Over the summer of 1961 I had become quite convinced that a number of prominent journalists were plotting to destroy me. There was, of course, no truth at all in this, but my suspicions had reached paranoid proportions. I telephoned one of these journalists, using an assumed name and purporting to be researching an article on that well-known P.R. man and philanthropist, Peter Thompson. I regaled him with a description of my humanitarian activities, hoping to persuade him to call off the (non-existent) campaign of extermination.

Subsequently, he discovered the rather flimsy little plot and threatened to expose me publicly. Having talked to my psychiatrist he in fact published the story in his paper, but avoided using my name. However, this piece was read by the President of the Institute of Public Relations (of which I was an associate member), who approached the paper's editor and got hold of my name. A Professional Practices Committee was set up to investigate my behaviour, and I was advised to offer my resignation from the Institute 'on the grounds of ill health'.

Following the usual pattern of my life, this wretched business was going on at precisely the same time as the publication of the Report of the Pakenham-Thompson Committee, which saw the light of day in the same summer (1961).

The Report, a ninety-two page document, was published by the National Council of Social Service. It made three main recommendations under fifteen heads.

The first recommended that there should be a department of the Home office 'devoted exclusively to after-care, under a director with status equal to that of a prison commissioner'. The second was that the work of the NADPAS (National Association of Discharged Prisoners' Aid Societies) should co-ordinate that of the Discharged Prisoners' Aid Society (DPAS) and local voluntary bodies with the statutory after-care of the central After-care Association, and that government grant-aid should be made available for certain important projects under their auspices (hostels, case-work, after-care, etc.).

The third recommendation, or set of recommendations, was concerned with the problems of employment and resettlement for discharged prisoners. The question of unstamped National Insurance cards – a long-standing handicap for the ex-prisoner – and the need for encouraging employers to take on ex-prisoners, in suitable circumstances, was central to our recommendations. We also suggested that after-care should begin three months *before* discharge, rather than after discharge.

The Report got tremendous publicity. Perhaps the most striking coverage of all was on the popular B.B.C. T.V. magazine programme, 'Tonight', where Cliff Michelmore interviewed Lord Pakenham. The item began with a close-up of my briefcase (the one stolen by John Fitzgibbon) and Cliff Michelmore taking the Report out of it and saying, 'Out of a briefcase came an enquiry . . .' All of the national papers carried major items, some of them very substantial, and I myself made five television appearances talking about the Committee's recommendations.

Not surprising, with all this publicity, I accumulated an enormous amount of background information, including hundreds of letters from ex-prisoners. Especially these tended to pour in after my television appearances, or after 'personal appearances' speaking about the Report up and down the country.

At around this time the Criminal Justice Bill was about to go to the Lords for its third reading, and I suggested to Lord Stonham that there should be an amendment to the Bill incorporating the three recommendations of the Pakenham-Thompson Committee. He said that if I drafted such an amendment he would put it down with Lady Wootton and Lord Longford, as Lord Pakenham was now known.

I went with Janet to see Gerald Gardiner, Q.C., at his home in Onslow Square – a ground floor flat. He showed me how such an amendment should be drafted, and later Bill Hewitt (C. H. Rolph of the *New Statesman*) helped me with the actual wording. Eventually this amendment was debated. I sat in the 'black box' as Lord Stonham's guest and followed the whole debate attentively. Here at last was the culmination of a concern begun through a stolen briefcase years before – and I could not help reflecting that the House of Lords was debating a subject and a set of propositions that I had been instrumental in bringing to public attention. Indeed, Lord Longford was kind enough to single me out for mention in his speech in the debate: 'I should like to pay tribute to all the members of that Committee,' he said, 'and in particular to a young idealist called Mr Thompson, without whom the thing would never have been started at all.'*

The amendment was narrowly defeated, but the debate had given the Committee's findings tremendous publicity, and several of them were subsequently incorporated into government legislation and administrative measures.

Not long after, I learnt from Lord Longford that Lord

* *Hansard*: House of Lords, 18 May 1961.

Montgomery proposed to make a speech in the Lords on the subject of the after-care of prisoners, and he suggested that I should phone him to offer help and advice. What I did not realise at first was how momentous an occasion this speech was to be. Although Lord Montgomery had sat in the Lords for fifteen years, this great war hero, one of the most admired men of our generation, had never made a speech. And now, for his long-waited maiden speech, he had chosen this, of all topics.

I rang him. He was at first a little surprised at my approach, until he discovered that it was on Lord Longford's instigation. Then he was most interested and eager to get all the information and help he could.

On the day of his maiden speech I had alerted the Press and fed them with advance information. I.T.N. wanted to film an interview with Lord Montgomery as he went into the House, but he declined the invitation – not surprisingly, in the circumstances. There was considerable interest in what he had to say and magnificent coverage in every national newspaper the next morning. Lord Pakenham (or the Earl of Longford, as he should now be called) remarked to me how surprising this was. I did not tell him that it was not fortuitous but the result of careful and painstaking public relations work in advance.

I was standing in the central lobby at the House after the debate, talking to William Compton Carr, M.P., when I saw Lord Montgomery. I excused myself and crossed the lobby to speak to him.

'Thank you, Lord Attlee,' I said, 'for supporting the Pakenham-Thompson Report.' (That very day I had met Earl Attlee at lunch.)

He looked at me distantly.

'Who are you?'

'I'm Peter Thompson,' I replied, 'the man behind the amendment you supported.'

He smiled. 'My name is Montgomery,' he said, not unpleasantly. 'I was glad to support the amendment. The whole after-care service is an absolute dog's breakfast.'

All of this concentration on the matter of after-care began to produce results, even though at first the Pakenham-Thompson Committee's recommendations were not accepted by the government. Before the end of 1961 – and not solely, let me emphasise, because of our work, but because of pressure from that and other sources – the Home Secretary set up a full-scale inquiry into the after-care of offenders. In due course its findings were published and accepted by the Home Office, and met in most respects the very needs to which the Pakenham-Thompson Committee had drawn attention. Perhaps the most important innovation was the setting up of a new body, NACRO (National Association for the Care and Resettlement of Offenders) to co-ordinate all after-care work in this field.

I have dealt with the results of the Pakenham-Thompson Committee in some detail because the whole episode was central to my life throughout a highly significant period. This work, important as it was of itself, gave a validity to 'Peter Thompson'. Without it, I felt I might have disappeared altogether, destroyed by malign forces or simply deprived of any meaning or significance. I needed the Pakenham-Thompson Committee as much as the ex-prisoners, but for very different reasons. I do not think that devalues my contribution to it, but represents a considered evaluation of my state of mind at that time.

In the autumn of 1961 I lost my job. My firm had stood by me splendidly throughout the affair that led to my resignation from the I.P.R., but a letter which I was foolish enough to write to the trade paper, *Advertiser's Weekly,* defending the (anonymous) P.R. man attacked in the Press report, proved the last straw. With genuine reluctance, I felt, they asked me to leave the firm.

Within a few weeks our first child – a boy – was born. 1961, this year of contrasts, moved on into its autumn. I was unemployed, a father for the first time, publicly recognised for my work for ex-prisoners, but privately tortured by an illness that was now mounting in intensity. The past months had seen triumph and failure, light and shade. The next chapter of my life was probably its happiest, as I shall relate, but from then on it was to be darkness, darkness all the way.

Chapter 3

The arrival of the baby threw my already strained mind into total confusion. Frankly, I was in no state to accept the responsibilities of parenthood. I was frightened of this baby; of what his arrival would do to me and what harm I might cause him.

Part of this was due to an odd, almost psychic conviction I had had for many years that I would die before I was thirty. In many ways this had acted as a spur in the past. I could not bear delays over such things as setting up the Pakenham-Thompson Committee, because I felt that in the end I might die without seeing the task completed. I was now twenty-eight and, as I looked at my baby son, I was appalled to think that within two years he would lose his father. I cannot describe how powerful this conviction about death had become.

However, worse even than my fear of dying was the sudden eruption of a new kind of psychotic fantasy in my mind, in which I carried out acts of indescribable violence, laying waste people and property, wreaking an odd, twisted vengeance on society. I think psychiatrists would call it 'defensive aggression'. I felt society was attacking me to destroy me, and the sudden turn of events (out of work, becoming a father, problems in marriage) heightened this. So I fought back. It was like a fight for survival. My night driving increased, and on my drives these appalling fantasies of violence swept over me, hunched there alone in the car. It is hard to convey the cold horror of it all in the coinage of rational language.

Janet became pregnant again in the spring of 1962 – which meant that we faced bringing up two children and paying the rent of our flat out of a gross salary of six pounds a week, my earnings as a kitchen porter – the only job I had been able to get and keep since leaving the P.R. firm.

However, Janet saw an advertisement in the *Daily Telegraph* for a well-known and international firm who wanted an experienced P.R. executive to open and control a new P.R. division in the firm. She sent off for application forms, and I put in for the job.

At the interview I was told that no one would be considered for the job who had not submitted in advance a total P.R. programme for the firm, fully costed and applied. They gave me a fortnight to attempt this. As an added test of initiative, I was informed that no one in the firm would be permitted to provide me with any information whatsoever. I said that this would be difficult – I did not reveal that I was currently working as a kitchen porter in a hotel – but agreed to attempt it. That began one of the most hectic fortnights in my life.

Janet was magnificent. Although by now seven months pregnant, she would spend hours every day at the *Financial Times* perusing company records, building up a dossier on this particular firm's operations. This information she analysed and sytematised, so that I was able to take to work with me each day at the Dorchester a bulky file of material which I could use as the basis of my proposed P.R. programme. Every spare moment at work – tea breaks, lunch hour and any odd moments of inactivity – would be spent on the dossier. In ten days I had compiled a 20,000-word report, incorporating an analysis of the firm's operations and an outline of a total P.R. programme. I might add that it cost me fourteen pounds – more than two weeks' pay – just to get it typed. But it was ready for delivery well within the fortnight they had given me, though no one could have imagined the conditions under which it was produced.

Within three weeks of submitting this report I was appointed group public relations executive – by far the best job I had ever had, involving responsibility for the whole public relations operations of a really major industrial concern. My new employers discovered before my appointment that they were taking on a kitchen porter as a senior executive. They also knew about the incident which led to my resignation from the I.P.R. But they based their assessment on the document I had prepared and on my past P.R. work, and backed their judgment against the evidence of my one serious professional lapse. I was, of course, very grateful to them for the opportunity to get back into top-level P.R. work again.

For a while after I got this job, my psychotic fantasies, and my night driving, eased off. This was partly due to job satisfaction, partly to a happier situation at home. I had accepted responsibility towards my son, and now a second son had arrived as well. I was seeing my psychiatrist every week, and he certainly felt I was getting better.

I tackled my new work with enthusiasm, and also got a second wind on the after-care of prisoners. In 1962 I launched a movement called 'The Society of Character Underwriters'. This was designed to help ex-prisoners in their search for decent employment, by providing them with substantial referees and guarantors. The Pakenham-Thompson Committee had reported that the chief difficulty for the ex-prisoner lay in keeping in employment and settling down to a job. I had come to the conclusion that this was linked with the reluctance of employers – understandable in many ways – to trust a man who had failed in the past. So the work they offered was often menial or required little responsibility or initiative. Strong references and the backing of reputable guarantors might, I felt, overcome this; hence my efforts to launch this new organisation.

All of this happened in a period of about twelve months which, I suppose, was one of the calmest of my life. But it proved to be only the calm before the storm. By the second half of 1963 I was running into serious mental trouble again. I could see the danger signals, but felt powerless to avoid the inevitable. It was the pressure of circumstances that once again began to undermine the thin defences which I could raise against psychosis.

I had taken on too much, I could see that. My job was very demanding, physically and emotionally. My home life was balancing on a slender knife edge. My charity work had really overwhelmed me – and this was now a major emotional problem.

What had happened was quite simple. Through allowing myself to be presented as an 'expert' in the subject, I had become a sort of refuge for ex-prisoners in trouble. The number of them turning to me for help had risen appreciably. This in itself would not have been disastrous if I could have avoided getting emotionally involved in their problems. But I could not. No matter how hard I tried to remain objective and uninvolved, inevitably I found myself desperately caught up in a man's situation, worrying about his problems and identifying myself with his situation. Again, an emotionally mature person might have been able to cope, but for someone like me it was quite disastrous.

I began to have fearful dreams and nightmares, some of them too horrible to describe. I also began to get addicted – almost literally – to horror films. I would comb London to find one I had not seen, in order to drink in for a couple of hours the ugly fantasies of a make-believe world and find some kind of catharsis in the violence and shedding of blood that tended to pervade them.

More than ever, too, I was haunted by 'spirits'. I could not sleep at all without a light on, my bedroom door locked and a pistol under my pillow. My night driving once again assumed dominant proportions. Sometimes, when driving, I would be so sure that the spirits or demons were about to invade the car that I would stop, switch on all the lights inside and outside and try to purge away the powers of darkness with the sheer volume of light. Not surprisingly, relationships with Janet deteriorated, and all the gains of the past two years disappeared in the course of a month or two.

I tried my old device of warding off the fantasy world by getting involved more deeply in the real one. In a sense, I was missing the Pakenham-Thompson Committee, and I suppose I felt the Society of Character Underwriters might fulfil a similar purpose for me, as well as benefitting a really needy group of people.

I had learnt from my solicitor, Rex Cowan, of a doctor in California who had launched a Society of Character Underwriters for ex-prisoners, and I assumed – wrongly, as it transpired – that he was operating an insurance scheme, literally 'underwriting' employers for the financial risks involved in employing discharged prisoners. This seemed an excellent idea, especially for 'white collar' workers, who were the ones experiencing the greatest difficulty in getting suitable jobs.

I approached a number of insurance experts, and the premium level needed to make a scheme viable was carefully calculated. We found that employers were very interested in the scheme, and felt that the premiums could be met out of the ex-prisoner's earnings. Employers would be insured up to £500 should an ex-prisoner on their staff involve them in financial loss. When we were ready to put our plan into operation, *The Times* gave a full column to the proposed new society.

In my own personal life I was becoming more and more seriously ill, though I could still disguise this from almost everybody, except for a few very close associates. My problems were aggravated by the shoals of desperate letters from ex-prisoners which arrived when the Society of Character Underwriters began to achieve national publicity.

It was crazy really – a perfect illustration of the saying of Jesus about the blind leading the blind. Although barely able to carry the weight of my own problems, I was unable to avoid deliberately incurring the burdens of others as well. I could see the inconsistency but felt incapable of doing anything about it. It was like a vicious and unbreakable circle of cause and effect. I saw myself in them, and by some trick of the mind felt that if I could help them I would also be helping myself. In the event, I did, I believe, help a number of ex-prisoners, but I all but destroyed myself.

In 1963 I met Ann, and this was an event of tremendous importance in my life. I met her at my secretary's flat, and we took an instant liking for each other.

I was thirty at the time, and Ann was twenty-five. She was slightly above average height for a woman, dark, with long dark hair, a tanned complexion and a slim figure. I cannot explain our mutual attraction, but it was very powerful. Unknown to Janet, we took to meeting, going to parties together, and even sometimes spending the night together on the roof of the Queen's Building at London Airport, watching the planes landing and taking off, and having breakfast together before going off to our respective offices.

I am not very proud of this episode, looking back, but there was so much more to my relationship with Ann than simply a squalid 'affair'. This is all of a part with my abandonment of long-held principles in other areas – truthfulness, for example. I honestly believe that it was all part of my illness –

a compulsive urge to act, from time to time, completely *against* the 'image' I usually presented to the world. But my friendship with Ann was not 'promiscuous'. Wrong as it undeniably was, it represented a genuine and very beautiful meeting of minds and personalities; and for me Ann was a nurse, not a 'mistress'. It was a costly relationship in many ways, because Ann's friends strongly disapproved of her association with me, and I dared not introduce her into my usual social circle. So we had to create yet another circle of friends, where we were accepted and welcomed, and that is what we did.

But that meant that I was now trying to maintain four sets of friends and acquaintances: those connected with my home, Janet and our relatives; those concerned with my social work; those I met through my work; and those Ann and I now cultivated who were not in touch with our friends and could accept us without question. It was, to put it mildly, a bit of a strain.

I was able to tell Ann about my mental troubles more freely than anyone except my psychiatrist, and I think she knew how ill I was. She once found a rifle in my car, and I told her it was there to frighten off the 'spirits'. She also knew all about my night driving and literally nursed me through bad spells. From 1963 to 1965 this close friendship persisted. We saw each other regularly and were, I suppose, by any normal standard of judgment, deeply in love.

On one occasion, in the heat of the moment, Ann made a remark that was very disturbing to me. We were on a day trip to Le Touquet, in France, and were having a pretty heated argument about something. Obviously I was being irrationally emotional about it, because suddenly she blurted, 'Oh, if only you were normal. . . .'

As soon as she had said it she regretted it, but the words could not be unsaid. This incident was, so far as I can recall, the first occasion ever on which I realised that my mental illness was beginning to 'show'. Until then I had been able to reassure myself that, though I and my psychiatrist knew I was ill, my symptoms were not apparent to the lay eye. Even though I had confided in Ann, until then she had never revealed that she knew I was not 'normal'. And she was absolutely right.

That was in 1964 – a year in which, at a time of great mental stress, I had a rather violent baptism in the stormy sea of industrial relationships, being involved in settling a strike of our firm's van drivers in the Midlands.

But everything to do with my work and my humanitarian activities was a great strain – not surprisingly, seeing that I spent most of the hours which other people spent in bed driving the streets of London and the Home Counties in my car, fighting a secret and lonely battle against the invisible spirits which were threatening to destroy me.

The night car rides were nightmarish. Although I could not see the 'spirits', I knew they were there, as real – indeed, *more* real – than I was. I would keep the interior light switched on, and the windows tightly closed, and drive relentlessly through the darkness in my mobile prison, in a futile attempt to get away from them. Then, sometimes as dawn was breaking, I would return home utterly exhausted and collapse into my bed for a couple of hours' sleep. So it was not surprising that I was acting in rather a strange way at work. Paranoid suspicions made me unwilling to trust anybody, though I retained my affection for my chairman. I was sure that my downfall was being plotted by faceless men in the shadows.

The remarkable thing is that, in this state of mind, I could have carried through some quite ambitious P.R. projects. In a way, they indicate how I had managed to divorce day from night, real world from fantasy, and preserve at all costs a sane and successful appearance for society, while being desperately ill mentally. All of this is important later on, because in one way I was too successful at disguising the degree of my illness, and many people insisted on judging my actions by the criteria of normality.

At any rate, desperately worried and afraid, I went to my psychiatrist whom I had been seeing regularly for several years. I told him that I was carrying guns and knives and having fearful fantasies of violence. But he did not think I was ill enough to warrant admission to a mental hospital.

Ann was my constant companion and support at that time. She spent hours and hours with me when I was depressed. One night I was in Reading, on one of my nocturnal drives, when I had a very serious attack of depression and collapsed weeping in my car. I managed to find a phone and ring Ann, who drove out to Berkshire to collect me and take me back to her flat. I really believe that she was the main reason why I was able to maintain a sane and fairly normal posture during the day, but I leant upon her very hard and it must have been an awful strain for her.

Chapter 4

In 1965 a chain of events began which led on to the major crisis of my life. They began in the area of my work and reflected just this irresponsibility which broke through into my 'normal' life from time to time. The first was not my fault, but led to a breakdown of a relationship which had meant a great deal to me.

I was, as Group P.R. executive, responsible for the Press arrangements at the company's annual general meeting. On this occasion it was held at the Dorchester, and a Press conference was laid on, with the Company chairman in the chair. A journalist asked why there had been such short notice about a transfer of shares. The actual reason was that the firm handling our financial P.R. was short of messengers, and the literature had not been delivered in time. However, the chairman, who was unaware of this, looked at me and then gave an obvious 'cover-up' answer which, in effect, put the blame on me. I thought that closed the incident, but I was wrong.

A fortnight later I went to him to ask for a rise. It was a fact that I was finding it hard to make ends meet – not surprisngly, in view of the kind of life I was leading. However, when I had put my request the chairman replied that the boot was on the other foot and that he had been thinking seriously about dismissing me. He then mentioned the incident at the annual meeting. I tried to explain that it was not my fault (which was true), but he countered that it was typical of my inefficient administrative methods (which was also true). He then said that, at the suggestion of another executive, he had decided not to dismiss me, but to send me on a course in management and administration, and he would arrange for me to meet a management consultant.

I was grateful for the remission of sentence, but I think this was the first blow at the root of a personal relationship with the chairman which had meant very much to me in terms of stability and confidence. I felt he appreciated my loyalty and enthusiasm, but now I realised that he was also aware of my weak points. My administration *was* bad, I could not deny it: largely due to an inability to concentrate on details.

Not long after, I accompanied him to a conference in Great Yarmouth. He was due to appear also on a B.B.C. regional programme which featured leading figures in British industry, to answer questions about the industrial problems and potentialities of East Anglia. I had prepared a 5,000-word brief for him, which set out information on almost any conceivable topic the interviewer might raise, but five minutes before the programme I discovered that the chairman had not even read it.

Incredibly, I flew off the handle completely and, in front of some startled company executives, I told their chairman that he was inefficient, incompetent and did not have the company's interests at heart. I added a few choice adjectives, too. It was like an eloquent plea for instant dismissal.

In fact, he threw back his head and laughed. He patted me on the shoulder, saying, 'Peter, you've got spirit!' – and he also promised to read through the brief before the programme. That was, of course, an impossible task in the time, but he absorbed enough information to get through the interview very successfully.

By now my depressions were becoming suicidal, and events entered a crucial phase. I was aware that, for all that he might feel I had 'spirit', my boss no longer had much confidence in me, and I was terrified I might lose my job. I had a heavy mortgage, a wife and two children, and frankly the responsibility was beyond me. I would spend my nights weeping in Ann's arms – often at London Airport on the roof of the Queen's Building – and my days in continual fear of espionage, betrayal and dismissal. It was all utterly horrible, and it could not go on for long without a disaster occurring.

On Friday, February 5, 1965, Ann phoned me at about ten o'clock in the morning to say that she was going away for the weekend with another man, to stay with a couple at their parents' home. For a long time she had felt uneasy about our relationship, but it was still a terrible and unexpected blow. Shortly afterwards I tried to see my chairman, but he would not talk to me.

I went back to my office in a state of shock. What I had feared for years was suddenly coming true. I was convinced (wrongly, as it transpired) that I was about to lose my job, and I just could not face that kind of crisis without Ann to support me. In the course of a mere hour I felt that the two people I depended on – my employer and my closest friend – had turned against me. I sat at my desk, bewildered and afraid. I knew how hard it would be for me to get another decent job. After all, I had recently applied for a top P.R. job and been interviewed, only to lose any chance of getting it through the intervention of another P.R. man who remembered the impersonation affair. Whichever way I turned, there seemed no escape.

I began to write a letter to Janet. I cannot remember in detail what I wrote, but I know that I told her that I could not face the future without a job, and that the insurances and so on should be enough to provide for her and the children.

I had been stockpiling my supplies of Librium, which my psychiatrist had prescribed for me, keeping them back for just some such moment as this, and now I got out the bottle. I took thirty Librium tablets, and a few others which I had on me, for good measure. I left the letter on my desk in an envelope addressed to Janet, waited for an hour in my office to let the tablets take effect, and then intended to go to the pub across the road to take a couple of whiskies in order to activate the drugs.

In fact, I never got there. I collapsed in the road outside our offices in the City and was soon surrounded by colleagues who had found the empty bottle and the letter on my desk and put two and two together. An ambulance was called, and I was taken to St Bartholomew's Hospital.

I was able to tell the ambulance men what I had taken, and they worked very hard all the way to the hospital to keep me awake. There I was given three enormous glasses of an emetic and eventually vomited violently. From then on, of course, I began to improve slowly, but I lost consciousness and was wheeled into a private ward.

The next thing I can recall is being examined by a psychiatrist. He told me that my firm had rung through telling me that I need not go back to my office. At the time I assumed they meant that in view of my illness I need not worry about getting back to work. He had talked to my own psychiatrist, who had told him that he would like to see me on Monday – clearly implying that he expected me to be discharged from hospital. The hospital doctor told me early on Saturday – less than twenty-four hours after my suicide attempt – that I was to leave the hospital that morning. He also said that he felt the message from my firm meant that I was not to return until I was well again.

Janet came to collect me, and told the doctor that she could not accept responsibility for me. She said that she knew

I would run away and she would not be able to stop me. In that she was absolutely right.

As we left the hospital I told her that I wanted to collect my car from the office. She begged me not to, knowing that if I did I would drive off. However, I went to the office. Instead of simply collecting my car, I went inside and ransacked three offices looking for confidential files, trying to find a non-existent report on my activities and shortcomings. Needless to say, I could not find it, but I removed several case-loads of files and loaded them into the back of my car, along with several suits and other personal belongings from the office, despite Janet's strong protests. The car, incidentally, was a Ford Consul belonging to the firm.

We went home and I spent the afternoon painting. At six o'clock the hospital psychiatrist rang to see if I was all right, and I assured him that I was. I did not tell him that I had ransacked three offices since I last saw him.

In the evening, trying to be helpful, Janet took me to a cinema in Putney. Unfortunately, there could not have been a worse choice of film. It was about a 'bird-man' in a cage, and it completely disorientated me. I left Janet in the cinema, ran outside, jumped in my car and drove off. I did not return home until three o'clock in the morning.

I spent Sunday painting pictures. My mother visited me and remarked to Janet on the strangeness of the paintings. They were, as I recall, my attempts to put into visual form the spirits that haunted me, and I believe they were very ugly and disturbing to see.

At about five o'clock Janet said that she was going to ask George Kerr to come and talk to me. George was an old friend of ours from Wednesday Club days at All Souls, but on one or two occasions in the past – for the best motives, I am sure – he had actually locked me in rooms in our home. Naturally, when Janet said she was going to fetch George, I assumed the same thing was going to happen again. With

E

the awful impression still vivid in my mind of the bird-man in the film fluttering desperately as a captive in his cage, I went completely to pieces.

I ran upstairs to my filing cabinet, took out a gun and some knives, and – wearing carpet slippers on my feet, without a jacket or a tie – dashed out to my car and drove off. I had very little petrol, so I went to a local garage and handed over my cuff links in exchange for a tankful. I then drove off. The time was about seven o'clock.

A girl hitched a lift from me, somewhere in the southern suburbs, and I picked her up and drove her home. She was an Australian, I remember, and we talked for about half an hour, which was the time it took me to reach her address. I also gave a lift to an elderly man and poured out my problems to him.

Soon after – at about nine o'clock, in pitch darkness – three girls thumbed a lift as I was driving through a wooded area near Esher. Because of all the files and clothes on the back seat they agreed to squash on to the bench front seat. They were foreign girls who could speak very little English. They indicated that they wanted to go to Kingston. The oldest of the three, who was about nineteen and had fair hair, seemed, to my utterly confused mind, to be a middle-aged woman with grey hair. My driving, they later reported, was wildly erratic. Sometimes I would swing out over the crown of the road, and cars kept on hooting at me. The girls, of course, were frightened by this.

I drove off up a side turning into some woods, but it proved to be a cul-de-sac. I turned the car round and headed back towards the main road. Then I stopped, switched on the interior lights – my headlights were full on as well – and asked them to look at a map for me. Of course, they did not understand what I was saying.

The oldest girl, whom I have described, was sitting furthest from me. I became convinced that she was an older woman and that she was about to attack me. In my state of mind she looked like the woman who had fostered me when I was very young – a woman who had often beaten me viciously. I picked up a knife from the carpet by my feet to defend myself and warned them not to touch me.

Understandably, at this the girls panicked and tried to get out of the car. I cannot remember exactly what happened, but there was some sort of a struggle and two of the girls were injured. Eventually they struggled out of the car and ran away screaming, leaving me slumped in the driver's seat, weeping hysterically, the car lights full on.

Then I started up the engine and turned the car off the road between the trees, driving desperately through the undergrowth. I thought I heard dogs and stopped my car in a muddy patch, sounding my hooter to attract attention. I wanted to be found, but in fact there was no one there.

When I tried to drive on, I found my wheels had sunk into the mud and I could not get the car to move. I desperately pulled suits and coats off the back seat and wedged them under the back wheels to get some grip. At last, the car moved, and I drove off wildly at a ridiculous speed, through the woods, skidding around trees and bushes, until eventually I ended up with the front half of the car in a deep stream. I tried to pull down a wooden fence to put under the wheels, but I could not. Obviously I was not going to be able to move the car. Almost without realising it, I had waded chest-deep into the freezing water of the stream and now, as I climbed out, I was covered in thick mud and water. I had lost my slippers and socks.

I saw a light through the trees and decided to go for help. I fought my way through the undergrowth and came to the door of a small house. I rang the bell, and two elderly ladies opened it. I must have looked a terrifying sight, hair dishevelled, dripping wet, mud and blood-stained. I told them I had had a crash and that my car had overturned, and asked if I could use their phone. Although they were obviously apprehensive, they let me do so. I phoned the Esher police, choosing my words carefully so as to avoid frightening the ladies, who were listening. I said that there had been an accident, and would they please come and pick me up.

I then tried to phone my home, but Janet was out, so I rang the Putney police to ask them to contact the Esher police and then inform Janet. I was still on the phone when the police car arrived. I saw that it was driving away – they did not know which house I was in, only the location of my car. I ran out into the road shouting after them, and they stopped and picked me up. From all of this, it will be obvious that from the moment of the incident I wanted to be taken into custody. That is important in the light of later events.

At Esher police station I was seen by a police surgeon because I said I had bumped my head. At that point the police did not, in fact, know anything about the incident with the girls and were treating my case as a motor accident. However, I now told them what had happened, and the police checked with a local hospital where the girls were being treated.

I asked to be allowed to speak to a solicitor, but they would not let me. Instead they put me in a police cell and interrogaged me until 4 a.m. I was still in the wet, muddy clothes in which I was arrested, and I was left like that all night, with only a wooden seat to sleep on with a single blanket. In the morning I told a C.I.D. superintendent who came in to question me that I had thrown the knives and guns into the stream near my car. He told me that I was to appear in court that morning (Monday). Later I was driven to Kingston Magistrates' Court and put in a cell to await the hearing. By then, Janet had been able to arrange for me to be legally represented, and she and my mother were in court.

The girls – they were Danish *au pair* girls, I discovered – were asked to identify me. My solicitor pleaded 'not guilty' for technical, legal reasons – a plea which produced cries of protest, I remember, from the public gallery. The magistrate said that he would like medical reports, and I was put back in the cell at the court. Apparently, I started banging my head on the wall of the cell until I was bleeding, so the police moved me into another cell where some young hooligans were awaiting trial, and made me stand in the middle of the room. Possibly my state of mind can be visualised from that incident. I was distressed and shocked, suffering from acute depression and mentally confused.

Soon after that, I was interviewed by some Scotland Yard officers. It slowly dawned on me that they were probing far beyond this present case. The previous night I had been shown photographs of some women and asked if I had ever seen them before. I answered truthfully that I had. In my confusion, I did not add that I had only seen them in the newspapers. Now the Yard officers were pushing me hard about these women, going back over dates a year or more earlier and asking where I had been on certain nights. Only slowly did I realise that they thought that they might have stumbled across the killer in the notorious and unsolved 'nude murders' which had attracted enormous publicity.

Later I learnt that they went to my firm, and also to Ann, to check on my whereabouts on the dates of these murders. Fortunately for me, Ann had kept a diary, which showed that I had been with her on most of the nights in question, and my firm were able to prove that on the occasion of the sixth murder I was addressing 120 senior executives and directors at a business conference – which, as alibis go, is a reasonable one. Reluctantly, I felt, the police were compelled to accept that once again they had failed to find this elusive criminal who – in point of fact – was never apprehended, though I believe the case was finally and rather mysteriously 'closed' in 1970.

Anyone could see, as I stood in that cell, that I was ill. I had a violent headache, I was shivering uncontrollably, and my mind was completely disorientated. I had never, at any stage, made the slightest attempt to resist or even avoid arrest. Indeed, to all intents and purposes I had given myself up. Yet now I was to face one of the most horrible experiences of my life, during the journey from Kingston Court to Brixton Prison, where I was to stay on remand. I was led up from the cells by a couple of police officers, along with other people on remand, and put into what is often known as a 'meat wagon'. It is a sort of mobile prison, with twelve tiny cells, just big enough for one man to sit in, six each side. I was put into one of these cubicles and the door was locked. There was barely room to move. There was a double glazed window of frosted glass, and between the panes – I learnt later – was a capsule of gas which would be released if the glass were broken and would render the occupant instantly unconscious.

I was terrified. It is not hard to imagine my state of mind – it was the bird-man come true. I felt stifled and hemmed in, confused and panic-stricken. I began to cry and scream, pounding on the door. Eventually someone took some notice, and a policeman opened the door. He could see the state I was in, and very thoughtfully said he would leave the door unlocked. He also offered me a cigarette, but in fact I was not, at that time, a smoker.

We made our way first to Wandsworth Prison, where we all had to get out. Some were to stay here, but the rest of us were transferred to another wagon. A policeman grabbed me and held my arm behind my back, frogmarching me with a quite needless show of force to the waiting vehicle.

Our next stop was Brixton Prison, where I was to stay on remand. If I had known then how long that was to be I believe I should have done something desperate. In fact, I was barely aware of what was happening. The whole thing seemed like some kind of awful, inevitable nightmare in which I had been cast for a leading role.

I was taken to prison reception, which is, on any account, a very peculiar experience. I was still in the clothes in which I had been arrested – mud-stained and torn. I was still, incredibly, without shoes or socks. It is as if the whole object of the exercise of arrest and prosecution is to dehumanise you and take away any last remnants of self-respect. At least I was now able to get rid of those clothes and put on clean, dry, prison clothes (not uniform, of course), shoes and socks. I also had a bath – under strict supervision. Then I was locked in a tiny cell – no bigger than four feet by three – along with two other men on remand. There was not even room to sit down on the floor, yet we stayed there for four hours, from 2 p.m. to 6 p.m.

The other two – who were up for theft – began to fill me in on prison life. As old hands, they obviously felt they ought to help out a new boy. I was grateful for one piece of advice which proved very valuable. 'Say you're depressed,' they told me, 'it's the only way to get out of being locked up twenty-three hours a day.'

Eventually I saw the prison doctor, who examined me cursorily, presumably to see that I was clear of infectious diseases or bugs. When he had finished, he asked me if there was anything I wanted to tell him.

'Yes,' I said, 'I'm feeling depressed.'

Whereupon, exactly as my cell-mates had prophesied, he arranged for me to be put in the hospital block of the prison.

This block is in a separate wing of the prison. There are two general wards for men on remand – one for those charged with a first offence or a capital charge, and one for those who have already been in prison. The former have much tighter security. There are also, as I was to discover, single hospital 'cells' on the ground floor of the block.

I was put in Ward 2 with other men up on their first

charge and with several men on murder charges. It was quite a while before I really took in my surroundings. Indeed, not until I saw an evening paper in the ward that night did I fully realise either what I had done, or that I, the prison reformer and champion of the ex-prisoner, was now in prison myself. It was an appalling shock to read the details of my case and be forced to accept that the person it was describing was me. Strangely, seeing it in print made it real and actual in a way that living through it had never done.

The ward was rectangular, with room for twenty beds. There was a bathroom and toilet – with locked razors provided – a few chairs and tables where cards and dominoes were played interminably, and a television set which was switched on at 6 p.m. and off at 9 p.m. The windows were barred and had no curtains, and the wood block floor was completely bare. We spent a good part of each day sweeping and polishing it. Twenty-four hours a day a prison officer sat by an alarm bell which he sounded in the event of an emergency.

All of that may sound very rational and unalarming, and in many ways it is. But when one recalls that this is the very best accommodation a prison has to offer and that the men kept here on remand have not yet been tried, let alone found guilty of any offence, it puts a different complexion on it. The worst aspect, for me at any rate, was the feeling of helpless isolation. Suddenly you seemed to have no rights; suddenly you were being regarded as less than a human being. You got the feeling that no matter how loud you were to shout – literally or metaphorically – no one would hear or raise a finger to help. Now that is probably an unfair comment. I met then, and have met since, kind and sympathetic prison officers and administrators. But isolated warm-hearted individuals cannot transform a cold and inhuman system into anything better.

The next day Ann visited me – men on remand are not

restricted, as convicted men are, to one visitor a month. She told me something, the full significance of which only dawned on me much later. Apparently on Friday afternoon, when I was in Bart's Hospital, she had phoned me at my office to say that she had decided not to go away for the weekend with this 'other man' after all. My secretary had told her that I was not there. Ann had then rung Janet, who had no idea where I was, but felt something was possibly wrong, and began to make enquiries, which eventually led her to the hospital. The fact is that, if Ann had got through to me, or if my secretary had told her that I was in hospital, one of my most serious anxieties would have been resolved, and it is at least possible that the whole sordid business of Sunday night would never have happened.

On Wednesday Janet visited me. I had been told that Lord Longford was also proposing to visit me the same day, but I got a message in the evening to say he was not coming after all. All the message actually meant was that he could not get to the prison that evening, but my jaundiced mind interpreted it as meaning that he had decided against visiting me *at all*.

This was the most devastating blow of all. For several years my work with Lord Longford had been a kind of raft of credibility to which I had clung whatever else had gone wrong. Peter Thompson might make mistakes, might be desperately ill mentally, might act irresponsibly, or even violently; but at one point and in one area he had managed to pay back part of the debt: he had, at least, the Pakenham-Thompson Committee to his 'credit'. Of that raft of credibility my friendship with Lord Longford was a major element. And now, I thought, it had gone. He had turned away from me. I had screamed for help, and deaf ears were being offered to my cries. A great wave of depression swept over me – perhaps the bitterest I had ever experienced.

I went to the bathroom, filled the bath with water and

climbed into it, fully clothed. My intention was to drown myself. For several hideous seconds I swallowed what seemed to be pints and pints of water, gasping and gulping at the same time. Then there was a flurry of hands and I was dragged, dripping and weeping, from the bath, flung on the floor and given artificial respiration.

From there I was carried to the ground floor of the block, stripped of all my clothes and locked in a padded cell. Words simply cannot describe what followed. I am told I spent three hours in this cell. It seemed like an eternity. The most awful part of it was the total absence of noise, or even echo. I screamed and pounded on the walls and door, but no one could hear, and even my own noises were strangely muffled. There were virtually no openings at all in the padded walls. Even the peep-hole in the cell door was padded. The tiny window of thick glass was high on one wall, and the only real source of light in the room was a bulb set in a recess in the ceiling. The only item of 'furniture' was a plastic chamber-pot.

Eventually the Governor came to see me. He asked me why I had tried to kill myself, and I told him about Lord Longford. He was sympathetic – but what could he do? The Governor was followed by a prison doctor, who told me that they were going to put me in a single hospital cell and give me some medicine which would put me deeply to sleep within thirty seconds. He thought I would feel better when I woke up.

As a matter of fact, I had not had a proper spell of sleep for about a week. During the nights leading up to my suicide attempt I had been out driving, my pre-dawn attempts at sleep plagued by a recurring and terrifying nightmare. In this, I was in a mental hospital. A nurse asked, 'Why is he here, he's normal?' To which a doctor would reply, 'Yes, but if you ask him such-and-such a question, he will turn violent.' Put like that, it sounds fairly harmless, but to me it had the most threatening and destructive overtones, representing very precisely the two parts of my life which I had fought so long to keep apart finally coming together in a violent explosion.

So I welcomed the offer of an induced sleep. I was taken to a cell where there was a mattress on the floor. I was given a canvas shirt and put between canvas sheets. Then I was given a blue glass containing some liquid. I drank it and, I learnt later, was asleep within seconds. That was about 7 p.m., and I did not wake until noon the next day. I felt much better physically, though still mentally depressed.

I was moved back to the ward and kept under observation. My solicitor came to see me and told me they were not objecting to remand, in my own interests – but I understood and cared very little at that stage about the legal machinery.

On the Friday I was shown a letter that had come to me from the Secretary of my firm. It had been written and posted on the Wednesday following my first court appearance, and put in writing the notice of dismissal they had so expeditiously sent to Bart's Hospital on the very afternoon of my suicide attempt. I am going to quote it in full.

Dear Mr Thompson,
On Friday, the 5th February, I sent a message through the staff of St Bartholomew's Hospital to you to the effect that you would not be required to report back to the office as the Company had decided to terminate your employment. The Company has now considered your actions further and has decided that they were in breach of the duties of your employment and constituted misconduct. On the grounds that these actions were injurious to the Company, I have been instructed to advise you that your employment has been terminated summarily without notice. Your salary has been calculated up to and including Saturday February 6. I enclose a P45 and your National Insurance

card and salary slip. No transfer has yet been made to your bank account pending the ratification of certain sums which appear to be due by you to the Company. It appears that you owe the Company £41. 1s. 3d in respect of petrol sold to you, that there are I.O.U.'s amounting to £6. 0s. 0d, and I hold a Promissory Note in respect of the Expenses float advanced to you of £10. In addition to these we have received a Restaurant Account of £30. 3s. 6d in respect of which you have so far submitted no Expense claim. In the circumstances it seems reasonable that no transfers to your bank account should be made until these matters can be more thoroughly investigated and until you have had the opportunity to render to the Company a claim for your expenses for the period from October 23, 1964 until the date of the termination of your employment.

Yours faithfully,

etc. etc.

I already knew I was dismissed, of course, and I hardly expected the company to feel well-disposed towards an employee who had latterly caused them so much trouble. But they, more than anybody almost, must have realised that I was desperately ill, and that I would have many things to worry about at that moment. There was, one notices, no mention of appreciation for my past services to the firm, which had not been entirely unsuccessful.

Among my visitors later that week were Lord Longford and C. H. Rolph, another member of the Pakenham-Thompson Committee, who wrote an article in the *New Statesman* about my circumstances, which Sir Frank Soskice (then Home Secretary) later told him was one of the most moving things he had ever read.* Janet and Ann – often travelling together in Ann's car – also visited me regularly.

* See Appendix.

Ill as I was, my 'professional' interest in prison matters had not disappeared. There was a certain morbid fascination for a prison reformer about actually being in prison. I might add that nothing I had read or been told by others had conveyed to me the precise air of dereliction and human indignity that hung over the whole set-up.

One example of this was the so-called 'airing courts' or 'recreational periods'. I was aware, of course, that prisoners were allowed a short daily period of exercise in the open air, during which they could walk around an enclosed quadrangle, under the close supervision of prison officers. In the case of Brixton, however, any psychological or hygienic advantage of this ruling was completely offset by the fact that the prisoners being 'aired' had to pick their way past piles of human excreta thrown out of their cell windows during the night by residents of B wing, which overlooked the quadrangle. As no attempt, to my knowledge, was made throughout the two months I was there to clear up this appailling mess, the stench can be imagined. Any notion of 'airing' was plainly ridiculous.

The facts themselves are unpleasant enough. But worse, to my mind, is the effect of such dehumanising factors on the residents – staff and prisoners. Treated like animals, men begin to behave like animals. The effect of this crudity and ugliness on a sensitive person is to destroy his spirit; on a more robust character, it simply creates deep resentment, bitterness and aggression.

I believe the prison authorities would claim that there was no way of preventing the prisoners in B wing from emptying their chamber-pots out of their windows during the night – it was, of course, almost impossible to identify the culprits. But, surely, a few sessions spent clearing away the mess in the quadrangle by the residents of B wing would, at the very least, have discouraged the practice?

A quite different example of the way in which even men

on remand are treated in an impersonal, thoughtless way is the whole stupid business of their weekly court appearance. The law quite rightly says that an accused person cannot be detained without trial for more than a week without appearing in court. For me this meant a weekly trip to court in a meat wagon, a brief appearance during which the police would ask for a further period of remand, which was automatically granted, being unopposed by my lawyers, and a return journey to the prison.

That was all a bit tedious, but no worse. What followed, however, was barely credible. Each week I was then treated as though Brixton Prison had never seen me before. I had the horrible lengthy wait in the tiny cell – up to four hours – another medical examination and all the formalities of being admitted to prison again! Not only that, but I would be put in a different bed and regarded as a new admission. All of this rigmarole was carried out every time a man appeared in court on remand, even when it was perfectly obvious to everybody that he would be returning to the prison the same day.

The food in Brixton was appalling. Even in the remand blocks it was picked out of trays by hand and eaten from tin plates. No sugar was provided for drinks, so a modest supply to sweeten my tea would cost me fourteen shillings a pound in 'barter' values. The price was paid in tobacco. The diet was basic, to say the least, unappetising and not even very nourishing.

I made time during these weeks on remand to talk to several of my fellow residents. These were all, of course, also men on remand. They were not yet, legally at least, prisoners. Ten men in our ward were on capital murder charges – under the interim rules at that time some categories of murder carried the death penalty while others did not. Each of these men faced possible execution for his crime. In view of my interest in the question of capital punishment, I asked each whether the thought of the penalty involved had at any stage deterred him from committing the offence. Each of them, in widely varying circumstances, claimed that the thought never entered his head; and I believe them. One of them, incidentally, confessed his guilt to me, but was acquitted in court for lack of evidence. Another, who had kicked a young lad to death, was found guilty of manslaughter but was actually detained for a shorter period than I eventually was!

There were two spies in our ward, as well: one an army sergeant who had sold information to a Middle Eastern government. For this he received sixty pounds from the foreign embassy and ten years from a British court – not a very good bargain. The other was an employee in the Defence Ministry who dealt in coded messages transmitted through music to and from the Soviet Union. He claimed that he was a double agent, working to uncover a Soviet plot, and asked me to get Lord Longford to intervene on his behalf, but I did not believe him and neither did Lord Longford. He was paid £5,000 for the secrets, and got twenty years.

One other man on remand became a very good friend and had a profound and lasting effect on my life. His name was Don, and he was three years younger than myself. He was a keen and enthusiastic Christian, the first one I had met and talked to at length for some time.

As I have recounted, from the time of my marriage my disenchantment with evangelical Christianity had grown. For a time Janet continued as a practising Christian, but latterly – perhaps under pressure of events – she had given it up too. Apart from isolated moments of need, I had not prayed, opened a Bible or even seriously thought of God for several years, and I had given up church-going completely.

This represented a very big turn-around for a person who had always had a strong religious inclination. I am not sure how much it was a result of my mental illness, or whether it was a result of its results, so to speak. What I am sure of is that my behaviour over the previous two years was so directly contrary to everything I had believed and upheld up to then that it could only truly be explained in terms of mental breakdown.

But other factors had contributed to my turning away from Christianity, especially what seemed to me judgmental attitudes by Christians; a lack of interest on their part in matters that seemed to me important and vital, like the care of society's outcasts; and also my long standing anxiety about and guilt over the matter of masturbation.

Don helped me, more than anyone else had ever done, to put these things into perspective. Although (or perhaps because) he was himself mentally ill, he seemed to have an insight and a Christian concern that was real. We talked together, and he helped me face my objections to Christianity realistically and to see them for what they were. We took to praying together and, for the first time for years, I began to feel the warmth of real faith flowing back into my life. I asked to see the chaplain, and two or three times a week we would go to the chapel and pray. This was a great comfort in a time of desperate anxiety. It was as though God had waited until disaster had crashed around my ears before coming back to me.

One day the Governor and the Prison Medical Officer were touring the wards when the medical officer noticed a book on my locker. It was *Streams in the Desert,* a devotional classic. He picked it up and told me he had a copy, too, and read part of it every day. He was a Christian, and I began to feel I was not completely without friends, not completely isolated.

At about the same time, Dr T. C. N. Gibbens, of the Forensic Psychiatric Department at the Royal Maudsley Hospital, came to examine me for the prosecution. He spent two and a half hours with me, before deciding to advise the Director of Public Prosecutions that I was not criminal, but mentally ill, and suitable for treatment under Section 60 of the Mental Health Act. This provided for up to a year's detention for treatment in a mental hospital. I was also taken to a hospital at Wimbledon for E.E.G. (electro-encephalograph) tests. I entered and left the hospital handcuffed and was very conscious of the glares and stares of bystanders, as though I were some sort of criminal exhibit.

As my defence were also pressing for a 'Section 60' decision, they agreed with the prosecution to enter a plea of guilty. I was happy about this because I felt I *was* guilty as charged, and my new Christian convictions made it increasingly difficult for me to claim I was not.

In fact, during this stay in Brixton my conscience began to come alive again. It was rather like watching Sleeping Beauty wake up. I could see, as I had not seen for years, how I had hurt people and treated them badly. I knew that my relationship with Ann was wrong, too, though frankly I lacked the strength of character to end something that was a major crutch for me.

I even discussed ways of making some reparation to the girls I had attacked: I felt this as a heavy obligation. I talked this over with a man who was to become a very good friend – Dr Ted Gurney, a medical missionary who had come to see me as a result of a phone call by the Principal of the women's Bible College Janet had attended. He could see how ill I was, and both then and later was a wonderfully reliable and practical counsellor to me.

Janet and the children, of course, were facing the inevitable financial problems following my arrest. One of the executives at my firm proved a good friend to them and to me, taking a friendly interest. Largely because of him the company agreed to make a modest but helpful *ex gratia* payment to Janet, and I believe they waived some of the items I owed them – which goes some way, I suppose, to off-set

F

that rather heartless letter from the Secretary. This friend also visited Janet almost every day while I was in Brixton.

As I have mentioned earlier, I had lectured on several occasions to prison officers about rehabilitation and after-care, arguing my usual case that rehabilitation should begin the day a man is sentenced, not the day he leaves prison. I must admit this view was usually received with some cynicism, but now, watching prison officers at work, it was my turn to be cynical. Prison service seems too often to attract entirely the wrong kind of man – a man without ambition or sensitivity, but who likes to be vested with absolute authority in his own limited realm. A good example of the sort of person I am describing led to a vicious piece of violence.

In our ward there was a prisoner who was seriously disturbed mentally: a fact which should have been obvious to anybody, no matter how unintelligent. Yet one of the warders took great pains to taunt this man, tease him and do his best to provoke him. Finally, the patient's control snapped and he attacked the warder, raining blows on him. The warder shouted to the rest of us to ring the alarm bell, but nobody moved. Appalled as I was to see a man being beaten up, I could not help but feel there was an element of justice in it. By the time other warders arrived and the prisoner was overpowered, the first officer was quite seriously injured. As I have said, the moral seems to be that if you treat people like animals, they will behave like animals.

Just to correct the balance and put the record straight, I must add a word about Mr Jenkins. He, too, was a prison officer at Brixton. I met him just before my trial. He had noticed some missionary pamphlets on my locker and asked me about them. We got talking, and I discovered that he, too, was a practising Christian, with a brother serving as a missionary in Singapore. I told him how I had found a degree of peace with myself, largely through pleading guilty and facing up to the realities of my situation. This contact, together with Don and the Principal Medical Officer, proved to me the return of God into my situation. I look back on Brixton, not exactly with pleasure, but at least as something of a turning point in my life.

However, the dominant thought in my mind at this time was the trial, which was to take place on a Monday in April, 1965. Despite the confidence of my legal advisors, I was apprehensive about its outcome. One man in the ward had said (perhaps as a joke – I do not know) that I could get up to fourteen years in prison for what I had done, and that remark haunted me. I hoped to be committed as a compulsory patient to a mental hospital or, better still, be sent to Grendon Psychiatric Prison, and that was what my defence expected. Indeed, Janet had approached a friend of mine, Bob Taylor, who was Director of Prison Administration, to see if this could be arranged. However, I knew that the Crown was asking for committal to Broadmoor, a prospect that filled me with horror – especially as my shocked mind had confused it with Dartmoor. So I awaited my trial with great apprehension.

Chapter 5

On the morning of my trial I was woken very early because there was a lot to do before we left the prison. We were required to take all our belongings with us, of course, as many would be sent to prisons in distant parts of Britain, and perhaps some of those on remand would be acquitted and go home after the hearing. For myself, I had collected a large number of books and papers, as well as what were officially called 'personal effects', and all that the prison provided to carry them in were large paper bags. By the time I had cleared my locker it looked like Christmas.

But it didn't feel like Christmas. There was a joky nervousness among those of us up for trial, and a cold horror deep in the pit of my stomach at the thought of spending the next few years incarcerated in some lonely, mist-shrouded place of doom in the middle of the moors.

Breakfast was served at seven, but I did not feel like eating. Then we were led out to a quadrangle where we were ringed by prison officers to await the transport. Our possessions were taken from us, and then we were marched, each man handcuffed to another, into a green bus with barred windows, which was to take us to court. Our drive through the wet, grey streets of London did nothing to lift my spirits. The dismal weather exactly matched my mood. I was obsessed with the thought of Broadmoor, and the image I had of it as a dire place of isolation and retribution.

We pulled up alongside a door of the Central Criminal Court at the Old Bailey and were led in and down some steps into a kind of well directly underneath the court. Here there were a number of single cells, each about six feet by four. For a little while I shared one with another man from Brixton, a postman who was charged with murdering his wife and her lover; but soon he was led away into court and I was on my own.

It is almost impossible to convey the aura of the security arrangements at the Old Bailey, yet it is just this that turns a legal system into a kind of mental torture of the accused. That is no exaggeration. Unless you can feel the impersonality, the ugliness, the air of gloom and despair, you cannot understand what it is that breaks a man and leaves him permanently crippled.

No one expects fitted carpets and armchairs, I suppose, but it is hard to see why dark grey stone walls, clanging echoes, iron-studded doors and plain wooden tables nailed to the floor are so inevitably associated with 'justice'. The whole thing is like a medieval dungeon. I spent three hours alone in the cell, with no natural light and no one even to speak to. During that time my already confused mind explored all the most terrifying possible outcomes until what would have been a nerve-wracking ordeal for a person who was mentally well became for me a horrible and extended torture.

At last there were footsteps and, with a great creaking of hinges – I am not exaggerating, it was like something out of *The Count of Monte Cristo* – the huge thick door swung open. The moment had arrived. I was led out of the cell through a door in the wall and up about fifty steep steps. At the top of these was a trap door, and I was escorted through this and straight up into the dock.

Behind me and rather below, because the dock was raised, sat the public, including, I quickly noticed, my mother, Janet and Ann. To my left was the witness box and ahead sat the judge – Judge Lyle – in lonely splendour. I had seen it before at the trial of a friend, who was acquitted. Casting my mind back to that occasion, I was beginning to wish we had opted for trial by jury (which would have meant pleading 'not guilty').

The case opened with a short speech by the prosecution, which seemed to be at great pains to present me as an unstable, unreliable person. They had approached my employers as far back as 1960 to discover that! Various exhibits – a gun, knives and shoes – were laid out before the judge. The police evidence followed. This mainly had to do with the facts, which were not in dispute, but the inspector who had interviewed me at Esher volunteered the opinion that I was ill at the time of my arrest. The medical records were not read out in court, but had been studied by the judge. My own doctor appeared and surprised me by claiming that I was 'getting better' and suggesting I should be sent to an ordinary County Hospital, where he had been able to arrange a bed for me.

The proceedings were swift and very brief – perhaps ten minutes in all. It seemed amazing that it was for this that I had waited three months. Actually, I was unaware of the major item of evidence, which was the full psychiatric report by Dr Gibbens, including the E.E.G. results. This report stated categorically that I had a "well marked abnormality of emotional instability" and that "this condition is constitutional". The E.E.G. showed what the psychiatrist called an "unusual abnormality" (which is a delightful tautology!) of "a constitutional kind", with disturbance of a stable rhythm by "low voltage rhythmic two-a-second waves". He felt this abnormality would account for my present behaviour. Dr Gibbens found it "difficult to interpret" the changes in the last two years, with the emergence "and, to some extent, acting out of irrational impulses", but felt they "indicated a need for treatment in hospital" and that I was "suitable for an order under Section 60 of the Mental Health Act of 1959". Dr Calder from Brixton gave evidence in court to support all this, and told the judge that, in his opinion, I should be committed to Broadmoor and that there was a bed available for me. The judge asked him for how long he felt I should remain in Broadmoor, and Calder replied, "for a shortish period". That, later, became a very important comment.

My counsel – Ivor Richards, M.P. – then spoke briefly, referring to my social work and contrasting my usual behaviour with this completely uncharacteristic incident. Lord Longford, incidentally, had offered to give evidence and had obtained the Prime Minister's permission to do so (he was at the time Lord Privy Seal). I wanted him to appear, but Ivor Richards strongly advised against calling any public figures because of the press publicity it would arouse. Although I disagreed at the time, I must admit that in a remarkable way the case avoided the kind of publicity we feared. Although it was reported in the papers, none of them linked the 'Frederick Pierre Thompson' who was charged with the 'Peter Thompson' who had plagued their offices for years in the cause of the ex-prisoner. Needless to say, I was very grateful for that.

Finally, Judge Lyle spoke to me. He repeated the formal charges and asked me how I pleaded. I hesitated. He had said "grievous bodily harm *with intent*", and I had not realised that a phrase about 'intent' was involved. I was not at all sure that I had ever 'intended' grievous bodily harm. I glanced at my solicitor – Rex Cowan, a man I greatly love and respect – and I saw that he had gone white. I think he must have guessed that I was thinking about changing my plea.

The judge repeated the question and, to everyone's relief, I pleaded guilty. I suppose at the crunch I felt I could not go back on what I had agreed with my advisors, but it still seems to me inconsistent to allege that a man is guilty of wounding 'with intent' and then state that at the time he was mentally ill and acting irrationally. But the law is not for laymen, as I have learnt.

Now Judge Lyle spoke to me again. He asked me if I had any statement to make, and I said I had not. Then he summed up.

"There are other people who should bear responsibility for what has happened," he said. That sentence has stuck in my memory ever since. It appears to me as a fair and perceptive summary of the situation. If negligence is a form of sin, then others were guilty of sins of omission matching my sin of commission, but they did not stand in the dock as I did.

The judge then read out the charges in detail, with the court incredibly hushed. "Frederick Pierre Thompson," he said, "you will be detained in Broadmoor under Section 60 of the Mental Health Act of 1959, the period of your detention to be decided by other authorities."

So now I knew my fate. My advisors, friends and relatives were, I learnt later, reasonably relieved by the outcome, but for me it was like a sentence of doom. I had always thought I would die by the age of thirty. I was now in fact thirty-one, but it was as though my life had been squeezed out of me by the sheer force of my circumstances over the past two years, and this was the final sentence of death. Although it was not the fourteen-year prison stretch I had feared, the name 'Broadmoor' and the thought of what I imagined it to be appalled me.

I almost fell in the dock and had to be supported by two prison officers. Still dazed, I was led down through the trap-door and back to the gloomy nether regions of the building. Two brief moments of light were to pierce the darkness. By some extraordinary means, Ann had got permission for herself and my mother to see me before I was taken away to Broadmoor. This defied every rule of procedure in the book and was a moment of totally unexpected joy. And then – like another gentle reminder that God was back in business with me – one of the prison medical officers looked in on my cell, brought me a cup of tea from his mess, and told me he was a Methodist local preacher and had been praying for me.

I needed those little encouragements, because I was in the grip by now of an almost paralysing fear. If I had had the means, I have no doubt I would have killed myself, but I was stripped even of belt or braces. Two burly warders came for me, I was handcuffed to them and led out to a van which was to take me and other men to our various destinations. We dropped off several men at Brixton and then, still handcuffed, the drive to Broadmoor began.

Broadmoor Hospital is about thirty-two miles from London, near Crowthorne, in Berkshire, and I suppose the journey took a little over an hour. As we approached it, one of my guards remarked that we were nearly there. I was baffled.

'But I don't understand,' I said. 'Where are the moors and the ponies?'

He laughed. 'This isn't Dartmoor,' he said, 'it's Broadmoor.'

I looked out at the fields and cottages of a typical stretch of the Home Counties, still very baffled.

'But what's Broadmoor, then?'

'Broadmoor,' he replied slowly, 'I'm sorry to tell you, is the most *infamous* criminal lunatic asylum in the world.'

By now the red brick walls of the institution came into view and above them the top storeys of the blocks of the building. Whatever else, even my disordered mind had to accept that this was not Dartmoor. I must add, for the record, that of course I knew rationally what Broadmoor was, and had done for years. You could hardly be engaged in penal reform work in Britain without knowing one of the most famous institutions connected with our penal system. But my illness had completely blotted out my grasp of rationality in some areas, including this.

We waited ten minutes outside the gates until a Broadmoor officer came out to meet us. I later learnt what a kind and thoughtful person he was, but he was a most terrifying sight. He was short and thick-set, wearing a long black tunic with a high collar – standard wear for Broadmoor staff at that time – and he had a dark beard. Another, almost equally unprepossessing officer appeared, a tall Maltese in identical gear. I must say he looked like Satan himself. The first officer – his name was Goswell – took one look at me and curtly told my escorts to take the handcuffs off me. They protested that they were told to put them on me, but he said I was mentally ill and they did not use handcuffs at Broadmoor – which was a welcome snippet of information in my state of mind.

The Broadmoor men led me into the 'waiting room' where I saw the duty medical officer. He looked through my papers.

"Only Section 60?" he commented at last – not to me, but to the prison officers who had brought me down. "Who was the judge?"

When they told him it was Judge Lyle he simply said, "Oh, him." I was very upset by the implications of that brief conversation, which I understood perfectly, despite the fact that I was feeling shocked and depressed.

I was then escorted by the two men in black tunics past several low buildings with iron gates and barred windows to a long three-storied building with bars everywhere. Here we came to a green door with heavy metal studs, and I was taken along a highly polished floor to a bathroom on the third floor. Here I was told to strip, while the male nurses present (I later learnt) kept an eye open for any identifying birthmarks or deformities. I bathed, dressed in pyjamas and slippers, and was taken to a small room with a high ceiling where I was told to get into bed. This was about 4 p.m.

I expected the nurses to shut and lock the door, but in fact they left it open – a nice piece of applied psychology, I felt, even if later in one's career at Broadmoor the doors were usually locked. It diminished the sense of being in a 'prison' and made the idea that this was a hospital, albeit of a special kind, much more credible, even though this was a maximum security block.

I was brought tea on a tray, with bread and jam, cheese and cakes – about as far from the 'Dartmoor' of my imagination, or even the Brixton of recent memory, as could be conceived. And then, miraculously, a figure I recognised passed my open door. It was Don, my Christian friend from Brixton, who had been sent to Broadmoor six weeks before me. After a chat with him and a prayer, I must say I felt more at peace than I had been for a long time. First impressions *are* important. As I shall explain, there are plenty of things at Broadmoor that are less than ideal, but this initial impression of care and consideration predisposed me to accept the place and to feel accepted. That, it seems to me, is worth a whole lorryload of handcuffs and window bars.

I discovered that I was actually in a room which was part of a ward. The ward, in fact, consisted of a day room (with a television), a recreation room (billiards and so on), a lavatory, a bathroom and individual rooms like mine. Normally these rooms were locked up at retiring time (about 9 p.m.) and unlocked at 7 a.m. For the rest of the day patients were free to move about the ward and had a stated period of recreation ('airing courts') outside as well.

On this first evening I was told I must stay in bed. Don assured me this was standard practice, but subsequently I adopted the normal routine of the admission block that I was now in. This combined maximum security with intense boredom. There were forty-two of us sharing a modest-sized day room, and there were not even enough chairs for us all to sit down! For a man like myself, accustomed to travel, to meet people and to *communicate,* this was the hardest part of my first few weeks in Broadmoor. Although there were newspapers in the ward, radio during the day and television in the evening, so that we knew what was going on, I still felt isolated from the world; and information about it only seemed to heighten that sense of being cut off from the world of men.

After several months in Broadmoor, following this daily routine of the 'new admissions', I was finding my severe depression returning. I had had no drugs and no psychotherapy at all. I was frequently in tears, even when visitors came in. I remember when George Goyder came on one occasion the visit ended with us both in tears. I sent a telegram to Ivor Richards to complain that I was getting no treatment and subsequently – whether as a direct result or not, I do not know – the Superintendent, Dr McGrath, took over my case. But he explicitly refused to give me drugs or treatment, saying I must "let things work themselves out". I learnt that he had told Janet I should be in Broadmoor a "very, very long time", which did nothing to improve my condition at the time.

Obviously, sharing a ward with other mentally ill patients – however well-intentioned the staff are – leads to many intolerable situations. One patient made a habit of washing in his own urine and then using a communal towel to dry himself. The permanent over-crowding and shortage of staff makes this even worse. At nights, twenty patients share one commode to a dormitory. On the two or three occasions a year when 'Berkshire Belly' strikes – an outbreak of diarrhoea and vomiting – the situation can be degrading. I remember a night when thirteen men were queuing to use the commode. By the time the last one used it, the thing was overflowing and the stench was appalling; and it was not even possible to open a window, for security reasons, nor wash one's hands. This kind of situation strips away one's last vestige of human dignity.

Sometimes patients were violent and provoked violence in the staff. There were occasional fights and rumpuses in the day room, and once I was beaten up by another patient. I think a major cause of this, too, was the severe overcrowding.

When my depressions were at their height I found a wonderful friend in one of the nurses, Alf Lister, a gentle and compassionate man. I remember him on one occasion sitting on the lavatory floor cradling my head in his lap as I wept uncontrollably. My violent fantasies had returned, too, as severely as ever, and it was obvious that I was going through a severe breakdown – possibly heading for the real 'crisis' of my illness.

I found the complete absence of privacy a heavy burden, though it may well have been good for me. Except for the hours of sleep, all of one's life was open to inspection. Baths were supervised by the staff, and all day long they kept an eye on us throughout the long months of the so-called 'admission' period.

Perhaps to counter this, I managed to start a debating society in the admission block (block one), modelled on the Hampstead and Bristol 'parliaments'. Forty out of forty-two was the average attendance and, as a result of the success of the debating society, the Departmental Nurse (D.N.) recommended to Dr McQuade, who had abandoned group therapy some years previously, that is could be restarted. It was, and worked well.

Chairing the debate was very difficult, especially for me, suffering as I was at that time from an acute depression. The whole situation was, of course, a perfect 'throw-back' to my behaviour before the 'incident', when I could cope with public activities and yet was in the grip of private emotional storms. I asked permission of 'the House' at the first meeting to expel from a debate any member who, after three warnings, refused to be co-operative, and the nurses supported that. It did not happen very often, though I did once expel a Lieutenant Commander, a man who was very ill, after three warnings. He protested loudly as he was escorted out by the nurses, but in fact he always attended the debates after that and was much more co-operative and constructive.

In my block – which was called 'admission', but also included all patients under the age of twenty-one – there was in fact a predominance of young people, some of whom had been there a long while. One young man had been in Broadmoor since the age of eleven. Most of the patients were reasonably stable. All admissions were put through an I.Q. test, and it appeared that the average I.Q. at Broadmoor is higher than the average I.Q. outside. The other admissions were a mixed bag. One of them came up to me and asked if I had ever "dined at Simpson's". I replied that I was sure he knew that you could only lunch at Simpson's and that obviously he was trying to catch me out. Actually, he did not know that fact and was not trying to trap me, so in effect I caught him out! At any rate, that was the start of a deep and real friendship. He was a dark, heavily-built Welshman, a school teacher. There was a surgeon among the patients, a barrister, a Lieutenant Commander and other service officers, school teachers and other professional people, as well as artisans.

One has to have spent three months in the admission block before one can have 'privileges'. These include such things as having a radio in your room at night, going to the hospital church or to the sports field. I spent a good deal of my time polishing floors, and I also enrolled for a large number of classes which were held in a special 'school room' in the admission block. I studied German, French, Mathematics, Geography, History, English Language and Literature: and I kept that up for three and a half years at Broadmoor. Very few patients made use of these classes – the average attendance was ten – but I enjoyed them, I must say. My classes were all taken by the same teacher, Mr Williams, a tall, fuzzy-haired Welshman who had been a naval officer during the war. The odd thing about his lessons was that whatever the subject, even Mathematics or German, Wales managed to invade it somewhere. He was the incarnation of all Nationalists.

Perhaps this would be the right point in the narrative to describe the lay-out of Broadmoor. As I have already explained, the hospital is enclosed by a red brick wall which runs along all four sides – probably the best part of a mile in all. Inside the wall stand all the hospital buildings, open spaces, airing courts and playing fields.

The external appearance of the place is, I should say, superior to the average hospital and greatly superior to most prisons. Broadmoor is *not* of course, a prison, and not every patient, by any means, is an offender. Nevertheless, all are people needing a high degree of security because of 'dangerous, violent or criminal propensities'. Hence the wall and hence the many locked gates, barred windows and so on.

Coming in through the front door – straight off the road – one enters 'reception'. This room in turn opens on to a small quadrangle surrounded by offices, including those of the doctors, senior nursing staff, administrators and the like. There is also a large, wooden double gate to the road outside from this quadrangle, through which vans and lorries can enter. Tribunals and other 'hearings' also take place in an office off this quadrangle. To get into the main part of the premises, it is necessary to go through corridors in this office block, which lead into open spaces to its right and left. Immediately behind the quadrangle is the hospital's central meeting hall, with the chapel on the first floor above it. Behind that stand blocks 3 and 4.

All the hospital blocks are three storeys high and of similar design. There are seven blocks, each for a different category of patient. Block 3, for example, includes geriatric patients, and block 4, where I spent my second four months at Broadmoor, is for patients moving on from the admission block (block 1).

The workshops and blocks 1 and 2 are to the left of the entrance quadrangle. Block 2 contains patients on 'full parole', which I shall explain later. To the right are blocks 5 (semi-parole patients, where I lived for several years) and 6 (maximum security for seriously violent patients) and an airing court; and beyond them, further to the right, are handicraft centres and block 7 (for those who are near to being mentally disturbed).

Behind and beyond blocks 3 and 4 – which also contain the Superintendent's office and the patients' canteen – is a large grassy area; and still further are gardens with trees, backed by an enormous twenty feet high wall. This was built in 1968 at a cost, I believe, of £90,000, and simply serves to separate the playing fields from the rest of the premises.

The women's hospital is located away to the left as you look from blocks 3 and 4 towards the playing fields.

The buildings were erected in 1891 in Victorian red brick. Floors are parquet wood or lino (well polished by generations of patients paid, during my time, six shillings, a week for their labour). The hospital was intended to accommodate 450 patients, but during my stay there were about 730.

Overcrowding, as I have already said, was a major problem. Indeed, the Parliamentary Estimates Committee Report in 1967/8 used quite emotive language in describing conditions at Broadmoor.

"The sub-committee were appalled to see for themselves the extent of the overcrowding in the century-old Broadmoor building," they wrote. "Their feelings are shared by officials of the Ministry of Health: 'We were all shocked,' said a witness, 'when we first saw Broadmoor' . . . By present day standards the hospital is not adequate for more than 500 male patients. . . .

"As a result, there is in Broadmoor a day room with thirty-five beds crowded into it, a medical ward which patients have to use as an overflow dining room, a corridor used for the same purpose, and seven beds placed in a corridor. Staff rooms have had to be turned into accommodation for patients. . . .

"The added pressure of work is considerable. . . . The effect on nursing staff morale was made startlingly plain to the sub-committee – 'We really do not do much more than a farmer would do for his animals. We are attending to their basic bodily needs; we are maintaining observation and discipline, but we are certainly not doing the job that the hospital should be doing'."*

The Committee rightly made it clear that all this was in no way a reflection upon the staff, "the value of whose work under such conditions is even greater than it would otherwise be". I would agree with that for, with certain exceptions, the nursing staff at Broadmoor do a fine job in very trying circumstances. One of the biggest problems, however, is the shortage of trained mental nurses. A small minority of the 300 'nurses' on the staff are State Registered or Registered Mental Nurses. Some are State Enrolled (assistant) nurses, but many are unqualified and some are very young – under twenty, in some cases. It was often these younger or unqualified men who, perhaps unwittingly, were the cause of some of the friction and tension on the wards.

In this setting I had to cope with a severe recession in my illness, as I have said. One among so many, I felt hopelessly rejected and alone. Delayed shock over the trial, the continuing rift with Janet, and what I saw as the absence of adequate medical support added to this depression. During those first months in Broadmoor I seemed to spend half of

* Second Report from the Estimates Committee, 1967/8, p. ix.

every waking day in tears and, if it had not been for people like Alf Lister and Paddy O'Connor, I do not like to think what would have become of me.

Paddy O'Connor was a large but gentle Irishman. Discovering that I wished to read my Bible in the privacy of my bedroom in the early hours of the morning, he arranged to switch on my light earlier than everyone else's, at six a.m. In fact, my Christian faith, new-found at Brixton, stood me in good stead, though it was sorely tested. I got permission, although not yet due for 'privileges', to attend church, but wept bitterly all through the services and had the privilege withdrawn. I think the trouble was that the thought of God's purity and love seemed so remote from this strange, sick world of the hospital, with hundreds of disturbed and confused people all round me. I was very wrong to feel like that, but in the chapel I was like a small child weeping for a well-loved but absent father. Prayer and Bible reading were, however, genuine elements of my daily routine, and I leant very heavily on these spiritual experiences. I also often prayed with Don, and this helped a great deal.

Meanwhile, quite a lot was going on outside, some of it unknown to me but concerned with my case. For one thing, there was a long double column article by David Roxan about me in the *News of the World* on 18 April – the Sunday after my trial. It was headed by a picture of me with Lord Longford taken during a meeting connected with the Pakenham-Thompson Committee. The article was sympathetic and accurate. Roxan told how I had tried to get in touch with him by phone on the day before what he called my "senseless attack", but he was out of London. "When I called back," he wrote, "I couldn't reach him. If I had, that attack might never have taken place." I had forgotten ringing him – he was, of course, one of my old press contacts – but his story confirms my own impression that I was searching around for help all through that ill-fated weekend.

According to the *News of the World,* Sir Peter Rawlinson, former Solicitor-General (and now Attorney General) and a member of the Pakenham-Thompson Committee, had "offered to help", but when Janet wrote to him he replied that the newspaper must have misunderstood him.

I was also anxious to make some practical reparation to the girls I had attacked. Dr Gurney, assisted by Mr William Deedes, M.P., did his best to discover the whereabouts of the girls, in the hope that we could make some financial arrangements, at least as a token of reparation. I had become very convinced about the importance of this. Indeed, I should like to see prisoners and detainees paid a living wage so that they can support their families and also make reparation to those they have injured or whose property they have damaged or stolen. This seems to me to represent a thoroughly Christian response to the criminal by the public, and to the public by the criminal. But the authorities – especially the police – were very unhelpful, and we had to drop the idea. Later, my doctor in Broadmoor told me that at the time of the attack the girls were not 'people' at all to me, and reparation would not be relevant or advisable.

Janet visited me every Saturday, and Ann on Sundays, which actually exceeded the strict limitation of seven weekend visits a month (we were allowed any number of visits on weekdays), but the Superintendent allowed me the necessary extra weekend visits. Partly unknown to me, both of the 'women in my life' were re-thinking their positions in regard to me, and it would be only a matter of time before the double blow fell. Ann paid a visit to Dr McGrath early in my stay at Broadmoor to ask him what would be the best – or least harmful – point to break the news that she would not be seeing me again. She was apparently under tremendous pressure from her relatives and friends. Janet was contemplating divorce.

I was allowed to write only two letters a week which, for an enthusiastic correspondent like me, was very irksome – especially as I was still chairman of the Society of Character Underwriters! I wished to write to my children, my mother and many friends as well. This situation led to my first burst of 'barrack-room lawyer' activity. I approached the Superintendent and suggested that it would be sensible if newly admitted patients were allowed to write up to four letters a week for a stated period, so that they could let everyone know where they were, and then revert to the 'ration' of two letters a week.

Dr McGrath refused to alter the rule. I said that I would approach the Management. "I am the Management," he told me. Faced with that I shelved my complaint, and also an appeal against my committal to Broadmoor which I had been considering. I felt that McGrath, who had told me he would oppose any such appeal strenuously, would make sure it failed. But on the letters question all was not finished, and the matter came up again later.

At about this time, having used up my two letters for the week, I foolishly smuggled a letter to my mother-in-law out of the hospital. It was a completely harmless letter, simply inviting her to visit me, but she noticed the London postmark and reported to the Superintendent that I was sending letters out of Broadmoor. There was a fearful row over this, and the authorities tried hard to find out which of my visitors had co-operated in breaking the rules. It was certainly regarded as a serious offence. The reason for the ban, incidentally, was that all outgoing mail from patients had to be censored – this was in accordance with Section 36 of the 1959 Mental Health Act, which gave people the right to refuse to receive letters from patients in special hospitals like Broadmoor. It was considered that more than two letters a week from each patient would put an intolerable strain on the censorship machinery.

While I was in the admission block I met a man involved

in an escape from Moss-side, Birmingham – a hospital of a similar kind to Broadmoor, to which he was transferred after recapture. The escape was one of the most ingeniously planned I have ever come across. Apparently, in the part of Moss-side where he was working there were a number of doors which were unused, but had the standard security locks common to the rest of the hospital. During one working day he unscrewed one of these locks and smuggled it out through one of his visitors. A key was made and smuggled back in, and one night ten patients escaped simply by unlocking the door and walking through it. Obviously the man who planned such an escape was not unintelligent. Apparently, he was not very ill, either, because soon after his transfer to Broadmoor he was discharged.

A man called Bob, an ex-prisoner whom I had helped to find employment some time before, read about my case in the *News of the World* and turned up quite unexpectedly one Sunday to visit me. Not only that, but he came to see me every month for four and a half years, driving up from Bournemouth and bringing me fruit, cigarettes and cakes.

Before I left the admission block, I reached a decision I had been toying with for some time. I had been feeling increasingly guilty about my association with Ann, and my new Christian enthusiasms heightened this. I was also aware that something pretty drastic would have to be done, and quickly, if my marriage was not to be destroyed completely.

So I asked Ann not to come and see me any more. It was a fearful and painful decision to make, for she had been a nurse and a sympathetic, understanding friend to me rather than a 'lover'. It was only then that she told me that she had discussed with my doctor the best time to tell me that she wished to stop seeing me. We were both heartbroken and sat through the visit in tears, but the decision was taken.

I had an interview with Dr McGrath at this point, and told him what had happened with Ann and Janet. It was a very emotional interview. I vividly remember lying on the floor of his office, crying and kicking the floor with my heels. McGrath is heavily built, with deep, round shoulders and black hair going grey. He stood over me as I lay there and talked very gently to me, often calling me 'son'. This word had a positively magical effect on me, especially when he also began telling me about his own daughter and of how she had gone off to a party. This conversation lasted all of an hour and mostly dealt with domestic trivialities, but it was very therapeutic for me. It was as though he were taking me into his family. At a subsequent interview he explained to me that Broadmoor was a crutch or walking stick to help me cope with a disability. When I had learned to cope, he said, I could throw it away for someone else to use.

At about the same time Dr Gurney, on a visit, made a remark that stuck in my mind and was a great help in times of discouragement. He said that I would leave Broadmoor when it was God's time for me to leave, and when that time came no one would be able to prevent it. In the event, he was absolutely right.

However, by the end of my time in the admission block I was beginning to settle down in Broadmoor. Helped by the routine, the discipline that created a sense of security, and by the fact that one's problems were confined to a tiny, recognisable and strictly limited environment, I found I could come to terms with them in a way I had not done for years. I felt – wrongly, as it transpired – that the crisis in my mental illness was over at last. The violent fantasies and the fits of depression began to grow less frequent and less powerful. I was not well, by a very long way, and one more serious recession lay ahead, but it was true that I was at least getting better, which was something.

I was then transferred to block 4, which is the second stage of the admission process – a sort of intermediate step before transfer to one or other of the 'permanent' wards. I first had to spend a couple of weeks under observation in a medical inspection ward on the ground floor, and here a rather unpleasant but revealing incident occurred.

One of the patients in the ward – there were about fifteen of us – was a very tall, strong fellow called Paddy. He was a quite seriously disturbed man. At night a nurse was actually locked in the ward with us, an alarm button at the ready in case of an emergency. At about two o'clock one morning Paddy got out of his bed and made his way quietly – but peacefully – towards this nurse. The nurse panicked and pressed the alarm button, but was then able to persuade Paddy to get back into bed. However, after a few seconds the ward door burst open and four nurses practically threw themselves into the ward. They got Paddy out of bed again and indicated that they wanted him to leave the ward with them, presumably to put him in a ward on his own. One of them unlocked the door again, and they let Paddy go through first.

At that moment a very young, unqualified nurse arrived rather late on the scene, just in time to see Paddy coming at him out of the open ward door, apparently making his escape. He threw himself at Paddy, who resisted pretty violently. The other nurses joined in and, by the time the whole non-event was sorted out, one of the nurses had a broken nose, there was blood everywhere, and several other nurses had bruises and cuts.

I watched all of this horrified. It was all so totally unnecessary and was caused, I am convinced, by the employment of young, inexperienced 'nurses'. An older, more experienced man would not have jumped to such alarming conclusions on such slender evidence. Staffing at Broadmoor is a terrible problem, of course, but many of these touchy younger men should never be allowed within twenty miles of a mental hospital.

After this we were moved up into the top floor ward of

block 4. This had a bad reputation in Broadmoor, and lived up to it. The dormitory and day room were dreafully overcrowded. Often seventy men would jostle for room to move in the day room, where it was standing room only most of the time. The dormitory too, was over-crowded, and there was a lot of homosexuality going on quite openly. There were serious staff problems, too. I can safely say that the four months I spent in block 4 at Broadmoor were the most miserable of my life, not even exceeded by R.A.F. Bridgnorth, which had held the nausea award until then.

While there I managed to get a 'job' as a room cleaner, which relieved the boredom and earned me six shillings a week. I was now under a different doctor and, for the first time since my admission, I was given a drug – sodium amytal – to help me sleep at nights. Incidentally, it frequently took three and a half weeks to see a doctor after putting in an application and often up to three months.

Lady Cripps, who regarded herself as my 'godmother', came to see me, and was surprised to find that patients at Broadmoor were transferred from one doctor to another, with consequent and often drastic changes of treatment. After her visit she made a formal complaint, and I believe that soon afterwards the system was changed, and patients generally stayed with the same doctor throughout their time at Broadmoor, even if they were no longer in his block.

I found block 4 very depressing, and my marital situation plagued my mind. George Goyder arranged a meeting between Janet and me to discuss a possible reconciliation. We duly met and both agreed that we had acted in an un-Christian way to each other. It was a very frank and constructive meeting, and at the end of it we agreed to try a reconciliation, if only for the sake of our children. But it lasted only a month or two.

The only bright spots about life in block 4 were the games of chess and bridge. I learnt to play bridge, taught by two very brilliant players, Reg, a school teacher, and Ellis, who was a real character. Ellis had a jaundiced look about him. His clothes never seemed to fit him, his hair was thinning, he had very bad teeth, he was sometimes unpredictable; but essentially he was a very likeable man. I remember once losing a contract at Culbertson bridge when playing with Ellis. He leapt up, grabbed my cards, waved them under my nose, swore eloquently, and then picked up the entire card table and hurled it at me. I had never thought of bridge as a blood sport before. It was probably the most popular pastime at Broadmoor, with up to nine schools of bridge going on at a time in a day room. The game was taken seriously, too seriously perhaps, with cheating – secret signals and so on – quite common, and occasional flare-ups between players. I suppose success at bridge was some kind of compensation for more fundamental failures in life.

There was no shortage of leisure activities for the patients, though the more popular pursuits tended to get overcrowded. There was, in addition to bridge, chess, billiards and table tennis indoors; and outdoors, according to the season, there was soccer, cricket, tennis, bowls and basketball. There were recognised clubs for most of these games, and teams from 'outside' played us at soccer, cricket and bowls. Actually, the hospital's bowls team had the exceptional privilege of being allowed to play an occasional 'away' fixture, but selection was on trustworthiness as much as playing ability! The level of ability at the various games varied considerably, though there were a number of brilliant performers.

One of the most brilliant of all was a school teacher, Ginger, with whom I often played chess. He was in his mid-thirties, had been in Broadmoor eight years – for arson – and had an I.Q. of 163. He was the most outstanding chess player I have ever met – and I have been playing chess since my boyhood. He would play with his back to the board, relying entirely on his fantastic memory to keep track of the moves, and still beat me every time. In fact, sometimes he would even correct my moves, although I could see the pieces on the board and he could not.

Another brilliant man in the same ward was a Pole, an engineer, who used to sit quietly in a corner doing calculus and advanced mathematics on rolls of toilet paper. For some confused reason he would never do any work in Broadmoor: he was under the impression it somehow 'helped the Government'.

Also during my stay in block 4 I became chairman of the Patients' Escape Committee. Needless to say, this was not recognised by the authorities. I had no desire to escape myself, but my miserable experiences in block 4 made me sympathise with men who had been there the best part of their lives and, unless they managed to escape, would be there the rest of their lives as well. Looking back, I can understand that people outside would be appalled to think that I was plotting the escape of men who had been put under maximum security because of their record of violence. But it all looks different from the inside, believe me, when you are working and eating and sharing your days with a man who looks and acts normally – at least, normally by Broadmoor standards. In the community of the disturbed, who *is* 'normal'? Not only that, but my experience in block 4, the crude behaviour of some of the staff and the squalid conditions drove any rational assessment of our situation out of my mind. I became a well known rebel and a leader and spokesman for the 'opposition'. That is probably why I was elected chairman of the Escape Committee, which held its meetings during the 'airing courts' and represented all the blocks in the hospital.

However, my association with the Committee was quite short-lived. One day, a patient approached me during the recreation period to report that he was planning an escape and, towards that end, he was manufacturing a bomb. Anywhere else, under conditions of total security, one could have regarded that claim as an idle boast. But with the odd Ph.D and research scientist scattered around the wards it was all too likely to be a genuine threat.

At any rate, I told him he must stop making the bomb – it could endanger the lives of the patients as well as the staff. Escaping, I told him, was one thing, but wounding or killing to achieve it was another. I threatened that if he did not stop making the bomb I should feel bound to report him. However, he refused and said that he did not believe I would report him.

I then wrote to the chief male nurse and told him I had reason to suppose that a patient was manufacturing a bomb in the hospital. He sent for me within ten minutes, and I saw him in complete privacy. I explained that I had no intention of naming the patient concerned, but that there was no doubt in my mind about the seriousness of his intentions. I suggested that he should search all the lockers in a particular block.

He countered this by saying that he would mention the name of three suspects. I did not agree to this, but he went ahead and named them. I did my level best not to reveal by so much as a twitch of a muscle which, if any, of them was the man involved, but when he had finished saying the three names he paused and added, "in fact, it's so-and-so, isn't it?" – and he was absolutely right!

We agreed that he should search all the patients' lockers, including mine. I suggested that it would be as well to confiscate all used or spare electric batteries, and even to check on the batteries in patients' radios and also certain chemical detergents. As it happened, no bomb, nor even a part of a bomb, was found, but I still believe he intended to make one and knew how to. The man concerned was a qualified chemist. More recently, of course, there have been newspaper stories about bombs being made by Broadmoor patients and while brilliant and inventive minds have little else to extend them, and while patients like the one I have described have access to library books about explosives, the possibility of a hideous accident in the hospital can never be discounted.

By now I must admit I had become the complete 'barrack-room lawyer' – something one of the doctors had sternly warned me against soon after my admission. I had my typewriter with me, and as well as using it to type such things as lists of questions and answers for panel games on Sunday evenings in the ward, I employed it to fight real or imagined grievances on the part of the other patients. In view of this the nurses tended to pick on me, but they dared not interfere with my activities.

I kept my typewriter and stationery on a table in the day room, and patients would come to me for help in drafting submissions to tribunals, letters to M.P.'s, lawyers and so on. It was well known that handwritten letters from mental hospitals are habitually ignored, but a typewritten and well-phrased letter at least gets read. I also prepared various submissions to the National Council for Civil Liberties.

In my own case, my lawyers and influential friends like C. H. Rolph, Lady Cripps and Lord Longford were doing their best to get me transferred to a county hospital, but to no avail. So the physician was not able to heal himself, but I think I did a fair job for some of the others.

During the last part of my four miserable months in block 4, things were somewhat lightened by a new friendship, and with a woman. Normally one could only meet the patients in the women's hospital at such things as dances and whist drives, which were not open to me yet. But I had a part as an understudy in the play 'Dear Charles', being put on by the patients' drama society. They were public performances, incidentally, and the standard was very high for an amateur production. At the twice-weekly rehearsals I met a young woman called Sheila, and we became very friendly. At one stage, when it became obvious that Janet was going to try for a divorce, we even talked of getting married. Sheila looked remarkably like Ann, I should explain, and my friendship for her was clearly an attempt to 'transfer' my dependence on Ann, who had now separated from me, to a substitute. This was not a permanent solution, nor even, as it happened, a very lasting relationship, but it does illustrate my need for a sympathetic 'nurse-figure' to lean on during these years.

Chapter 6

At last I said a glad farewell to the noxious block 4 and made my way as a semi-parole patient to block 5. Here I came under the immediate care of Dr Udwin, who was to play a big part in my treatment.

It was a relief to be out of the 'admission' blocks, and I welcomed the comparative freedom of block 5. Patients here could move about pretty freely and were able to attend dances, whist drives and other social functions in the hospital. We were also encouraged to take up one or other of the various handicrafts that were available to us and for which we were paid at a modest rate. I took up marquetry.

As I was feeling somewhat better and more secure, I suppose I should have been able to expect from now on a gradual but definite improvement to the point at which I might reasonably have expected to achieve my discharge. However, one dark cloud hung over it all – the breakdown of my marriage. And before I was to get well, the cloudburst was going to break over my head.

Towards the end of 1965 and about a month after I had been moved to block 5, Janet wrote to Dr McQuade and told him that she was going to divorce me. Although I had feared this for a long while and knew for a fact that she had approached some of my friends for evidence to use against me, I had never been able to accept that it could really happen. So the news, when it was broken to me, was an appalling shock.

I broke down completely. I was put under constant observation and given heavy sedation. I entered a black and dismal period which was, in fact, the emotional crisis of my whole illness. During this time many important things happened, but I was so confused that I find it hard to recall events accurately. I was not violent, but became completely withdrawn. I could not be bothered to wash, cut my finger nails, shave or clean my teeth, but simply sat for hours trembling and shaking while waves of depression broke over me. It was just as well that at that time I was in a place of maximum security, or I would certainly have committed suicide.

Dr Udwin saw me three times a week. He explained to me that the Pakenham-Thompson Committee and my other public achievements were my sole crutch in life. I had used them to 'earn' a place in society. He intended, he said, to strip away my façades and pretences, over a period of time, break down my disordered personality and then slowly rebuild it. As part of this we agreed never to mention the Pakenham-Thompson Committee during these sessions. I went on seeing him regularly for about eighteen months, and I must say he fulfilled that brief to the letter.

But for the present I was in the grip of real despair. For a time I could not even get a solicitor to represent me over the divorce. In the end George Goyder found me one, and this was a great relief. I could do nothing but leave things in his hands.

The routine in block 5 was fairly leisurely, and when events in the outside world permitted it I found the environment generally helpful. We rose at seven and shaved by seven-thirty. Hot water for tea was then available in the kitchen until ten-to-eight, when there was a 'voluntary' recreation period, which meant you could walk around the pleasant, tree-lined airing court until breakfast at eight-fifteen. The food was starchy and uninteresting. Breakfast, for example, would consist of tea, porridge, one rasher of bacon and half a slice of fried bread. But it was distinctly better than at Brixton.

After breakfast there was nothing to do until nine, when work began. Then at nine the gardeners were called out, to work in the enormous kitchen gardens; and after that others would leave to work in the shoe shops, tailors' shops, laundry and so on; and others, including me, would go off to handicrafts.

At ten-fifteen there was a tea break (we brewed our own with tea we had bought out of our 'earnings'), and then work continued until twelve. At noon we were escorted back to our block for lunch. A typical lunch would be a piece of beef, two potatoes and a spoonful of greens, followed by a small helping of pudding. Work began again at two o'clock until four-fifteen. Tea was at four-thirty, and after that the time was our own until bed at a quarter to nine. Boredom during this period was quite bad, though there was television: I.T.V. on the first floor, B.B.C. on the second floor.

I found I was really quite good at marquetry. I specialised in portraits, which is fairly rare, and had two of my efforts – one of Ian Smith and the other of General de Gaulle – exhibited in Read House, Piccadilly, and I actually won two Koestler awards for my work. Although I was paid for working in handicrafts, the hospital gained nothing from what I produced; but to offset that they did very well out of the work of the carpenters (who made all the furniture) and the tailors (who made all the hospital uniforms). The money I was paid was simply an incentive. Those who did not work in this way were required to do other jobs, such as cleaning out the lavatories, polishing floors and so on. I was also allowed eleven shillings a week National Insurance money.

In fact, the work at Broadmoor was the main thing that gave any real meaning or purpose to our existences. Non-working periods – holidays, for example – were universally loathed. Even Christmas was regarded by most of us as simply a time when we had nothing to do but hang around the block.

There were, of course, some pleasant aspects of Christmas, especially for the family men. Apart from visits, and in most cases presents, we were allowed to gamble with tokens for money vouchers which could be spent at the canteen over the Christmas period. Mind you, with a two-ounce tin of tobacco costing seventy-two of these tokens, you had to be remarkably fortunate – or cunning – to get much joy out of the concession.

The hospital was decorated for Christmas, of course, and there was a carol service and Christmas dinner. The League of Friends of the Hospital provided a parcel for each patient. But my main memory of Christmas in Broadmoor is simply of a tense, emotional time, with more weeping and depression than usual. I suppose it was the sheer contrast between what we knew 'inside' and what we remembered of 'outside'. It was, as I have said, generally a pleasure to get back to the usual routine of work again.

During my first few months in block 5 I had one frightening experience involving physical violence. For the second time in under a year, I was attacked by another patient. I believe he had made a derogatory remark about my case and I had threatened to report him. At this he attacked me quite violently.

I did in fact go to Dr Udwin to report him, and even threatened to take out a private summons for assault, but Udwin, whom I respected very much, talked me out of it. The man in question, unbelievably, was due for discharge in a few weeks, and Dr Udwin felt that I would be so unpopular with the other patients if his discharge were postponed that I should have to be transferred to a security block for my own safety. In fact most of the patients supported my complaint, but nevertheless I took his advice and the man was duly discharged.

During all this time my mother came down from London to visit me every week, and she kept this up all the time I was in Broadmoor. 'Outside' contacts like this are very important to patients, if only to put the rather intense and 'close-range' relationships of Broadmoor into perspective.

I made many friends there, and some I still visit once a month and hear from. Charles was one. He was the man who had asked me, back in admission, if I had ever dined at Simpson's. He was quite a character; he was very prominent in our debating society and always began his contribution by announcing solemnly: "I am Charles So-and-so," as though his identity might be in some doubt. But he was marvellously kind. In fact, all through my stay at Broadmoor he made my morning tea and my evening supper for me. We were very close.

Then there was 'the Duke'. He was a highly intelligent man, about 5′ 9″ tall, with a rather pointed face; but his most distinctive features was his meticulous tidiness. In Broadmoor this was more of an achievement than elsewhere, I might add. He was my bridge partner during my last years in Broadmoor. He was rather touchy and quick to take offence if he thought he had been slighted. His particular interest was marquetry. He was reproducing the designs of the Bayeux Tapestry in marquetry and had actually got his work planned for five years ahead. One day he burst into my room while I was praying – a slightly annoying habit of his. However, I invited him to join me. He did, and from then on we often prayed together, and a distinctly 'spiritual' dimension entered into our relationship.

Fred was another very gifted patient, a brilliant painter. From a small colour transparency he did a large canvas portrait of my children. He once told me that he learnt to pray through painting, his mind being led on from the beauty of art to the perfection of creation in God. This was, I believe, a true 'conversion' for him, and he, too, joined me sometimes for prayer and Bible study.

Another man, Ernie, was a sort of depressing by-word among Broadmoor patients – not that he was a depressing person, but his circumstances were. For years Ernie had been one of the most cheerful and 'normal' patients in the hospital. He had been active at football and cricket, a leading light in all the social activities, and an influence for stability and good humour among staff and patients. Some time before I was admitted to Broadmoor he was due for a Tribunal. This was an arrangement to enable patients to have their detentions in Broadmoor reviewed periodically. Discharge from Broadmoor could only come either by a 'responsible medical officer' or through a 'Mental Health Review Tribunal'. According to the Estimates Committee Report, "the procedure involves interviewing the responsible medical officer and normally the patient" and a Tribunal "may direct an immediate discharge". At Broadmoor – in direct contrast to its 'sister' hospitals at Rampton and Moss-side – only a minority of patients are discharged by Tribunals (31 out of 179 from 1961-7).* Despite this, Ernie, and just about everybody else in the hospital, thought that he would be discharged by the Tribunal, having behaved in a co-operative and socially adjusted way for several years since his admission.

In fact he was turned down, and was never the same man again. When I first met him he was unshaven, unwashed and untidy. He looked, and was, cowed and beaten.

It would not be exaggerating to say that the Tribunal system is apparently designed to create the maximum possible

* Report of the Estimates Committee, 1967–8.

distress and sense of grievance on the part of the patient. An Appendix to a Government Report on the Special Hospitals explained the situation very well.

> At Broadmoor, a Tribunal would very rarely wish to discharge a patient against the opinion of the doctors concerned; but there are a fair number of cases where they would like to recommend a transfer, but are powerless to do this. The most they can do is unofficially to urge the responsible medical officer to consider a transfer in the near future. The purpose of the Tribunal is therefore largely defeated in such cases.
>
> Another defect is that the Tribunal must take a "once for all" decision (i.e. until the patient is again entitled to apply) which must be carried out at once; it cannot look forward and say, for instance, that the patient should be discharged in six months' time if there has been no change in his condition. The decision, moreover, is communicated to the patient as a bald "yes or no" statement, and the Tribunal therefore must appear to the patient as a cold, impersonal body, with no real interest in his future.*

Now that was exactly what I felt when my first Tribunal, in 1966, turned me down. I realise now that their decision was probably the correct one, but the effect of it was depressing. This Tribunal came at a time when I was going through the bad patch I have already mentioned. I was paranoid, suspicious, withdrawn and depressed. The immediate trigger for this setback was undoubtedly the divorce case which Janet was now pressing ahead with, while I felt powerless to do anything, confined to Broadmoor and unable to take any real steps to counter it.

As in the past, I was still able to maintain some sort of an image of competence, organising activities, representing pati-

*Appendix I to Second Report of the Estimates Committee 1967–8, p. 297.

ents, and doing very good quality work in the workshops. As before, helping other people was the raft to which I clung. But I was ill, more ill than I cared to admit, and certainly not fit for discharge at that moment.

In fact a second medical opinion was taken at about this time, when Derek Miller, of the Tavistock Institute, came down to examine me. Miller, who was a friend of Lord Donaldson and C. H. Rolph, was sometimes employed at Broadmoor to provide a second opinion on cases. He told them that I was very ill, and that at this point he could neither recommend a discharge from Broadmoor nor transfer to a county hospital. He felt neither course would be in my own best interest.

Lord Longford also sent me an interesting visitor, his secretary, Angela Lambert. She was a very able and knowledgeable woman, who had read Politics and Philosophy at Oxford and offered to help me with patients' cases, complaints, correspondence with government departments and so on. As it happened, although mail was censored, letters from solicitors, government offices and the House of Commons were not. Yet letters from Lord Longford's office, in the Lords, were censored. The only way we could find round this ruling was for mail from him to be posted in House of Commons envelopes and franked there.

At about this time – early in 1966 – there was an epidemic of razor-slashing of coats and jackets at Broadmoor, and in the process my own coat, a good and quite new one, was cut from top to bottom. I was very annoyed and called in the police. They took statements, but told me that there was nothing else they could do, short of interviewing all 700 patients, and that I would simply have to accept that it was done by a mentally sick person. Strangely enough, as a result of this incident, my prestige among the patients rose sky-high. They were delighted that one of their number had had the effrontery to by-pass the hospital authorities and go direct to the police.

Still, the staff got their own back on me in a rather amusing way. I had a small kitchen garden patch to tend. One day a nurse asked me what I intended to do to keep the frost out of my potatoes. I admitted that I had no idea. He said: "Have you ever thought of anti-freeze?" It seemed a good idea, so I put in for a couple of gallons and could never understand why the stuff never turned up – or why several of the staff found the subject so amusing. The incident also demonstrates, I think, two things: the indifference of some of the staff to their patients' illnesses; and the extent of my own mental disturbance. I should certainly have known my leg was being pulled if I had been well.

Just as in earlier years, the worse my illness became, the more I struggled to assert my individuality in other ways. Like a drowning man with a lifebelt, I clung to my own rationality with a desperate grasp. And one of the methods of demonstrating that rationality was to fight some complex legal or social cause. I suppose the Polish man doing calculus on rolls of toilet paper in the corner of the day room was engaged in much the same sort of exercise in his own chosen realm.

At any rate, a chance remark by a friend in the kitchen, Jock, set me off on another typical Thompsonian P.R. campaign – and it was waged right through the period when my illness was at its peak: roughly July to December 1966. I had repeated to him what McGrath had told me when I first raised the question of patients' letters – that he was 'the Management' at Broadmoor. Jock assured me that that was not the case. There was a management committee in London.

That remark really got me going. I felt I knew something about persuading a committee to change its procedures. I found out the name of the secretary of the committee – it was the Ministry of Health's 'Special Hospitals Management

Committee' – and drafted a letter setting out the case for a revision of the rule that patients at Broadmoor could post only two letters a week. The secretary, a Mr Bolton, replied saying that the Committee could see no reason to change their rule – which undoubtedly reflected the view of the senior staff at Broadmoor.

I had only regarded my letter as the first skirmish in what might have to be a protracted campaign. I think I might have been quite disappointed if the committee had given in too quickly. At any rate, I then approached Lord Donaldson, this time with a fully argued, statistically supported case. He in turn wrote to the Health Minister, Kenneth Robinson, drawing his attention to my arguments. I had, as it happened, had a slight acquaintance with Mr Robinson just before the previous General Election, when he agreed to take part in a meeting I was planning in connection with one of my P.R. exercises in the laundry business, but in the end he had had to cry off because of parliamentary pressure on his time.

I cannot categorically say that my campaign was responsible, but within three months an announcement appeared on the ward notice boards to the effect that in future patients could send letters without any restriction at all on their frequency. Censorship, of course, remained. At the same time, Dr Udwin sent a message to me by a nurse to let me know the decision was nothing to do with my efforts. What he did not explain, if that were the case, was how he knew I had made any efforts! Certainly Lord Donaldson thought we had won the battle. He wrote to me saying that the result was "a flag for the Donaldson-Thompson Committee"! Personally I found the relaxation of the letters rule a great practical help. On one memorable occasion before I left Broadmoor I posted ninety-six letters in one day.

Lord Donaldson also sent me the draft of his maiden speech in the Lords, and invited my comments on it. I took the liberty of amending it where I thought he had been overoptimistic about the future of the prison service and, when I read the reports of his speech in the paper, I had the satisfaction of seeing that he had incorporated my amendments. I do not imagine that many maiden speeches in the House of Lords have been 'vetted' by a Broadmoor patient.

While all this was going on I was put on drugs again – barbiturates – and also moved to another dormitory, probably because of the occasion when I was attacked. This was a much smaller but less crowded room, with twelve beds instead of twenty-six. I was still finding great help from prayer and from Bible study. The latter was considerably aided by Janet's entire library of commentaries and study aids, which she had given me 'because she would not be needing them again' – having renounced her Christian faith. In the summer I would sometimes wake at first light and sit on my bed studying the Bible from as early as three a.m. until the doors were unlocked at seven.

Yet, despite this, my relationships with the staff, and even my fellow-patients, became worse than they had been at any time during my stay in Broadmoor. I was very paranoid and deeply suspicious of everybody. I remember once tearing back the curtain in the day room which separated the television watchers from the rest of us, and shouting at the innocent T.V. fans: "Stop talking about me!" Fortunately such behaviour was tolerated by patients in Broadmoor far better than in everyday life.

I also had one appalling period of fantasy. I had been given sleeping drugs to take 'whenever I felt the need'. One night when I had taken one of the pills I awoke in the middle of the night from a very deep sleep. A cold wave of horror swept over me, and I heard Janet screaming. I knew, with awful certainty, why she was screaming.

In 1964 Janet had been pregnant. Through having to work in order to support my penal reform activities (as I saw it), she had a miscarriage. She was taken ill at night, and I could not find a doctor to attend her. She was in pain, and screamed as I tried in a panic to get help for her. A doctor finally came, but it was too late. She lost the child. The foetus was male, and the doctor said it was perfect.

Now the horror of that occasion returned as I sat on my bed in a Broadmoor dormitory, and the guilt of it overwhelmed me. I wept and rocked to and fro, moaning that I was a murderer. A friend invited me to lie on his bed and tried to console me, but I was beyond it. For days I could think of nothing else. I told my doctor that I was guilty of murder, and nobody was able to persuade me otherwise. The person who helped me most at this stage, I think, was Mrs Paton, the hospital's resident psychiatric social worker. She was a motherly, warm-hearted person, and she did her best to convince me that I had not committed murder, nor anything like it. Janet had had an unfortunate but fairly common *medical* mishap. But it was a month or two before the awful sense of guilt began to leave me.

I was not fit to think about important issues, let alone take serious, rational decisions. This complicated the matter of the divorce on which Janet had set her heart. Indeed, Dr Udwin at once stage seriously considered putting me under the protection of the Courts. By this I would have surrendered my legal rights to the Courts, but they would have acted on my behalf. I think he was worried that the strain of the divorce proceedings would make my illness even more critical than it now was. But my solicitors advised against this course of action.

My unhappy relationship with Janet was mirrored, as I have said, in unhappy relationships inside the hospital, too. I felt I was being criticised and attacked, and an outbreak of anonymous letters, with myself as one of the unlucky recipients, did nothing to help matters. About eighteen patients received them and, as they were very abusive and dealt with alleged 'sex' offences (which my offence, of course, was not),

I imagine they were sent to a selected group. I was very disturbed by the letters, and for the second time went over the management's head and called in the police.

Once again they were unable to help. Their attitude seemed to be that in a mental hospital you should expect to receive sick letters from sick people – and, in any case, what could they do about it?

As it turned out, this was to be the last time a Broadmoor patient would be able to call in the police. The Chief Constable of Berkshire wrote to the Ministry of Health invoking section 36 of the Mental Health Act and asking that in future no letters or complaints from Broadmoor patients should come to him.

Broadmoor figured in the news quite a bit at that time (the second half of 1966), largely through a daring and almost successful escape by one of the patients, Tony. At that time security was fairly lax during the airing courts. No security staff were present while we were exercising ourselves in the enclosed courts, but numbers were checked on entering and leaving. There was also no roll call at night.

While we were strolling around the court, Tony apparently pulled a bench up to the high wall which surrounded it, climbed on to the top and dropped down the other side – all without being seen. He then made off down the road and began to try to hitch a lift. Broadmoor patients do not wear any 'uniform', but the suits provided are so outstandingly ill-fitting that one would be less conspicuous dressed in arrow-printed overalls. Nevertheless, Tony got a lift and began to think that he had a real chance of getting as far as London undetected.

Unfortunately for him, the person who had given him a lift was a Broadmoor nurse, who had recognised him. The nurse stopped his car on some pretext and went to phone the hospital. While he was away, Tony recognised his 'official'

Broadmoor bag and decided the time had come to change transport. He ran away into some fields.

However, the alarm had now been given, and the full Broadmoor escape man-hunt was in operation. There was a certain awful routine about a Broadmoor escape. The police would be called back from off-duty; the officer cadets at Sandhurst would be mustered, issued with clubs, and sent out to track down the miscreant; tracker dogs would howl all through the night; and the local M.P., Mr van Straubenzee, would complain at Westminster about these dangerous inmates on his constituents' doorsteps.

The full ritual was invoked on this occasion, and within a couple of days Tony was brought back to Broadmoor again. As usual, the papers were full of it, but it was a two-day wonder and soon forgotten. However, it was not so soon forgotten by the management. Security in general was tightened, a nightly roll call was instituted, and since then there has not been a single escape from Broadmoor.

Mind you, there were still loopholes in the internal security arrangements. On one occasion I was working in the central hall area and had to pass along a connecting corridor. I noticed that a 'push bar' on a pair of doors was riding high – only a push would have been needed to open them and get into a high security area. I notified the Chief Mental Nurse, and within thirty minutes the entire pair of doors had been stripped down and refurbished. Strangely enough, no one seemed very grateful to me for drawing attention to this chink in the security armour. Indeed, Dr Udwin contented himself with the remark that it was the duty of parole patients to conduct themselves in a 'trustworthy manner'.

Another internal security breakdown concerned a group of seriously disturbed patients from block 6 who managed to get out on to the roof of their block and stayed there for a couple of days, throwing slates at anyone who tried to approach them. Apparently they claimed to be protesting about conditions in the block, but the response of the authorities, once they had been recaptured, was simply to tighten up security. If they had been parole patients, they would have lost their parole status; but as they were not there was no punishment which they could be given except to increase general security. Indeed, one could say that at Broadmoor security equals punishment, and punishment equals security. No other sanction remains to the authorities.

I was no longer chairman of the Escape Committee, as it happened. After the explosives' incident I decided I could not actively support escapes which might put lives at risk. But, like everyone else at Broadmoor, I was pleased when a fellow-patient managed to outwit our guards and get away from the place. I realise now how shortsighted and even irrational such a feeling of pleasure really is. Many of the patients undoubtedly were violent and dangerous people. But such is the community of suffering, we saw each other in quite a different light. It was the world outside that was cruel, violent and aggressive. It was hard to imagine one's Broadmoor friends as brutal or dangerous. Most of them were gentle, even fearful men. I suppose this is consistent with the illnesses that had brought them to the place. So we stood together, a strange, motley band, outcasts of society and yet forming a strange society of our own in which many of the values of the outside world were turned upside down. I can honestly say that it never occurred to me that Broadmoor escapees might be a menace to innocent residents of the district. They seemed to be more menaced than menacing in the setting where I saw them.

In any case, I was again grappling with violence in my own mind. I managed to make a knife in the workshops, and carried it with me everywhere. All the old fantasies came flooding back, and once again defensive aggression took over.

However, there was one difference between my circumstances now and my circumstances two or three years earlier:

Broadmoor security. When I mentioned to the Departmental Nurse that I was carrying a knife, he asked me to show it to him. When he saw it he realised how pathetic my state of mind was, for my 'knife' – with which I meant to scare off the evil forces again seeking to destroy me – was one nail protruding from a plastic pen. The worst injury it could have inflicted would have been a minor scratch. Yet to me it was as potent as Excalibur. The nurse smiled and suggested I gave it to him, and I handed it over.

Three men at Broadmoor were a great support and encouragement to me at this time, and they were all connected with the workshop. Jack Barber – a very tall, heavy man – was head of handicrafts. He was a sharp man, but one who bore no grudges. Right to the end of my stay I do not think he ever really *liked* me, and yet he put up with me. More than that, he helped me more than he realised. At this time, for instance, I would have frequent bouts of tears, often starting at about 9.30 in the morning and lasting perhaps a couple of hours. There was no immediate reason for them, beyond my general depression. On mornings when I arrived in handicrafts in tears, Jack would leave his office, saying: "I'm going to sit with Peter", and he would sit with me for up to two hours at a stretch, sometimes fetching me a cup of tea.

Frank Smith, who was also tall, was a 'craftsman' in the handicrafts section; and Jim Gale, a much shorter man, was in charge of Occupational Therapy. Both of them, too, were very helpful and encouraging at this stage. Frank believed my cure was to 'take me out of myself'. He once doused me with water from a hose, and on another occasion put wood cuttings in my tea. I cannot say I always appreciated his style of humour, but I did appreciate his interest in my welfare.

Chapter 7

At the end of 1966 a representative of Janet's solicitors came to Broadmoor to get my signature on a document. It was an admission of my adultery and would pave the way for Janet to obtain the divorce she had set her heart on. Mainly because of my fear that if I refused, my whole medical history might be made public in a divorce court, I voluntarily provided Janet with evidence she could never have obtained in any other way, and signed the paper. I also agreed that our house should be sold to pay the costs of the case. I was led back to my block in tears.

I had another Mental Health Review Tribunal at the end of 1966, in the hope of getting my discharge from Broadmoor. Dr Udwin was totally opposed to my discharge (correctly, viewing it with hindsight), and the Tribunal supported his view. This came at the height of my depression over the divorce, and the result was yet another crushing blow to me.

However, from the beginning of 1967 I began to get better again. It was a slow process, as will be seen, and I still had the actual divorce proceedings hanging over me, but Broadmoor's 'walking stick' was doing its job and, by leaning heavily on it, I began to see a gradual, infinitely slow, but quite definite improvement. This was marked officially by my being given my 'green parole' card which allowed me to move fairly freely round the rear blocks of the hospital and then, within a month, the top 'red parole' card. I was given this because I had taken on a new job, working in the administration of the handicrafts section, which involved frequent trips to the front quadrangle, where articles made in the workshops were stored before being sold. I also found that singing in the hospital choir, which I now did regularly, had a very therapeutic effect on me. Apart from that, I also enjoyed it!

I was particularly fortunate to get those two important upgradings in my parole, because only just before I had been involved in a fight which – for the one and only time – I had initiated. It was in the kitchen, and in the scuffle I had a tooth loosened. (Soon after I persuaded a friend in handicrafts to pull it out with a pair of pliers.)

At this time there had been quite an outbreak of violence in block 5, and Dr McGrath had ordered that all patients involved in fights should be reported to him. Transfer to the security wing – block 6 – looked inevitable for me. Dr Udwin took statements from me and from the other patient involved and reported the incident to the Superintendent . . . but we heard no more about it. I sighed with relief and made a mental note to keep out of trouble in future.

Escapes and violence at Broadmoor are undoubtedly infectious and, following Tony's escape, there were several abortive attempts to emulate him. The most spectacular one I have mentioned briefly already. It was by two patients in the security block 6, which adjoined our block. These men were in a room on the ground floor. One night they broke through the ceiling of their room into the room above, then through the ceiling of that room to the top floor, and finally – incredibly – through that ceiling on to the roof. They were seriously disturbed patients, and began shouting and throwing slates from the roof at anybody they managed to see. We were all moved out of our rooms on the third floor of block 5 and, with the thuds and bangs from the roof overhead ringing in our ears, carried our mattresses down to the day room where forty of us spent the rest of the night and the following night. The would-be escapers stayed on the roof for two days, and after their recapture wire mesh was incorporated in all ceilings to prevent anyone else following their example and escaping 'upwards'.

One really typical flash of the old Peter Thompson emerged in 1967. It was as though I was allowed one successful P.R. campaign per annum in Broadmoor. The *Daily Express* had run a story which described Broadmoor as 'the Berkshire institution for 900 insane criminals'. I wrote to the Editor, Mr Derek Marks, pointing out that it was nothing of the kind, but he refused to publish an apology or a correction.

Not at all daunted, I then took the matter up with the Press Council. They adjudicated on the matter on July 25, 1967, and found that "when the mistake was pointed out a correction should have been published", and the complaint was upheld. The report of the adjudication in the *UK Press Gazette* mentioned that the complaint was made by "Mr Peter Thompson, writing from Broadmoor" – a very nice way, I felt, of describing my status! The incident helped considerably to publicise the change in status of Broadmoor since it had been taken over by the Ministry of Health from the Home Office in 1949. The *UK Press Gazette,* for instance, recorded the fact that only a very small percentage of Broadmoor's inmates could correctly be described as 'criminally insane', and quoted a Ministry of Health official as saying that the correct description of the 775 people then resident in the hospital was 'patients'. The Editor of the *Daily Express* told the Press Council that he had now given instructions that the word 'criminal' must not in future be used in any "general description of Broadmoor or of the patients".

At about the same time the late night news on B.B.C. radio

made a similarly inaccurate reference to Broadmoor. Again I wrote and protested, and my letter was read out after the news bulletin a few days later, as an apology.

I had written to the godfather of my youngest child, a solicitor, Philip Stunt, who was an old friend from All Souls days, saying that I very much wanted to meet and establish a deeper friendship with Christians from the 'outside' world. He mentioned this to the Rector of All Souls, John Stott, who approached a master at a well known public school. This man was not able to visit me, but he put a friend of his, Peter Waghorn – a housemaster at Wellington College – in touch with me; and so began a friendship that was very, very precious to me. Peter visited me once a week throughout the remainder of my stay at Broadmoor, and was more help to me than I can ever possibly describe.

The divorce proceedings, which had been dragging on for some time, were completed in 1967. So far as I was concerned, the results were pretty disastrous. I received a bill for £220 towards the costs, and no arrangements at all were made for me to see my children. The sale of our house produced a very small sum after paying off mortgages and so on, and I found myself left with only £75 towards the sum asked for by Janet's solicitors. I wrote and asked if I might keep ten pounds, as this was the only money I had in the world, apart from a weekly income of six shillings, but they replied that she had already been generous to a fault and insisted that I hand over the whole sum.

This left the matter of the children unresolved. George Goyder arranged a sort of 'lay tribunal' in an attempt to come to an amicable agreement about my seeing them, and C. H. Rolph and the Rev. Bruce Reed agreed to act as arbitrators.

Janet had been given custody of the children by the court, and my solicitors had not at that time made any application for access to them. This 'tribunal', of course, had only moral authority. It had no legal force at all. In the event the adjudicators decided that I should be allowed to see the children once every three months, and this was agreed. At this point, I had not seen the children for over eighteen months, but from then on I saw them for a couple of hours every quarter while I remained in Broadmoor.

At about this time Lord Longford and Lady Cripps, who never ceased to take an interest in me, went to see the Broadmoor Management Committee in London, to find out whether I could be transferred to a county hospital. Dr McGrath strongly opposed this, but I felt that from then on my case was regarded in a rather more sympathetic light at Broadmoor itself. I should say here that Lady Cripps, who regards herself as my 'godmother', was a tremendous source of strength and encouragement to me all through my time in Broadmoor. Although in her seventies, she was one of my most faithful correspondents, writing me many warm and inspiring letters full of her own deep Christian faith. She told me that she prayed for me every day while I was in hospital.

I took up chess seriously and began to play in matches against teams from outside Broadmoor, including Reading University. I was usually on table two or three. This was a real breath of the world outside, and very welcome. I also began to have regular visits from Victor Hall, who was preceptor at Newbold Theological College. So, with Peter coming every week, I had no grounds for complaint about any absence of visitors.

The final escape incident of my stay at Broadmoor occurred at about this time, and I had a small finger in the pie. I was working in handicrafts one day when I saw a patient snatch an ironing board and use it to climb on to a hut roof and from there on to a wall behind the block. This was an *internal* wall. I ran into the chief male nurse's office and gave the alarm. Within minutes, the man had been brought down from the wall and was being led away to a security ward. It was all rather a non-event. Imagine our surprise, then, when the *Daily Mirror* ran a story the next morning about a Broadmoor patient seen running along an outside wall and causing a full-scale security alert. It was, perhaps, an example of the emotive way in which news about Broadmoor is usually reported.

I did not take that one up with the paper – a rare lapse on my part. But I was back in full flood in my 'barrack room chambers', dispensing free advice, drafting letters and generally making myself a major thorn in the administration's side. I waged a battle with the Ministry of Health about magazines for prisoners, and helped several patients in block 2 write letters to their M.P.s complaining that they had not seen a psychiatrist for long periods.

I also began to write a regular column on political matters in the Broadmoor *Chronicle,* over the pen-name 'Backbencher'. I was particularly fascinated by American politics and read over thirty books on the subject. The *Chronicle* was the Broadmoor patients' own magazine, although the Superintendent was 'Managing Editor' and could censor articles of which he disapproved. However, the Editor – a tall, extrovert, very able man – and all the contributors were patients. It was duplicated, about thirty pages each month, with a two-colour cover, with regular features on hospital affairs, stories, reports and a column on political affairs. This last was my responsibility and, with the help of a regular supply of *The Economist,* the *New Statesman* and the *Spectator* provided free by their publishers, I contributed my 700 words a month for the last eighteen months of my stay in Broadmoor.

The 'authorities' were not very happy about my stream of high-ranking visitors. One can hardly blame the Superintendent for feeling that his problems in running the hospital were multiplied by the frequent visits of such influential figures in the penal reform world as Lord Longford, Lord Donaldson, Lady Cripps, C. H. Rolph or Bob Taylor (Director of Prison Administration). But, of course, there was nothing that could be done to forbid it.

Another visitor of rather a different kind was Peter Oxley, who was introduced to me by the Rev. Bruce Reed of Christian Teamwork. He was a sales director, and when he came our sole topic of conversation was business and economics. He felt this was the contribution he could make – not to discuss my health or my case, but to broaden my interest in the world outside. I am sure he was completely right, too.

Also at this stage I began a long campaign, still uncompleted, to get my case reviewed. I wrote to Laurence Pavitt, M.P., chairman of the Commons Health Committee, and Eric Moonman, M.P., asking for an investigation into my medical and psychiatric treatment during the period leading up to February 1965. Mr Pavitt was sympathetic, but felt there was not much he could do. I filed his letter, regarding it as simply marking the start of a campaign that would probably take years to achieve its object.

I made my first trip outside Broadmoor for over two years in the summer of 1967. I was in the hospital's bowls team, and we used to play a couple of 'away' fixtures in the locality. The strange thing is that as soon as we left the familiar setting of the hospital I felt very afraid and could not get back inside quickly enough. We passed some children in a field, I remember, and I kicked their ball back to them. A small boy of about eight warned his even smaller friends as they collected the ball: "Don't talk to them – they're lunatics!"

Broadmoor was obviously more important to me than I had realised. As I got better, so I was able to see how much the security, the routine and the orderliness of Broadmoor meant to a man like me. I *was* getting better, of that there was now no doubt, but it would be some time before I could throw my 'walking stick' away.

1968 was, in fact, the year that yielded the first solid evidences that I was beginning to make a recovery. All my social activities continued – I started a 'Monday Club' for groups to discuss the topics we should later be tackling in the debating society, which was now well established on a hospital-wide basis – but in addition I found my relationships with the staff were improving. As well as the men I have mentioned, I began to build firm friendships with several of the senior nurses: men like Deputy Chief Male Nurse Allen Lee, Bert Wright, Reg Sheppard, Bill Kingdom and Harold Lee.

I was also much helped by a rather strange but touching relationship which I had established with one of the women patients, whom I will call 'Sosca'. Her story is a very remarkable one.

Sosca was born in Hong Kong and deserted by her parents at the age of six months. Brought up in a convent, she went to live in an orphanage in Saigon, Vietnam, at the age of twelve; eventually worked for an airline company; and finally married a sergeant in the British army. He brought her to England – the first time she had seen the land of her own nationality. However, the marriage was bitterly unhappy, there was a good deal of violence in the relationship, and she ended up in Broadmoor.

A short, rather plump woman a couple of years older than me, Sosca was a real source of strength. I met her at dances and other activities, and in between we corresponded with each other. She was discharged a couple of years before I was, and from the time of her discharge sent me a pound a week to supplement my meagre pocket money in Broadmoor. At one point, she more than anyone or anything else, stood between me and suicide.

Two rather strange battles of words kept me busy pretty

well throughout 1968, taking my mind off other matters. The first concerned the *Daily Telegraph* and the second, the establishment of a patients' committee.

William Deedes, an M.P. for whom I have the greatest admiration, and who had done a great deal over the years to help me, wrote an interesting and factual article on Special Hospitals in the *Daily Telegraph*. Unhappily, the paper headlined it 'Treating Our Insane Criminals', which incensed me. Rather hastily, I think, I wrote to the Editor complaining and, when I got no apology, referred the matter to the Press Council. However, this time they adjudicated in favour of the paper, though the Editor did accept a letter from me pointing out the inaccuracy of the headline to William Deedes' article.

I have always said that you cannot win them all, but in my life failures and success have usually come alternately. So it was in keeping with history that my next campaign should be very much more successful. I had been elected as a member of the hospital's social committee, which was responsible, with the senior staff, for organising the leisure activities and recreations of the patients. However, I felt that this committee's terms of reference were too restrictive to enable it to be what was badly needed at Broadmoor – a genuine voice for the patients' views on the running of the hospital. So I conceived the idea of a 'Patients' General Purposes Committee' and set about organising a careful P.R. campaign to promote it.

First I wrote an article for the Broadmoor *Chronicle* setting out the case for such a committee – especially to represent patients' views to the Management Committee on their quarterly visits. As Dr McGrath was 'Editor-in-Chief', I knew he had read, and presumably permitted, the article. The following month, at my instigation, the Editor wrote an editorial commending the idea. I then worked to get a general meeting at which the proposal for a General Purposes Committee could be discussed and voted upon. Eventually, such a meeting was held in the main hall. Dr McGrath, the Matron, the doctors and the chief male nurses were present to see the meeting approve the idea very warmly. But as we left, Dr McGrath said to me: "A typical P.R. campaign, Peter." Then he smiled, "But I'm not giving you a blank cheque."

I knew what he meant and was quite content. Under this pressure, he set up patients' committees in each block, who met once a month with the doctors on a Wednesday morning to discuss all aspects of hospital life, complaints, patients' welfare, food and so on. I felt we had really achieved something there, even though I had failed to get the direct contact I wanted with the Management Committee.

It was in 1968 that I uncovered one fact about myself of which I was previously completely unaware – that I was illegitimate. The discovery came about in a strange way. I had learnt of my father's death – I had neither seen nor heard from him throughout my stay in Broadmoor – and wrote to his solicitors enquiring about his estate. They replied that, owing to 'certain circumstances', I had no standing in the matter, and the estate (of £13,500) had gone to my uncle, Major George Thompson.

Baffled by the phrase about 'certain circumstances', I wrote demanding to know what these were, only to be told that at the time of my father's 'marriage' to my mother he was already married to someone else; which made me and my sister illegitimate. It was little consolation to know that sundry drill sergeants, warders and mental nurses had been quite correct in their mode of address to me over the years.

From the middle of 1968 I had been having treatment not only from Dr Udwin but also from a brilliant and charming young Greek doctor whom I had first met when I had kidney pains. We got on very well together, and I had great confidence in him. Apart from a serious bout of pleurisy late in 1968 – which was a completely physical illness – my health continued to improve, and I looked forward eagerly to the chance of another tribunal the following year.

My Christian faith flourished in Broadmoor as never before. At one time I organised a 'prayer vigil' for nine o'clock each evening, when patients would pause and silently remember each other in prayer before going to sleep. I also tried to get a 'Christian Union' started for men who wanted to study the Bible and pray together. However, the chaplain was advised that such a thing "wouldn't work in Broadmoor" and permission was refused. Nevertheless, two or three of us did meet regularly for Bible study and prayer.

With regard to getting out of Broadmoor I was ambivalent. I applied for a tribunal each year, but was frankly not at all sure how I would have fared in the world outside. I really wanted to win my case at the tribunal to clear myself of the stigma which I felt committal to Broadmoor carried. It was a kind of intellectual exercise – a challenge like a game of chess, that had to be won. But in my more honest moments I knew that I was probably happier inside than I would be outside.

So I prepared my case for the 1969 Tribunal with mixed feelings, though I desperately wanted to establish my *right* to release. When it came to the crunch, it seemed that I was going to have to do it on my own. Twice I had persuaded my 'supporters' to travel down and give evidence, and twice it had been to no avail. Now, apparently, they had decided it was all an empty ritual. They had lost faith in the Tribunal, and so I lost faith in it, too. The list of people who could not or would not appear for me got longer, and my hopes grew thinner every day. I became almost hysterical over it, feeling as I had read Gerald Brooke felt in a Soviet prison – trapped, hopeless and isolated. No patient could ever have approached a Tribunal with less enthusiasm or less hope.

And yet I won my case! Indeed, the Broadmoor authorities, with indecent haste, gave me just twenty-four hours to leave the place once the Tribunal's findings were released. It may be that a letter Judge Lyle wrote to the Tribunal influenced their decision: I do not know. I was bewildered, amazed and elated all at once. It was almost as though the hospital administration, piqued that I should obtain my discharge against their advice, were taking it out on me by throwing me on to the street, or into the arms of a hostile world, unprepared and unaided.

In fact, I appealed, and my discharge was delayed for one week. Three senior Christian friends – Nevill, the chairman of a merchant bank; Bruce Reed, director of the Grubb Institute of Behavioural Studies; and George Goyder – agreed to act as my 'guardians'. I was given ten pounds by a charity for discharged prisoners, and the clothes I was wearing on admission were returned to me. My personal effects – boxes and boxes of them – were piled up beside me at the main gate as I was ushered through it.

Everything had happened so suddenly and unexpectedly that I had simply not been able to take it in. Here I was, on a late summer afternoon in 1969, standing outside the gates of Broadmoor, blinking like a frightened animal at the sheer spaciousness of the world before me, and yet inwardly – if I were honest – longing to run back inside again.

Which brings us, as it were, full circle to where this book began. The questions asked then remain largely unanswered. What happened to me has been related. Why it happened has emerged incidentally. In a final chapter, however, I want to describe the effect this experience had on me, viewed from the point of view of a return to 'normal' life; and then to probe a little more deeply into the wider implications of a story which may have happened to me, but has relevance to every human being who cares about mental health and social justice.

Chapter 8

I was met at the gates of Broadmoor by Peter Waghorn, and we loaded my gear into his car. We drove back to Wellington College and had tea there. Dr Gurney had come down to drive me back to London, having found me a room in a hostel in south London run by a Christian organisation. As we made our way towards London, I became terrified at the speed we were travelling and urged him to go more slowly. The significant fact here is that Dr Gurney is the mildest and most cautious of drivers and had probably not exceeded 40 m.p.h. at that point! But I was feeling very insecure without my 'walking stick' and very conscious that I had been suddenly cut off from a community that, with all its faults, was purpose-built to shield people like me from forces with which they could not cope.

Not only that, but, because I had had the audacity to achieve discharge through a Tribunal – a comparative rarity at Broadmoor – I was automatically deprived of even the minimal 'follow-up' procedures offered in the usual case. At the hostel – an institution, like Broadmoor, but strange to me and rather stark – I was overcome with loneliness and more than a hint of depression.

I had to arrange to 'sign on' with a National Health doctor and re-establish contact with my psychiatrist. I got no help at all from Broadmoor. Dr Udwin told me that this was my own fault because I had left through a Tribunal. It was almost as though I had done something illegal or irresponsible – to use a procedure laid down by the Ministry of Health itself!

Fortunately, a number of my friends, including my 'guardians' stood by me. Nevill got me a senior management job in the City, arranging the 'decentralisation' of a merchant bank. This assignment involved visiting thirty-five towns and development areas, interviewing mayors and town clerks, drawing up assessments of housing, schools, transport and so on, and then advising the bank on the most suitable locations. It was rather more demanding, intellectually and emotionally, than pushing a wheelbarrow, which was my last assignment at Broadmoor, just two weeks earlier. It is probably as well that the various civic dignitaries were unaware of that.

Few patients discharged from Broadmoor have had this priceless advantage of influential friends to get them work suited to their abilities. Without them, I should probably still be washing up in a transport cafe somewhere. However, various people warned me off the P.R. field, memories being long, although the National Institute of Industrial Psychology gave 'Public Relations' as the right field for me, after extensive psychological tests, and also showed that my ability had not been impaired by mental illness.

Another temporary job – on the 'fringe' of P.R. – followed with a semi-political organisation, 'Aims of Industry', but a permanent post seemed as far away as ever. It was at this point of desperation, with loneliness and a feeling of isolation mounting, that I asked Broadmoor to take me back, but my request was turned down.

I am glad now that it was, for I can see these fears for

what they were. The walking stick – the crutch – had been taken away, and taken away abruptly. The first few steps without it were painful and nervous, but things began to improve. I found many of my former friends cold, hostile and judging. Had it not been for people like Nevill and two new friends, Ian, who was a broker, and Anthony, I think my newly rediscovered faith would have withered away in the frost. Later, I was helped by the vicar of a local church, who was experienced in clinical theology. Lord Longford and other old friends stood by me, but I was missing my home and family and often felt very lonely.

Still, I was able to see the children once a month – an arrangement now set up by the solicitors – and I also saw my mother most weekends. But relationships were more difficult than in Broadmoor. I lost one new friend, a young woman called Juliet to whom I had become deeply attached, when my Broadmoor background became known. This triggered off a minor depression, which ended with my going into the local police station in tears to get help. After the comparative calm and security of Broadmoor, I was finding it hard to retain the measure of inner tranquility that I had found there. In four years, the world 'outside' seemed to have become even more hectic and pressurised than before. So I followed up a suggestion by Dr Gurney that I should visit the 'surgery' of two men who specialised in divine healing, Ken Lock and the Rev. Michael Smith. They prayed and laid their hands on me, and I must say I became immediately conscious of a deep, inward peace such as I had not known for many years, perhaps ever: and this has stayed with me since.

Yet, despite these setbacks, I was slowly getting used to the pace and pressure of ordinary life again, and painfully picking up the threads of social and business life. I had discovered for myself how hard it is for a man with a 'record' – even if, like me, his record is not 'criminal' – to re-establish himself. Without my influential friends, I doubt whether I would have made it.

As it was, things changed for the better after a more or less permanent job was found for me – a post organising a huge national appeal on behalf of a well known international voluntary organisation. Lord Longford and Lady Monckton were indirectly responsible for this. At last I was back in a world I knew: a world of press releases, radio and television publicity and personal contacts.

Now one thing remained, and that was to have the whole handling of my case reviewed. I was not prepared to let it all slide into history as though it had never happened. I wanted to know the answers to questions that had never been properly faced. Why was I allowed to wander London with knives and guns, a *self-confessed* danger to society? Why was I discharged from hospital less than twenty-four hours after a suicide attempt? Why was nothing done to help me until *after* I had made a dangerous attack on three innocent people? Why was it that I alone had had to pay the penalty for all this, when others too, in Judge Lyle's words, 'shared the responsibility'?

It is these questions that I am determined to press, not to reopen old wounds, but because they raise profound questions about society's attitude to the mentally ill. It simply will not do to lock people like me away in Broadmoor and try to pretend we do not exist. At this moment hundreds, perhaps thousands of people every bit as disturbed and potentially as dangerous as I was are wandering our streets. It is not enough to feed them with tranquilisers and hope for the best. And it is not enough, when the worst rather than the best happens, to jump on them like social outcasts and hurl them into the outer darkness of our 'Special Hospitals'. My case, and others like it, raises all these questions, and I believe society must answer them.

Quite apart from the personal implications of all this,

which are considerable, a number of more general matters relating to our treatment and care of the dangerously mentally ill have also been raised in this book. The overcrowding at Broadmoor continues, and will continue until a new hospital is completed (economic squeezes permitting) in 1974. The eccentricities of the Tribunal system remain: a sort of lottery, with the sanity of human beings as the Big Prize. The recruitment of suitable nursing staff for Special Hospitals, the role of the patients in the hospitals' administration, the treatment of mentally sick men and women on remand in general prisons,* the absence of any adequate after-care for those discharged from Special Hospitals – especially under Tribunals – and the public embarrassment at encountering a 'man from Broadmoor': these are problems and attitudes that must be dealt with if we are to move out of the 'Bedlam' era into a new and more humane treatment of the mentally ill.

It is hard to change attitudes, but there are a number of practical steps which could be taken now that would ease the problems immediately, and in the long term might make for a change of attitude.

The first step would be to change the name of Broadmoor to 'Crowthorne Hospital'. Without such a change, the place will never live down the stigma of its days as a criminal lunatic asylum. It would cost virtually nothing, but it would be a great deal more than an empty gesture. After all, the names of the blocks in the hospital have already been changed from numbers to English counties (Kent, Dorset, Essex, etc.). Broadmoor is the only hospital in the area, and there would be no confusion if it were known, as the other Special Hospitals are, by its geographical name, 'Crowthorne'. Such a change would underline the change in the status and role of the hospital which occurred as a result of the 1959 Mental Health Act – when it ceased to be a criminal lunatic asylum

* See Appendix.

– but which has never really registered with the press or the public.

As a result of a letter of mine in the national press early in 1971 this question, and also the question of an overhaul of the whole system of after-care of patients discharged from mental and Special Hospitals, was raised in Parliament by Mrs Shirley Williams. The Secretary of State said that he had received suggestions 'from a former patient of one of the Special Hospitals' and was studying the existing services and their need for development. In fact, I had been granted a long and constructive interview with the Secretary of State for Health and Social Security, at which I had argued for reforms at Broadmoor, and had found Sir Keith a sympathetic listener. So perhaps something will be done.

Certainly there simply must be set up a national system for the rehabilitation and after-care of patients from the Special Hospitals. My case is not typical, for two reasons. I was discharged by a Tribunal, so the normal after-care was denied me. But this consists solely in finding the discharged patient a job (usually menial) and somewhere to live (usually a hostel). On the other hand, I had the advantage of influential friends who found suitable work for me: and I might also mention the generosity of the Institute of Public Relations who gave me money to buy a suit, and of another advertising charity, who gave me five pounds a week, mostly in Luncheon Vouchers, for the first few weeks after my discharge. People like Lord Donaldson, Alan Eden-Green (of British Oxygen) and Basil Saunders (of the Wellcome Foundation) – as well as my long-standing supporters – enabled me to survive the trauma of being abandoned like a new-born baby in a strange and hostile environment.

Let me illustrate how hard this can be. From 250 letters seeking a job sent out for me by a direct mail firm, I gained fifteen interviews. These letters made no mention of Broadmoor, but simply stated that I had been in hospital for four years. From 225 letters sent out by Apex – an agency which helps ex-prisoners to find jobs – I had only one interview. These letters referred to my detention in Broadmoor. As soon as Broadmoor is mentioned, most employers simply do not want to know any more. Perhaps that explains why one honours graduate who was discharged from Broadmoor after eleven years as a patient ended up working as a cleaner in a supermarket. But for my influential friends, I am sure I should have been in a similar situation.

My interest in the after-care of prisoners has been sharpened by my own experiences, for the two situations are directly comparable. Suggestions that the already over-stretched probation service could handle the situation seem to me quite unrealistic. The Pakenham-Thompson recommendations about after-care officers have never been implemented, but perhaps the time is now ripe to press the matter again. I raised this question in December, 1970, in a letter to the *Guardian*:

> I am distressed to see that the Probation Service is to be stretched even further to accommodate more parolees. In your columns in the early sixties you gave considerable attention to the Pakenham-Thompson Committee on 'The Problems of Ex-prisoners', of which I was co-chairman with Lord Longford. . . .
>
> You will recall that one of the main recommendations of the Pakenham-Thompson Committee was that, instead of weighing down the over-burdened Probation Officer, there should be a new body of people known as 'After-care Officers', complementing the Probation Service and designed to take away pressure from the Probation Officers. Lord Longford and I felt so strongly about this in the past that we even 'put down' an amendment to the 1961 Criminal Justice Bill, which was debated in the House of Lords. . . .

Alas, the amendment was defeated, but at that time considerable public opinion was in favour of 'After-care Officers' for the rehabilitation of prisoners.

A further practical step would be the establishment of 'halfway houses' for patients discharged from Special Hospitals. At present, county hospitals and voluntary hostels, like those of the Church Army, are used for this purpose, but clearly this is unsatisfactory. In such 'half-way houses' patients could adjust themselves to the differences between life 'inside' and life 'outside', and be spared the shock of the present abrupt transition.

But the most fundamental need in the treatment of the dangerously mentally ill person is a change of emphasis in the Special Hospitals. At the present, security and therapy are mixed up in a confusing and unhelpful way. Nurses are expected to act as security guards at one moment and as psychiatric counsellors the next. It simply cannot be done.

I believe Broadmoor should become a teaching hospital for psychiatrists and mental nurses. This would raise its medical status and the morale of the staff and patients. Administration, at every level from top to bottom, should be separated from medical care, so that the Superintendent is not deluged with day-to-day details of hospital routine, and the doctors and nurses are free to do the work for which they have been trained. I should like to see all nurses in Special Hospitals given psychiatric tests every few years to establish their emotional suitability to continue to work amongst mentally ill and disturbed patients; and the minimum age of nurses raised to twenty-five.

I was glad that I left behind me at Broadmoor a patients' committee, even though its terms of reference are limited. I should like to see a similar, or better, committee set up in every Special Hospital and prison. This is the great age of consultation. Everybody, from shop-floor workers to students, wants a say in the running of the body to which he belongs. Many of the tensions and much of the violence in prisons and Special Hospitals is caused, I am convinced, by frustration at the conditions, and at the apparent impossibility of the prisoners and patients being involved in any way in alleviating them.

I am sure that it was this kind of frustration that lay behind the notorious Parkhurst riots of July 1970, which were led by a man whom I had known as a good friend in Broadmoor until 1967. He was a warm, lovable person, as his Q.C. said in court, but frustration could provoke him to a violence that was contrary to his real nature. There is healing simply in being able to voice a grievance, let alone get it solved. Properly constituted and recognised prisoners' or patients' committees could take the heat out of many a potentially explosive situation.

All in all, my experiences in Broadmoor and since have convinced me that things are even worse than I had believed them to be as an enthusiastic and well-informed prison reformer. Our prisons and Special Hospitals are full to overflowing, and yet we give little time or attention either to preventing people from ending up in them,* or helping them to live in an acceptable way outside them once they have offended society. We are destroying men by neglect.

I have been fortunate to have influential friends and social contacts to help me circumstantially, and a faith in God and Christ to help me come to terms with myself. I hope that this book will make some small contribution to helping those many – including hundreds personally known to me – who lack both these advantages, and feel that society, too kind to kill them by the brutality of the past, has decided to kill them by a kind of apathy instead.

* It would be interesting to know the proportion of Special Hospital patients who had had psychiatric treatment *prior* to committing an offence. I feel sure these figures would underline the need for better preventive psychiatric treatment.

Appendix

Prison Without Trial

C. H. Rolph

On such figures as one can find, you are less likely to be wrongly arrested in this country than in almost any other. This of course is as it should be, since most foreigners deserve to be arrested every now and again; but we can be even prouder (still using our sense of comparison, I mean) when we contemplate the treatment of untried and unconvicted prisoners in some foreign jails and the length of time they have to spend in them. In England they are very unlucky if it is now as long as four months and the average seems to be five weeks. Professor Grygier of Toronto University says in the January *British Journal of Criminology* that in Nassau County, New York, jury cases in 1961 had taken from forty-four to sixty-eight months to come to trial, while in Boston they were waiting three years and in Chicago four or five, a good many of them in jail.

But even four months can seem an eternity to an innocent man who is in prison because the magistrates have refused him bail. Have you ever visited someone in a remand prison – visited him, not as his lawyer, doctor or other V.I.P. (who can see him in a relatively private room) but as a mere relative or friend? Every magistrate ought to do this at least once, and so should every M.P. Brixton Prison would do. The visiting conditions at Brixton are an outrage; and they persist only because, instead of coming to the knowledge of the right people, they are seen and endured only by those who must suppose them to be inevitable. To savour the full effect, the man you visit should be someone you have known for some years. You will wait with fifty to a hundred others in a room crowded with metal chairs, loud with indignant protests, and ringing with the shrieks of children. After a time a prison officer will open a door in the corner and, in the sudden hush, shout some names and numbers. Each name is that of a prisoner, each number that of a kind of polling booth to which he has just been marched. He is ready to receive visitors; and with a dozen others you shuffle in single file along a passage until you get to him. He is standing, collarless, on the other side of a thick glass window, the glass being bordered on each side by a vertical strip of close-meshed wire netting. There are no seats. You stand and look at each other through the glass. He is degraded, depersonalised, stripped of all self-esteem, muttering anxious things you can't hear. You shout at each other through the wire netting, putting mouth and ear to it alternately as you strive to beat conversations going on competitively in a dozen neighbouring booths. The twenty minutes soon go.

Every year in England and Wales 17,000 people who are locked away like this are then found to be undeserving of imprisonment – many, of course, because they are found not guilty. It seems a staggering number until you discover that in New York City alone the comparable figure is 75,000. But in New York, where the Vera Foundation is now undermining the iniquitous 'bail bondsman' business and getting people out on bail itself, something is at last being done about it because the problem is big enough to attract wider indignation.

Quite apart from the fact that he may be innocent – if that supreme consideration can for the moment be left out of account – the remand prisoner's lot is the unhappiest of all. His whole treatment takes its tone from the fact that, whoever else may contrive to escape, he simply mustn't, innocent or not. The prison authorities are charged with the job of holding him until the courts and 'the Crown' are ready for him. A 'remand' is usually, though not always, kept away from convicted prisoners; but among his fellow remands there are many old lags awaiting trial and some mental invalids under medical observation.

For misconduct he can be punished with all the prison rigours except flogging, he forfeits the right to wear his own clothes if he tries to escape, and the privilege (seldom used) of having his own food and books brought in at his own expense can be withdrawn at the Governor's discretion. What he can't have (and therefore can't lose) is the privilege of writing letters on something other than the squalid little rectangles of cheap ruled paper head 'Number.................. Name'.................. and (in the dreariest conceivable block capitals) the name and address of his prison. He is 'banged up in his cell' from 4 p.m. every day, and because he is not yet known to be guilty he can have none of the film shows and concerts by which the lot of the guilty is alleviated.

But in the official literature you have to search with some diligence for this kind of information about remand prisoners. The Annual Report of the Home Office Prison Department, for example, doesn't so much as mention them. When it was called the Prison Commission it often mentioned them, as it mentioned debtors, with some bitterness; they present the prison staffs with their worst problem. Nor do the Criminal Statistics acknowledge their existence. Even the late Sir Lionel Fox, chairman of the Prison Commission, gave them minimal attention in his book *The English Prison and Borstal Systems,* a seminal work in the literature of penology; but what he does say about remand prisoners is repeated, with little variation though without attribution in official publications like the Home Office pamphlet *Prisons and Borstals*:

> Since in all proper cases the courts will normally release an untried offender on bail, it must be assumed that, *in at any rate a great many cases,* courts have decided that detention is necessary either to ensure further appearance or to prevent interference with the course of justice.

Fox was a careful writer, and the words that have always interested me in this passage are those I have italicised. What about those implied other cases? I happen to know that Fox was always disturbed about them. They include, as well as the ones who might run away, or tamper with evidence or intimidate witnesses, those about whom the courts want medical reports (which could in fact be got without locking them up) and those whom the courts want to straighten up with 'a taste of prison', whether guilty or not.

Reprinted from the *New Statesman* April 23, 1965, by kind permission.
NOTE: C. H. Rolph wrote this article after visiting me while I was on remand in Brixton Prison.

P.T.

Epilogue

At my trial at the Old Bailey the Judge implied that there were others who should share the responsibility for what had happened'. I have left the reader of this book to reach his own conclusions as to whom the Judge might have had in mind. But for me there are two areas of responsibility – personal and social – that I have felt my case opens up, and since my discharge from Broadmoor I have begun to devote myself to seeing that they are not quietly forgotten.

The first of these areas was touched on in a footnote on page 143. My own case raises this question very sharply. If a significant number of patients sent to the Special Hospitals after committing serious offences had already been receiving psychiatric treatment, as I had been for many years, then should not questions be asked at the highest level about the nature of that treatment and its value as a preventative?

I met many patients in Broadmoor who, like myself, had put themselves in the hands of doctors and psychiatrists over long periods of time, but who were nevertheless able to commit apparently *unexpected* acts of violence. One young man committed a murder while an out-patient of a mental hospital from which he had been recently discharged. And I myself of course, injured three innocent girls within a few hours of being discharged from a hospital the day after an attempted suicide. If similar results followed from physical or surgical medicine, there would be an outcry and demands for an enquiry. Yet apparently it is felt acceptable, or at least unavoidable, in the sphere of psychiatric medicine.

I am, of course, aware of the difficulties. The mind cannot yet – and perhaps never will – be treated like an appendix or an infected tonsil. But plain common sense requires that all that can be done to lessen the unhappily large number of serious offences committed by people who are mentally ill, and known to be, should be done. Yet there is a widespread reluctance in official circles to see the extent of the problem or the seriousness of it.

For example, my own case has been persistently raised by Lord Stonham, a former Minister of State in the Home Office. In correspondence with Lord Aberdare, Minister of State at the Department of Health, he has urged a departmental enquiry into the circumstances surrounding my discharge from hospital so soon after a suicide attempt. They constitute, he wrote to Lord Aberdare, 'an appalling tragedy the consequences of which will be with him all his life'. Lord Stonham continued: 'I think that this could have been avoided if he had been detained for a few days in St Bartholomew's Hospital, instead of being discharged on the morning after his suicidal attempt . . . It was for this reason that I asked you to institute a departmental enquiry.' I simply want to establish the importance of *preventive* psychiatric treatment, and draw attention to its failure in this and, I am convinced, many other cases.

But official opposition to such an enquiry is very strong. 'Enquiries into these matters of clinical judgment would not be appropriate,' Lord Aberdare wrote. 'A clinical decision in respect of any patient is a matter for the individual doctor concerned with the patient's treatment.' I would agree. But surely where wider issues including public security and danger to innocent life are involved, those 'clinical decisions' become matters of public concern?

Not only that, but there is also an official reluctance to investigate the extent of the problem. William Deedes MP, a former Conservative Minister, wrote to the Secretary of State for Health and Social Security, Sir Keith Joseph, asking how many patients at Broadmoor were in the hands of a psychiatrist at the time of the offence (or whatever it was) for which they were detained there. Sir Keith felt that it would be very difficult to obtain this information, and declined to provide it.

But is it really so difficult? There are only 700 or so patients. Their medical records are to hand at the hospital. Surely it involves a few hours' work, at the most, to examine these documents and record quite simply whether or not the patient in question was undergoing psychiatric treatment before he was committed to Broadmoor? I believe this is a question that must be answered, both for the good of the patients and also for the security and safety of ordinary citizens.

The second area of responsibility which I feel my case opens up is the whole question of the after-care of patients discharged from the Special Hospitals. I have dealt with this in the final chapters of the book, but I believe fundamental issues are raised here about our attitude towards and treatment of the mentally ill. There is still a stigma attached to mental illness of any kind, especially when it comes to getting a job; but this is nothing compared to the stigma attached to having been a patient at Broadmoor or one of the other Special Hospitals. I have given examples of this, and in a way it is not at all surprising. One does not expect to walk out of Broadmoor and immediately be accepted back into society as thought nothing had happened.

But that is exactly what the authorities seem to expect. Even less is done for the patient discharged from Broadmoor than for the man discharged from prison, and heaven knows that is small enough. I talked about this in the House of Commons with Christopher Mayhew MP, a former Labour Minister and current Chairman of the National Association for Mental Health, who told me that there were 60,000 patients in mental hospitals who were almost cured, and certainly fit for discharge, but needing community care, who had to stay in hospital simply because there was nowhere for them to go and no one to care for them if they left hospital. That, I maintain, is a scandalous situation, if only because we can ill afford 60,000 hospital beds occupied by patients who do not really need them.

I have put to Sir Keith Joseph three reforms which I am convinced would help ease the situation, particularly where it is at its most acute, in the Special Hospitals. First, and most simple, I asked for the name 'Broadmoor' to be changed, because since the 1959 Mental Health Act it is no longer a criminal lunatic asylum. (I am assured that when the new building is completed it will be given a different name). Secondly, I asked for 'half-way' hostels for those discharged from hospital. Thirdly, I asked for a national organisation to be responsible for mental after-care. Subsequently I have had a letter from Sir Keith saying that the study of mental after-care is a continuing process, and that no special report on the subject is required. He also said that he would arrange to contact former patients of Broadmoor to find out if half-way hostels would have helped them.

I do not intend to let this campaign lapse. Many MPs and health experts have given me their support. Together our aim is to persuade the Minister that there is a need for these reforms, and that the need is urgent. My own case is a clear example of this.

I suppose there is a danger of turning a desire to 'clear my name' and justify my past behaviour into a moral crusade about mental health. I can only say that I do at least see the danger, and try to avoid it. There is more, much more, to all this than simply the Peter Thompson case. Hundreds, perhaps thousands of others are in a similar position, but lack the contacts or will to make their plight known. This campaign, and this book, could really be said to be an attempt to help them, and, more significantly, to help the countless greater number who, unless our preventative measures improve dramatically, are doomed to tread the same miserable and destructive path in the future.

$35.95

CW01655892

THE PLEASING HOURS

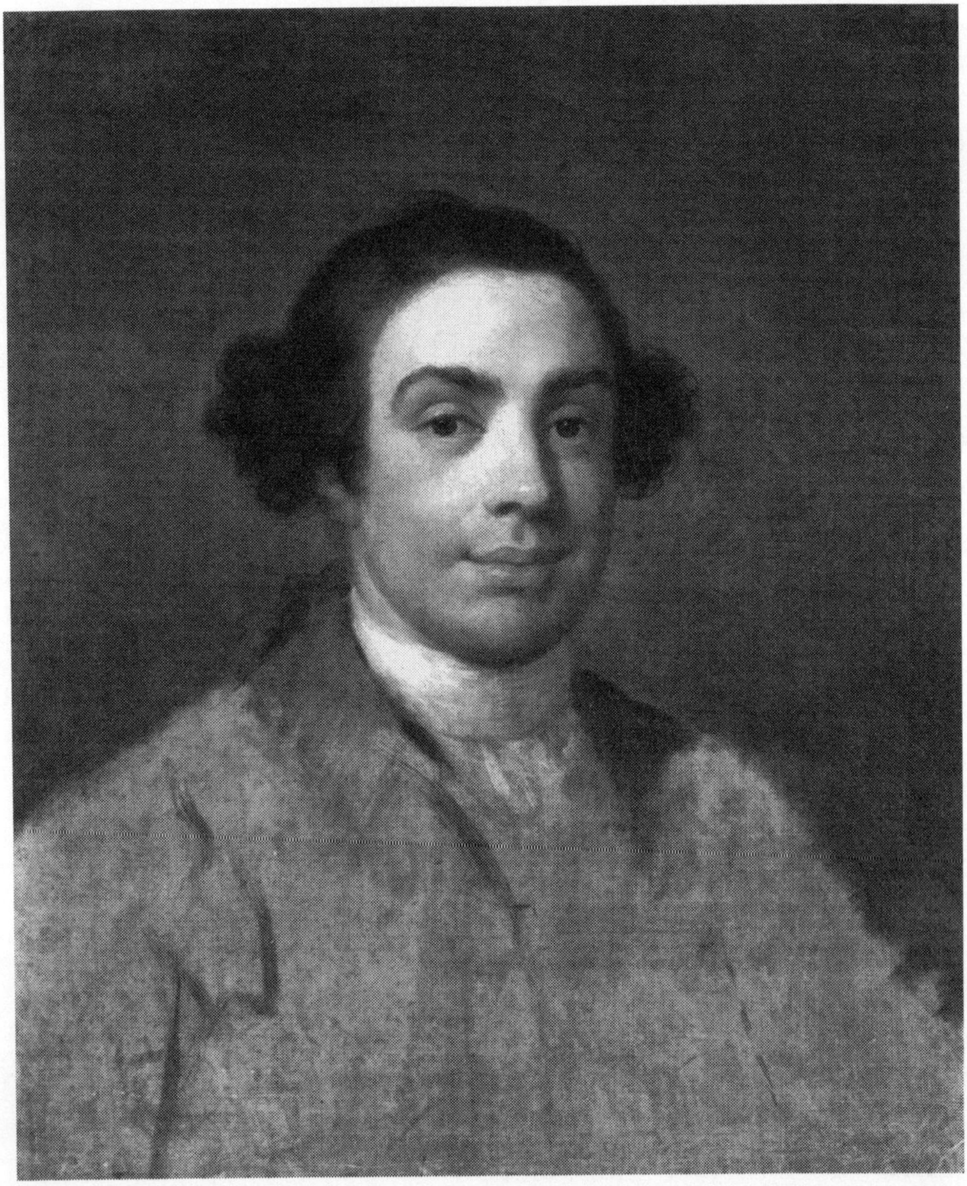

The Pleasing Hours

James Caulfeild, First Earl of Charlemont 1728-99

TRAVELLER, CONNOISSEUR AND PATRON OF THE ARTS IN IRELAND

Cynthia O'Connor

The Collins Press

PUBLISHED BY
The Collins Press, West Link Park, Doughcloyne, Wilton, Cork, 1999

British Library Cataloguing in Publication data.

ISBN: 1-898256-66-7

PRINTED BY MPG BOOKS, CORNWALL, UK

JACKET DESIGN BY
Uppercase Ltd.

BOOK DESIGN BY Jarlath Hayes/ORIGINATION BY Susan Waine

FOR ROBERT DAVIS-GOFF

FRONT JACKET PICTURE:
Thomas Roberts The Casino, Marino
Courtesy of Whitworth Art Gallery, Manchester

FRONTISPIECE:
Hogarth: Unfinished Portrait of Charlemont
Courtesy of Smith College Museum of Art, Northampton, Mass.

CONTENTS

The title *The Pleasing Hours* is taken from an anonymous Epistle addressed to Charlemont on his return from his travels to Ireland, which is, significantly, an adaption from Popes's *Epistle* to Lord Burlington. Pope's lines, as we may recall, read

> You too proceed, make falling arts your care,
> Erect new wonders, and the old repair,
> Jones and Palladio to themselves restore,
> And be whate'er Vitruvius was before …

Charlemont's anonymous versifier wrote:

> 'Tis, Yours, sir, to enjoy such Pleasing Hours,
> To make what Greece, what Rome can boast of, Ours
> to give to Arts success unknown before
> And fix the Graces on thy native shore.

ACKNOWLEDGEMENTS

For permission to publish extracts from the Charlemont MSS, I am indebted to the Council of the Royal Irish Academy. I wish to thank also the A.G. Leventis Foundation for allowing me to refer quoted passages from Charlemont's essays to *The Travels of Lord Charlemont in Greece & Turkey 1749*, edited by W.B. Stanford and E.J. Finopoulos, London 1984.

Without the persistent goading of the Knight of Glin and the advice and encouragement of Professor Michael McCarthy, this book would never have been completed. Michael McCarthy kindly read the first draft and suggested corrections. I also thank my daughter, Annabel Davis-Goff, for her rigorous editing at all stages. I have to admit to not being able to satisfy her every particular.

Over long years of research, I have received help and information from many and I hope none are, inadvertently, forgotten. At the beginning there was Sir Brinsley Ford, the late Professor Stanford and Mr Finopoulos, the Staffs of the Royal Irish Academy and the National Library of Ireland. I also wish to thank Dr Michael Wynne, Dr Edward Mc Parland and Patrick Bowe for helpful advice in the early stages and more recently also. As my research continued, I owed much to consultations with John O'Connell, David Griffin, Dr Niccola Figgis, Dr Theresa Watts and with John Redmill, who was working on the restoration of the Casino, conducted by the Office of Public Works at that time. Further credits will be found in the reference notes but I should like to mention here, Tom Duffy, who pointed out to me in good time that Charlemont's tutor, Edward Murphy, was not in holy orders, as has previously been assumed.

Illustrations are courtesy of the National Gallery of Ireland; the Whitworth Art Gallery, Manchester; the Lewis Walpole Library, Farmington, Connecticut; The Smith College Museum of Art, Northampton, Massachussetts and the Yale Centre for British Art, Paul Mellon Collection. John O'Connell supplied the photograph of the Greek stele as it was, when found at Marino, and Christies for the photographs of the Medal Cabinet on its discovery at the Elvedon Sale, Suffolk. The photograph of detail from one of Charlemont's letters to Chambers is reproduced, courtesy of the Royal Irish Academy. I also wish to thank John Redmill for the photographs of the Casino's interior detail.

PART ONE

The Levantine Voyage

1

'AWAKE, MY LORD, OR ... SLEEP FOR EVER'

James Caulfeild, 4th Viscount Charlemont, was barely eighteen years of age when, in the summer of 1746, he set out on his Grand Tour. Considering the outcome, a revolution in taste in his own country and the building of one of the western world's architectural masterpieces, his travels had an unpropitious start. Ostensibly, at least, still tied to his tutor's apron strings, he was, in his own words, being 'sent abroad'.[1]

Lord Chesterfield, acquainted from his Viceroyalty in Ireland with the young man and the circumstances, was tepid in his recommendation. 'I am ashamed,' he wrote in a letter to the British Minister Plenipotentiary at The Hague, 'to be so troublesome as I am often forced to be with my Irish recommendations for I am now obliged to mention Lord Charlemont, a young Irish nobleman of very good estate, who is or soon will be at the Hague.'[2] He added that nothing need be done for him except to tell him, he, Chesterfield, had mentioned him.

Philip Stanhope, Lord Chesterfield's natural son and the recipient of the famous letters, was on his way to Lausanne and was to pass through The Hague; Chesterfield, conversant with Dublin gossip as indeed with that at every court in Europe, and peculiarly sensitive about the shortcomings of his son, was wary of undesirable influence. It may not have been a coincidence when next the paths of the two young men were to cross, Chesterfield was particularly vehement in his warnings to Stanhope about the general ill-conduct and indecent behaviour of the British abroad.

Charlemont, as a minor, had been a ward of Court and while in Ireland Chesterfield had himself authorised a distribution of funds from the 'very good estate', a legacy of accumulated honours and vast acreage from four generations of Caulfeilds. The Caulfeilds, as Ulster planters from the times of Elizabeth and James I, had successfully withstood battle, seige, murder and attainder to establish themselves in the counties of Armagh and Tyrone. When in 1734 the 3rd Viscount died, Charlemont, as his eldest surviving son, had inherited the title. He was then only six years old.

Charlemont's mother had remarried in 1740; her new husband was her cousin Thomas Adderley. Three years later she had died in childbirth. Adderley had been appointed guardian of her three Caulfeild children – Charlemont, his sister Alicia and his younger brother Francis – and was also left with a surviving daughter of his own.

Following the death of his father, Charlemont, possibly a delicate child, had been much cossetted and was not sent to school. 'An unlucky choice of tutors', according to Charlemont himself, had done little to further his education and by the time he was fourteen, he was found to have 'little or no knowledge'. A new tutor, formerly the headmaster of a public academy, was then put in charge and was able to persuade him that to make up for lost time, he must sacrifice every amusement and give himself up to 'laborious and incessant study'.[3]

The tutor was Edward Murphy, a classical scholar with an edition of Lucian* to his credit. He was middle-aged, a widower, as far as we know without children, and he was prepared to devote himself entirely to the education of the young viscount. He was an amiable character, much given to enthusiasms and always riding some hobby horse or other. If his ways were eccentric, he was endearing and as Charlemont was diverted by his little oddities, and at the same time responded to the demands Murphy put upon him, a happy relationship developed.

For two whole years Charlemont studied by day and night. In later life he was to blame reading by candle-light for his weakened sight. His studies brought him by degrees, if not to the front rank of scholarship at least to a situation from which it was possible to proceed, or so Charlemont himself thought. Murphy's pride and enthusiasm swelled. Charlemont's diligence and learning began to be spoken of among Murphy's cronies, and William Dunkin, Swift's friend, composed some verses in Charlemont's honour.[4] Murphy, himself, believed it was not so much the extent of Charlemont's reading, but

* Lucian (*c.* 125- *c.* 190), Greek sophist and satirist, *Select Dialogues of Lucian*, with Latin translation and English notes, 1744 reprinted Dublin 1771.

his perception and understanding of it that on occasion surpassed men of celebrated learning.

When it began to be noticed in Dublin that Charlemont was no longer to be found, in the words of William Dunkin, 'sitting among sages or poring over musty pages', Murphy was at first only concerned for Charlemont's, and possibly his own, good name. He tried to 'soften the thing'[5] by putting out that Charlemont was unwell and needed amusement. When Charlemont was heard of sitting at play in wild company, Murphy defied cards or dice ever to get the better of so much sense and caution. But as 'the nervous disorders, extreme lassitude and flying into a great passion for nothing at all' increased and Charlemont continued to come in at one, two and three o'clock in the morning and to keep company with one, named only by Murphy as 'a scoundrel pimp', Murphy grew very anxious. It seemed to him inevitable that Charlemont must soon get 'a seasoning in taverns, stews and gaming sets', and that a certain companion whom he trusted and was very unguarded with, would be the first to betray him.[6]

Charlemont in later life referring back to this early friendship with Jack St Leger, claimed that even with him for his companion, he had kept his 'principles of morality unchanged', but this claim was made in a homily to his own son upon 'the frightful dissipation'[7] into which he, in turn it seems, had fallen!

Of Jack St Leger's subsequent and unprincipled career, we shall hear more, as he too went on the Grand Tour and Charlemont and he met again in Italy. Only one story has survived of St Leger in the early days in Dublin and that, by coincidence, is of a scene at the Theatre Royal during a performance of Dryden's *All for Love* at which Lord Chesterfield, then Viceroy, was present. It is told by George Anne Bellamy, the actress, that St Leger, being 'a little flushed with liquor' had taken 'the unallowable liberty' in expressing his approbation of her playing of Cleopatra by pressing his lips to her neck as she passed. Enraged by the insult and notwithstanding Lord Chesterfield's formal presence, she had struck St Leger. Amid the consternation that followed and her embarrassment, as much for her own unpremeditated retort as for St Leger's affront, Lord Chesterfield had risen to his feet and applauded her. Whereupon the whole audience followed suit and St Leger was sent for to make a public apology.[8]

Returning to Murphy's problems, we find that with all thought of Charlemont going to university put aside, nothing presented itself but the traditional solution. A Grand Tour had been envisaged in any case and it was necessary that he and Adderley put the plans forward. However, the young Charlemont showed that he did not care to leave Ireland just then. He displayed no open defiance, merely a lazy reluctance, which greatly taxed Murphy's powers of persuasion. When at last he agreed to leave, it was with the consciousness that he was being 'sent abroad'.

This was not really the case. Ostensibly responsible to his stepfather and guardian and paying lip-service to his tutor, Charlemont was not accountable to any one. Both men deferred to his rank, although one of Murphy's small eccentricities was his claim to descent from the kings of Leinster and on one occasion he was to go so far as to extend to a group of surprised, but amused, English aristocrats, his royal hand to be kissed![9] Adderley, while arranging credit for Charlemont with merchant bankers in Rotterdam and also in Paris, although England and France were at war, put no restrictions on Charlemont's spending.

When we consider these circumstances in the light of today's thinking, we find Charlemont, not just a lazy and pleasure-loving young man, but potentially a tragic figure, subjected to what we might regard as the two most destructive of opposing forces, deprivation of the most grievous kind in the death of both parents, and the over-compensation of material wealth and privilege. That the outcome was at this stage only slight signs of disturbance speaks for the equilibrity of his temperament as well as for the understanding and wisdom of Murphy, but it may explain why in later life he found what appeared to be trivial reasons to fall out with his stepfather and never speak to him again. One of the extraordinary factors of this story is that Francis Hardy, Charlemont's first biographer, who undertook to write the *Life* because he had constantly 'acted with him in public, and had the honour of being known to him in private life' never alludes to Adderley by name and mentions him but once as 'a gentleman connected with his Lordship'! [10]

It is Francis Hardy who tells us something about Charlemont's sojourn at The Hague. According to him Charlemont used often to relate how he attended the whole revolution, or tumult, which terminated in the establishment of the Prince of Orange as Stadtholder. Charlemont does not mention The Hague in his *Traveller's Essays* and the chief source of our information is, apart from Hardy, a letter written by Murphy to Charlemont from The Hague.

To understand what was happening at The Hague and thereafter, it is necessary to touch briefly on contemporary events. The tumult or revolution in Holland was a repercussion of the wider issues of the War of the Austrian Succession, which was still dragging on when Charlemont and Murphy arrived at The Hague. Marshal Saxe's victories since the battle of Fontenoy had placed the entire Barrier* of the Dutch in French hands. The invasion of Holland seemed imminent and the Dutch people, remembering the House of Orange (as indeed had Charlemont's forebears) as their stay in times of trouble, were beginning to clamour for the Prince of Orange to take over from the Stadtholders, their High Mightinesses of the States of Holland. This was, as Horace Walpole was later to remark tartly, because they had not given proper thought of how little qualified he was to re-establish their affairs. In England it was feared the Dutch might make a separate peace. Lord Chesterfield believed that their High Mightinesses were unwilling to do so, but advised sending fresh instructions and a new minister for fear their inclinations might yield to necessity. Little confidence was placed in the Prince of Orange. Married to George II's daughter, Princess Anne, he was referred to by his brother-in-law, the Duke of Cumberland, who had command of the Allied Forces, as his sister's baboon of a husband.

Chesterfield's counsel being taken, a new minister was sent and John Montagu, 4th Earl of Sandwich[11] arrived at The Hague in November. 'Well intentioned, with good capacity and natural caution'[12] was the character then given him by the prime minister, Henry Pelham, who thus deemed him well-fitted to represent England's interests at the conference at Breda and to conduct those delicate negotiations, which were to lead eventually to the Peace of Aix-la-Chapelle.

There was as yet no hint of the scandals of the future when Lord Sandwich's profligacy became a by-word, and when for his part in the prosecution of John Wilkes, one of his former companions of the orgies at Medmenham, he was to earn the traitor's soubriquet of the *Beggar's Opera*, Jemmy Twitcher.

Besides representing England's interests at Breda and at The Hague, Lord Sandwich was a first Lord of the Admiralty (he was a direct descendant of Pepys' patron, the 1st Earl), Colonel of two regiments and a Fellow of the Royal Society. His enemies, conceding his administrative ability, (which history does not), contributed his

*Corden of fortresses in Flanders: Tournai, Ghent, Bruges, Oudenaarde, Ostend.

political advance to his prowess at cricket and amateur theatricals, both of which the powerful Duke of Bedford, to whom he had attached himself, held in high regard. The many complexities of his character and appearance were perhaps a part of his fascination: he combined the charm of an easy manner with unprepossessing looks, cold eyes and angular features; he was very fond of music, but said to be insensible to harmony; he was good at games and yet so ungainly that one of his contemporaries remarked at his distant approach, 'I am sure it is my Lord Sandwich, for, if you observe, he is walking down both sides of the street at once!' [13]

The wicked Lord Sandwich is not referred to by Francis Hardy nor does Charlemont make any mention of him in his *Memoirs* or his *Traveller's Essays*, but Sandwich made an impression on Charlemont. He advised and influenced him throughout the winter of 1746-7 at The Hague. Later they were fellow members of the Society of Dilettanti. At the time Sandwich was beset by difficulties caused by his own distrust of the Dutch and the frequent altercations between the Austrian and Sardinian ministers at The Hague: Sandwich had more trouble with England's allies than her enemies. A secret meeting with the Spanish minister gave him an understanding of the position of the adversaries.

Meanwhile Charlemont whiled away the winter months in the agreeable company of the military in their winter quarters and showed no disposition to study or make plans for the future. Not that Murphy was unhappy about Charlemont's friends; he approved of Henry, Earl of Drumlanrig, Sir Thomas Kennedy Bt and the Hon. John Ward, but he feared Charlemont's idleness. However for the future Commander-in-Chief of the Irish Volunteers (as Charlemont was destined to be) these were stirring times. If Charlemont had but known it, there were lessons for him to be learned from Lord Drumlanrig, who was proposing to recruit in Scotland (a year after the Rising of 1745), a regiment of Scottish Protestants, for service with the Scots Brigade in Holland.[14]

Spring came and on 1 February the Duke of Cumberland embarked from Harwich. A week later he was in council with the Prince of Orange, the Commander of the Dutch forces, and, in the face of Marshal Saxe's successes, private animosities were forgotten. Sandwich's bargaining strength was reduced to relying on Austrian successes in Italy and British naval victories at Finistere and Belleisle. A raid under the command of General James Sinclair upon Port

L'Orient had been disastrous for a reason explained in Charlemont's presence when he met the General later at Turin. In the face of this and other 'disagreeable news' Sandwich felt his situation to be so delicate that he could not be too cautious about engaging upon any measure, or depending upon his own 'weak judgement' as he modestly wrote in his dispatches.[15]

However, at the first hint of the province of Zeeland (exposed so immediately to the danger and thus likely to be the most dispirited) acting in a resolute manner, Sandwich appealed to Whitehall for support. The arrival of a squadron and three battalions was timely and on 20 April Sandwich sent his despatch upon 'a great decisive victory in this country'.[16]

Nevertheless the revolution had not been anticipated and was as much a surprise to the Dutch Government as it was to Sandwich. It was purely by chance that Charlemont found himself a witness to the drama. Reluctant to part with his military friends, he had left The Hague for the camp at Tilburg, ostensibly to pay his respects to the Duke of Cumberland, who, as Hardy assures us, was not only very kind then, but throughout later life. Had not Murphy, left alone at The Hague, written to Charlemont a lengthy letter urging him to return, Charlemont would not have witnessed the event.

The tumult was a dramatic reactivation of an historical cause in an historic setting, and a repetition of that wave of feeling which had brought William III to power in 1672, when the mob had attacked the de Wittes and torn them limb from limb. Then, and on this occasion, there had been a vast and insistent crowd threatening death to all traitors. But this time it was a bloodless revolution and only one sympathiser with the French found it necessary to leave the country. He bore the hated name of de Witte.

On 3 May the Prince of Orange was declared Stadtholder of the province of Holland and shortly afterwards of all the provinces. The French were incensed and refused to treaty within the territory, proposing the removal of the congress to a neutral town in Germany. Sandwich was inclined to take a haughty attitude, but got no backing, and the congress was moved to Aix-la-Chapelle.

The letter, in the nature of a homily, which Murphy wrote to Charlemont at Tilburg and which had the effect of recalling him to The Hague, was dated 4 April. It recapitulated the ups and downs, the triumphs and disappointments of Charlemont's progress throughout the Dublin days. It told of Murphy's fears in the past and for the present and the future, but not in an orderly manner and it is evident that Murphy's thoughts were in turmoil. He regretted his sycophancy in the past and immediately resorted once more to flattery. He appears to have lost confidence in his own powers of persuasion and his appeals to Charlemont to amend his ways are directed through the medium of Lord Sandwich.

'Have you not noticed that Lord Sandwich also said to you some time ago – Turin is the best place – I spent 12 months there and am well acquainted! Palpable and most friendly advice in an almost distant yet home way, observing upon your indolence and deficiencies and offering impartial assistance to serve you'.

Murphy went on to quote Lady Sandwich: 'Does your Lordship think that your innocent indolence escapes notice even here? I think it does not. Did you not observe what my Lady Sandwich said to you one evening My Lord, said she, I think I never see you ride out and then she began to rate my Lord Sandwich for not riding out that morning.'[17]

Charlemont's military friends were held up for emulation and finally we have the irony of the excellent Murphy's view of Lord Sandwich as a veritable paragon. 'Observe you not Lord Drumlanrick, how knowing? See you not Mr Ward with his classics in his pocket and quoting his authors? Ken you not my Lord Sandwich playing tennis, playing his harpsicord and steering the navies and senates of Great Britain at 29 years of age? Could he do this without great acquisition of knowledge?'

If Murphy was smarting under the humiliation of bearleading a Grand Tour which in eight months had not got farther than Holland, erudition was still his priority and one feels that had Charlemont not put away his books and neglected all study, there would have been no homily. 'My Lord, mind such lectures or you are ruined... Awake, my Lord, or the lethargy will grow too strong for you and you will sleep for ever.'[18]

Such a whimsical appeal was not to be resisted. Charlemont returned to The Hague, witnessed the revolution and notified Adderley of his future plans. On 30 May 1747 Adderley wrote Charlemont that he thought it not improper that he should have unlimited credit and on the same day advised the merchant bankers that Lord Charlemont intends to set out speedily for Turin, 'Accept what bills his Lordship may draw'.[19]

Once it becomes evident that Charlemont took Lord Sandwich's advice about Turin, the question arises whether Sandwich was the prime mover of the plan for Charlemont's Levantine voyage. It seems likely, since in 1738 Sandwich had himself with three friends sailed around the Mediterranean,[20] searching for the lost sites of ancient cities, transcribing antique inscriptions, seeking for treasure and bringing back antiquities from Egypt and Greece; they had a draughtsman aboard to record the costumes and the wonders of the ancient world. Sandwich's voyage could have been the prototype of Charlemont's but for one small but significant deviation. Sandwich's draughtsman was Jean Etienne Liotard, a portrait painter and a skilful depictor of dress, whereas Charlemont hoped to take an architect to make plans of ancient buildings and to record architectural adornments and detail.

Support is given to the theory that Charlemont's voyage was charted by Lord Sandwich since plans began to go forward soon after Charlemont reached Turin. The momentous and costly decision must have already been made at The Hague. Because he was conscious that Sandwich, under the burden of his responsibilities had been generous with his time and attention, Charlemont appears to have felt himself beholden. Evidently he went to some trouble over a present which, unfortunately could not be accepted. Adderley wrote, 'As to ye box, I could wish it had been proper for yr Lordship to have presented it for my Lord Sandwich must have been pleased even with a faint resemblance of the original. I shall most gratefully receive it, but cannot on any accnt. think of laying the least expense on yr Lordship.'[21] Unfortuntely, nothing has so far come to light as to what the box was a copy of, nor why it could not be accepted.

NOTES

1. HMC, Rept. 13, App.pt.XIII (1894) p. 269.
2. Ibid, Rept. 14, App. pt. IX (1895) p. 149.
3. Ibid, Rept. 13, App. pt. XIII, p. 269.
4. M. Craig, *The Volunteer Earl*, London 1948, p. 31. Evidently Charlemont's fancy already ran on Greece and Rome.
5. HMC, Rept. 12, App. pt. X (1891) p. 178.
6. Ibid, p. 179.
7. Royal Irish Academy, Charlemont MSS, 12.R.18, no. 28.
8. G.A. Bellamy, *Apology for the Life of.....*, London 1785, 2nd ed. Vol. 1, p. 137.
9. RIA 12.R.21, no. 157.
10. F. Hardy, *Memoirs of the Political and Private Life of James Caulfield, Earl of Charlemont*, London 1818, p. 48.

11. DNB, Vol. XXXVIII, 1894, pp. 254-8.
12. HMC, Rept. 14, App. pt. IX, p. 149.
13. DNB p. 258.
14. J. Ferguson, *The Scots Brigade in Holland*, Edinburgh 1899, Vol. 2.
15. Public Records Office, London, Sp 84, 424-2.
16. Ibid.
17. HMC Rept. 12, App. pt. X, p. 178.
18. Ibid. p. 179
19 Ibid. p. 180
20. Ed. Rev. J. Cooke ed. *A Voyage performed by the late Earl of Sandwich round the Mediterranean in 1738 & 1739*, 2nd ed. London 1807.
21. HMC, Rept. 12, App. pt. X, p. 180.

2

TURIN

Leaving The Hague, Charlemont and Murphy travelled eastward and then south through Germany. The country made such a disagreeable impression Charlemont that his friend Lord Bruce of Tottenham was afterwards surprised at finding Germany and its climate not as 'detestable' as Charlemont had led him to believe.[1]

Years later Charlemont was to recall to Edmund Malone a haunting incident of that journey. 'Travelling through Germany I went three days journey out of my way to visit the source of the Danube, which takes its rise from a copious spring in the courtyard of the Prince or Landgrave of Furstenburg. My road lay through that immense tract known by the terrific name of the Black Forest, at the extremity of which the capital of the Landgrave is situate; and as I approached his residence, I was surprised and shocked to observe that most of the trees bordering the highway were hung with human limbs, so as to have the appearance of a shambles in a country of cannibals. Hands, feet, arms, legs and even heads were everywhere to be seen and my first idea was that some numerous gang of robbers had been taken and executed. I stopped the chaise and enquiring of the postilion into the nature and circumstances of these supposed banditti, was thus answered, "No sir, here we have no robbers; these limbs once belonged to certain desperados who were audacious enough to kill the Prince's game", and upon further enquiry I soon found that the hands and arms had murdered partridges and pheasants, that the legs had feloniously followed hares and the heads had been so abominably impious as to plot and execute the assassination of wild boars.'[2]

By which route Charlemont and Murphy continued on into Italy is not clear, but subsequent evidence of connections with Lyons and Charlemont's assurance to a French galley slave he met in the Greek Islands that he knew France, suggest they rejoined the more constant traffic by way of Lyons to cross the Alps at Mount Cenis. Charlemont however disdained, perhaps as too commonplace among Grand Tourists, all mention of the terrors of the mountain pass with the chaise dismembered and loaded upon pack mules and the travellers, wrapped in furs and carried by savage Alpine chairmen, shouting and quarrelling among themselves, strong as giants and nimble as goats, who showed a careless contempt for the awesome chasms so close to the narrow and rocky path.

Hardly less sublime than the heights would have been the slopes of the descent, under massive waterfalls, and then between larch trees and chestnuts until they reached Susa, where they would have rested a night before making the approach to Turin.

The road to Turin, a remarkably good one, ran between plantations of low mulberry trees with vines growing over them. The tracks between the plantations led away into the distance, suggesting those contrived vistas which so fascinated English taste. The road passed the royal hunting lodge at Rivoli.

The city gave an impression of being small and elegant in spite of the broad streets, the wide squares and the immense monumental royal edifices, and testified to the able town planning of three generations of the House of Savoy. In the old city the streets were dark and narrow, but in the new city they were clean and fresh. Clear water ran in the gutters or kennels, which were so unusually wide they created an obstacle for pedestrians. This did not deter the élite from going everywhere on foot, their chairs carried at a respectful distance to provide near shelter should sudden rain, or even hail or snow from the mountains, break in upon their perambulations. After dusk the streets were lit by *flambeaux*, compulsory to every chair and carriage.

His Sardinian Majesty's sense of order, his exacting punctuality and strict discipline pervaded the entire city. Charles Emmanuel's court moved with the clock, the same royal scenes at the same royal places at precisely the same time every day. Nevertheless the King was very easy and civil with the English, as was appropriate with the citizens of an allied country, and though it was necessary to be formally presented, once this had been accomplished through the British Chargé d'Affaires, a casual informality existed.

As with other Grand Tourists, Charlemont would have come furnished with letters of introduction, although at Turin these were hardly necessary. It was not like Rome where society ladies maintained a wall of reserve against English visitors. Madame St Gille, 'the famous Italian lady all our men are so fond of', made favourites of them and her assemblies were very like English ones, 'of the moderate kind, not a rout'.[3] Charlemont soon had entrée to the best houses and was received not only by Madame St Gille, but the Marchese Gorsegni and his daughter, Madame Richelini and the Marchese Moncreuil, the brother of the Duc de Richelieu.

The Academy at which Charlemont enrolled for a year was under royal supervision; Charlemont was to consider it 'the most desirable in Europe for being so intimately connected with the Court and so immediately under the inspection of the King himself.' Its governor was Count Salmour, a correspondent of Lord Chesterfield's; Salmour's son, a student in England, was a frequent visitor at Chesterfield House. As already mentioned, Chesterfield warned Philip Stanhope against his young countrymen at Turin, 'especially when they are in numbers together' as they were at the Academy. About Charlemont's Irish friend, Francis Pierpont Burton, the jolliest and noisiest of companions, Lord Chesterfield might have had some reason for complaint. But also at the Academy was the Prince Royal, Victor Amadeus, Duke of Savoy, who was two years Charlemont's senior. They became friends and, according to Hardy, in later years after he had inherited the throne, he would still enquire for Charlemont from visiting Englishmen and once sent a message that although his rank and situation had changed Charlemont would not find him altered.

Dancing, fencing and riding were a part of the Academy's curriculum. As for languages, Lord Sandwich had recommended Turin for French and Italian, but Tourists were inclined to complain that the Piedmontese spoke a language between, neither one nor the other. Yet the evidence points to Charlemont being fluent in both languages before the end of the year. From Dublin on 2 February 1748, barely four months after Charlemont's enrollment, Adderley wrote to assure him the Lord Chancellor 'a few days ago mentioned your Lordship with esteem and regard ... all accounts agree that my Lord Charlemont has been and is most deservedly esteemed since his having left the country'. A poem which Charlemont had written, perhaps as evidence of his application and diligence, had been circulated and given pleasure, it was implied, to the Lord Chancellor and to the Dean of Down.[4]

The days being given up to study, the evenings were spent in pleasure and the best company. Social life centred upon the Opera House where the boxes of the second and third storeys were rented for the season by persons of quality. Here the ladies held their *conversazioni* and liveried servants waited upon their mistresses and guests with coffee and iced water, and then withdrew to the amphitheatre to enjoy the performance until a signal from the boxes called for departure and the bringing up of carriages.

Charlemont, spellbound himself by opera, was astonished to find first here and then all over Italy that, in spite of the high regard for music, the audience chattered and played cards throughout the recitations. The pieces that bored them, and indeed the greater part of the performance, were marred by incessant noise. In the event of the King's presence some attempt was made to lessen the din. The Royal box occupied the centre of the house on the second storey and here too gambling went on during the performance; those card players, whose backs were to the stage, were able to watch the spectacle reflected in the mirrors of the closed doors at the back of the box. When the audience found something in the performance that particularly pleased them, their enthusiasm was extravagant and the whole house from the ordinary people in the pit, the ladies of easy virtue in their allotted row, the quality in their boxes and the bourgeois aloft, became ecstatic.

Hardy reminds us that Charles Emmanuel's court abounded with eminent personages. Contacts with the famous were a desired part of European travel. Charlemont formed what might be regarded as useful connections with the Marquis St Germain, future Ambassador to France, and with Count Perron, soon to go to England, and Count Osorio, Ambassador to Spain. These diplomatic appointments followed the signing of the Treaty of Aix-la-Chapelle, which came at the end of Charlemont's year at Turin.

In the meantime, although the war was virtually over, Charles Emmanuel was committed to honour, with a quota of troops, England's subsidies. This agreement was the reason for the presence at Turin of General Sir James Sinclair as Envoy Extraordinary and David Hume, who was acting as his secretary.

Sinclair, somewhat under a cloud due to the failure of the raid on Port L'Orient, found himself again in difficulty. His Majesty of Sardinia did not conceal his displeasure at the preliminaries being signed at Aix-la-Chapelle. On the subject of the raid, Hume, the General's loyal supporter, and Sinclair himself showed no embarrassment. Warming to the subject one day in Charlemont's presence, he related that being wholly unacquainted with the French coast, he had earnestly requested from the War Office a set of accurate maps by which he might direct the operation. The landing made good, he had then to march into a country of which he knew nothing and therefore took recourse to the maps, which he had not yet examined and which when unpacked, proved to be sea-charts![5]

It being thought that Sinclair's secretary should appear to be an officer, 'Hume was accordingly disguised in scarlet' and a wig *à la militaire*. This greatly added to his natural awkwardness for he wore his uniform 'like a grocer of the trained bands'. Charlemont's description of Hume is well-known: 'Nature, I believe, never formed any man more unlike his real character than David Hume. The powers of phisiognomy were baffled by his countenance; neither could the most skilful, in that science, pretend to discover the smallest trace of the faculties of his mind, in the unmeaning features of his visage. His face was broad and fat, his mouth wide, and without any other expression than that of imbecility. His eyes, vacant and spiritless, and the corpulence of his whole person was far better fitted to communicate the idea of a turtle-eating Alderman, than of a refined philosopher.'[6]

Hume had already published his *Treatise of Human Nature* with the third volume *Of Morals* and Charlemont had been prepared to meet an atheist, an affronter of religion and decency, but found not a monster but a man of the utmost sincerity and good-nature. To Charlemont he extended his friendship, manifested by his addressing him, not as 'My Lord' but 'Man' with a strong Scottish accent. It is not to Charlemont's credit nor to those of his set that they latched onto Hume as a butt for ridicule because he was too good-natured to resent this.

While Hume was at Turin 'he was affected by a most violent fever attended with its natural symptoms, delirium and raving. In the paroxisms of his disorder he often talked with much seeming perturbation of the Devil, of Hell and of Damnation, and one night, while his nurse-tender happened to be asleep, he rose from his bed and made towards a deep well, which was in the courtyard, with a design, as was supposed, to drown himself. Finding the back door locked, he rushed into a room where upon a couch, the gentlemen of the family, he well knew, used to deposit their swords, and here he was found by the servants who had been awakened by the noise he had made at the door in endeavouring to open it; he was then forcibly brought back to bed. This whimsical adventure was as may well be supposed, after his recovery, a subject of merriment among his friends, and we all agreed in laughing at the philosopher's fears and desperation. "Why you Boobies" said he and perhaps reasonably enough, "What would you have of a madman? Do you suppose philosophy to be proof against madness? The organization of my brain was impaired and I was as mad as any man in Bedlam".'[7]

The discomfiture of Hume, as witnessed by Charlemont from behind a curtain, when the 'old, fat philosopher plumped down upon his knees' and declared his passion to a beautiful young Contessa, to whom Charlemont was also paying court, does not make pretty reading. The Contessa dealt unkindly with him and he left the room with 'tears trickling down his flabby cheeks'.[8] Charlemont describes the scene at length in one of his political essays; because he had in the first place introduced Hume to the fair lady, he could not resist from acquainting Hume before their parting with the unwelcome news that he had witnessed the final humiliation, if not actually assisted in it. Yet Hume bore him no malice and met him in later years as a friend, and recorded in his *Life*, written when he was dying, that at Turin he had to wear scarlet and there was good company.

The Contessa was twenty-four years of age, five years older than Charlemont and married 'for some years, tho' hitherto childless, her husband being an old decrepit man, whom family convenience had compelled her to espouse'. Charlemont goes on to describe her as 'a lady of great beauty': 'her complexion was that of the most lovely brunette and her features, tho' sufficiently regular were rather beautiful from their extreme expression and animation than from their regularity. Her mind shone thro' her countenance with endless variety, and was a perpetual source of grace and beauty. Nature never formed anything more perfect than her shape and the Coan Painter,[9] instead of collecting the beauties of Greece might have framed his Venus from her alone ... The elegance and grace of her manner baffle all description ... Fitted by Nature for love and liberally endowed with every quality which can tend to inspire and participate the most ardent passion, she had been united in her earliest youth to a man, whose person, age and character were complete antidotes against every tender inclination and her heart was consequently left unoccupied, unguarded. Yet, tho' she had too much sensibility to be incapable of passion, her choice was however so guarded by good sense and judgement that her nicety and discernment rendered her conquest almost as difficult as if she had been naturally or rather unnaturally insensible. Such was the woman to whom I had the honour of paying my court and in whose company I regularly spent my evenings.'

Moreover she was learned, 'yet far from incurring any of those disgusting defects which study usually produces in female scholars, her genius, while tho' strong and bright, was truly feminine, had softened all the effects of her extensive acquirements into that modest and diffident exhibition of knowledge, unalarming to the fastidious pride of Man, by which alone the conversation of a woman pleases while it instructs and her hearers, who were always the wiser for what she said, far from being lessened in their own opinion, were induced to believe that they were teaching her, when in reality they themselves were being taught.'[10]

Cicisbeism* was, as Charlemont was to remark in other circumstances, 'a foolish and dangerous practice'. It seems as if on this, and on a future occasion in Rome, he bent the rules. When on the eve of Hume's departure with General Sinclair for Vienna, Charlemont drew Hume aside, Hume gave him 'a friendly and sensible admonition, which was now become very necessary' and of which in a short time he profited. '"Oh the jade" Hume commented with some agitation, "And did she serve me so. I cannot however be angry. It was indeed but strict Justice. Yet in revenge I will give you a piece of Advice, which, if you follow it, will make my vengeance more complete perhaps even than I would wish. You are young ... You are beloved. All that is precisely as it ought to be. Yet let me make one short observation in French also, though you well know it is not my talent. *Cueillez, Milord, les fleurs. Cueillez les fleurs. Mais ne vous faîtes pas jardinier*".'[11]

It was a warning, which, as Charlemont agreed, had become necessary, and in any case the end of his year's term at the Academy approached. Charlemont began to make plans for wintering in Rome and Naples before embarking upon a voyage to Constantinople in the spring.

Charlemont's invitation to his compatriot, Francis Pierpont Burton to join the expedition does not suggest a very serious approach; huge and rumbustious, Frank Burton was a jester, not a *savant*, but Charlemont knew what he was doing. There would be danger and hardship, it went without saying, and Burton was strong,

* A custom in Italy, whereby a married woman was attended in public by a professed gallant or *cavaliere servante.*

brave, loyal and unfailingly cheerful, 'the dear companion' of many hazardous adventures.

Then came the rub. Burton had with him his tutor, Alexander Scott, a genteel cleric who was responsible to Burton's uncle; the Rt. Hon. Henry Conyngham was evidently paying for his heir's European education. Scott was doubtful about an enterprise that went so far beyond the arranged itinerary and there was the question of money. Charlemont offered to lend Burton what was needed and Scott was for the moment over-ruled.

Talk began to circulate of the coming voyage and aroused considerable interest among the English and the Piedmontese. The Duke of Savoy took the matter to his father and got a sympathetic hearing. The King was prepared to give leave to one of his subjects to accompany the voyage as draughtsman and the choice fell on the Court architect, Giovanni Battista Borra.[12]

A rendezvous was set for March 1749 at Leghorn and Charlemont and Murphy, leaving Burton to complete his year at Turin, travelled south for the winter and to make the considerable and necessary preparations.

Charlemont's plans were destined for a reverse. The voyage, which was in any case to become historic in the annals of archaeology and Greek topography, lost its architect draughtsman; Borra defected, and at the final hour.

Charlemont was already at Leghorn when the news came. The details followed almost immediately in a letter dated 5 March from Charlemont's correspondent at Turin, C. Douglas, 'As to Squire Borra, I cannot describe to you how much he has lost himself in this place by his dropping his Constantinople project. The Duke cannot bear to hear his name mentioned and it is so very untrue that the King opposed his making the voyage that as late as five o'clock the Sunday evening when he took his leave of his Majesty, he banter'd him on his want of resolution and was glad to find he had mustered up courage enough to take a step which he assured him should turn out to his advantage, if he made the best of his time; besides this gracious encouragement from his Majesty, he ordered him to make duplicates of all the plans he took for you and to bring them to him, intimating he would make this likewise worth his pains.'

The explanation came a week later when Douglas wrote again, 'He gives it for a reason in town why he did not go that he was present when Mr Scott disputed and refused to set out before my Lord and Mr Burton gave an obligation for a sum of money, and it immediately struck him, he had no more reason to trust 'em any more than Mr Scott and from that time he determined not to go ...'[13]

Charlemont's anger can be gauged by his total dismissal of Scott as a contributory member of the expedition. His presence is barely recorded in the voluminous accounts of Charlemont's travels in Greece and Turkey, and the only individual mention of Scott was when in Alexandria he was struck in the chest by a stone thrown by an unfriendly native! Even then there was not a word of sympathy!

Meanwhile Charlemont having left Turin with everything settled, as he believed, was completing his preparations from Rome and Naples. He had chartered a 200 ton frigate, a French prize named *L'Aimable Vainqueur* with an English crew. There was a library of classical works and other books of reference to be put aboard, with a treasure chest in English silver and English cloth and pairs of pistols, gifts for the suspectedly avaricious Turks.

Although we know very little of the chronology of the events in Rome and Naples, it is evident that some time during those four months Charlemont ran across Jack St Leger, now on the Grand Tour. He also met James Stuart and that colourful expeditionary of future Palmyra fame, James Dawkins, and Charles Wentworth-Watson, Lord Malton, (future 2nd Marquis of Rockingham and twice prime minister of England).

Jack St Leger was bent upon a course of havoc. At Florence he had allowed Horace Mann, the British resident, to think him sole heir to his cousin, Lord Doneraile, a misapprehension Mann passed on to Cardinal Albani, who clandestinely acted for Mann in Rome. St Leger was in fact the son of Sir John St Leger by his second wife Letitia. Sir John, one time M.P. and Baron of the Exchequer, having died, was spared the embarrassment of his son's excesses. Lady St Leger was diverted by her son's escapades, and prone to run into exaggeration in recounting them to an incredulous Dublin audience. In Rome, St Leger had disputed with his French servant over wages and the man had appealed to the French Ambassador, who could get no satisfaction and had brought the matter to the courts. Mann and Albani both thought St Leger's behaviour contemptible and hinted as much, but he would take no advice except the practical one of making himself scarce for a time and departing for Naples. Meanwhile he had left his belongings with the Dutch Consul, Mr Born. The police had descended upon Born to seize St Leger's goods on account of the debt. Born was an under-cover agent for Mann and Albani and Mann were badly frightened. St Leger was told not to return to Rome, but this advice he also chose to ignore. What story St Leger told Charlemont we do not know and we hear nothing more of him until Charlemont returned from the voyage.[14]

Murphy had prepared himself for Rome with a special course of reading for his and Charlemont's study of the antiquities. The archaeological plum of that season was the obelisk dug up in the Campus Martius, which had been moved at the direction of the Pope, Benedict XIV, in its separate massive pieces to a nearby courtyard for examination. James Stuart had written a learned treatise in Latin; so pleased was the Pope with Stuart's *De Obelisco Caesaris Augusti* that he undertook to defray the expenses of publication, an unprecedented honour for a Protestant. This work Stuart dedicated to Lord Malton.

Stuart's reputation naturally ran high in Rome, and Charlemont could not have been otherwise than impressed with the proposal that Stuart and Nicholas Revett issued in Rome at the end of 1748. That proposal is now lost, but the extant version of 1751 gives us some idea of its content, which can be summed up in the following extract:

'Rome, who borrowed her arts and frequently her artificers from Greece, has by means of Serlio, Palladio ... and other ingenious men, preserved the memory of the most excellent sculptures and magnificent edifices which once adorned her ... But Athens, the mother of elegance and politeness, whose magnificence scarce yielded to Rome, and for the beauties of a correct style must be allowed to surpass her, as an original excels a copy, has been almost entirely neglected, and unless exact drawings from them be speedily made, all her fabrics, her temples, her palaces will drop into oblivion and posterity will have to reproach us ...'[15]

This was purposeful and heady stuff and Stuart and Revett, looking for support, were 'liberally assisted with money' by James Dawkins, Lord Malton and Charlemont.[16] A link had been formed between Charlemont's coming voyage and the proposed expeditions of Stuart and Revett to Athens, and Dawkins and Robert Wood to Palmyra; journeys which were to have a revolutionary effect upon taste in the promotion of Neo-Classicism in the kingdoms of England and Ireland.

Here, also in Rome, began Charlemont's lifelong friendship with Lord Malton, to whom after his death Charlemont was to dedicate the Rockingham library at Charlemont House. The young Malton, two years Charlemont's junior, was accompanied by a serving officer, Major James Forrester, who had been granted leave of absence by the King and the Duke of Cumberland for the express purpose of looking after him. Malton, whose noble appearance and bearing had first brought him to the notice of George II as the fifteen year-old colonel of one of the regiments raised by his father, at a review on Rotherham Common, was the hero, as everybody knew, of a spirited escapade. When the Young Pretender had turned north from Derby and immediate danger had receded in the south, the youthful colonel had written out a chit for himself to himself in a fictitious name and without a word to his family, had ridden off with a brace of pistols and one servant to join the Duke of Cumberland. On the third day he reached the camp and presented himself. A messenger from his father had out-ridden him, but the Duke received him sympathetically and sent back word to the Marquis of Rockingham that he would see that his son came to no harm.[17]

NOTES

1. HMC, Rept. 12, App. pt. X, p. 187.
2. HMC, Rept. 13, App. pt. VIII, pp. 308-9.
3. B. Fitzgerald ed. *Correspondence of Emily, Duchess of Leinster*, Dublin 1949, Vol. 1, p. 476.
4. HMC, Rept. 12, App. pt. X, p. 181. Robert Jocelyn, Dr. Patrick Delany.
5. Hardy, note to pp. 8-9.
6. Ibid, p. 8.
7. RIA, 12.R.7. p. 517.
8. Ibid, p. 507.
9. Apelles, whose Venus Anadyomene was considered his most perfect painting. Pliny and Ovid give Cos as his birthplace, hence Coan.
10. RIA, 12.R.7, pp. 499-503.
11. Ibid, p. 511.
12. See Olga Zoller, *Der Architekt und der Ingenieur Giovanni Battista Borra* (1713-1770). Bamberg 1996.
13. RIA, 12. R.9 nos. 7 and 8.
14. L. Lewis, *Connoisseurs and Secret Agents in 18th c. Rome*, London 1961, pp. 145-8.
15. D. Wiebenson, *Sources of Greek Revival Architecture*. London 1961, App. 1.
16. J. Woods ed. Stuart & Revett, *Antiquities of Athens*, Vol. IV, 1796, pp. xvii and xxiii.
17. G.H. Gutteridge, 'The Early Career of Lord Rockingham', University of California publications in History, No. 44, 1952, pp. 1-9.

3

MESSINA

L'Aimable Vainqueur sailed from Leghorn in early April 1749 with no draughtsman aboard. Throughout the eleven months' voyage Charlemont kept a journal, which has since disappeared; sadly, because although he made it the basis of his *Traveller's Essays*, written and re-written in later years, the spontaneity of his first unedited impressions must inevitably have been lost in the subsequent editing.

The *Essays* are in the main what we would today call sociological studies: *A Traveller's Essays/Containing an Account of Manners rather than Things/The Proper Business of Mankind is Man* ... and Charlemont stayed close to the text. He regretted his lack of experience at the time of the voyage and those 'avocations in search of antiquities, which were then my principal objects'.[1] Nevertheless, whenever he quotes directly from his journal we cannot but be impressed by the range and perception of his observations. Even in the most polished of the essays, he retains his youthful sense of fun. There are chronological gaps; there is no specific account of his travels in Egypt, nor thereafter of the years in Italy, but from other sources taken in conjunction with his own notes appended to essays on other subjects, it is possible to follow fairly closely the course of his travels.

We first catch a glimpse of him at Naples on the feast-day of St Januarius, witnessing with some Protestant scepticism, the miracle of the liquefaction of the saint's blood. Although conscious of his own heretical presence and alarmed by the frenzy of the huge crowd, he was gratified he, unlike Admiral Byng before him, had stood his ground and not been obliged to quit.[2]

Next we find the ship sailing between the Lipari Islands with a Sicilian priest whom they had picked up at Naples aboard, not being able in common charity to refuse him a passage to Messina. There was no cause to regret the civility. He turned out to be a whimsical character such as Charlemont took delight in, and provided the company with much amusement. He related many stories of miracles, some of them very surprising, but nobody doubted his sincerity, and as they passed under Vulcano, which was bellowing smoke, he informed them this was one of the mouths of hell. It was here that St Giulielmo had his vision of 'a certain impious king' being hurried towards the crater by 'the indignant spirits' of a bishop and a priest, who had suffered martyrdom at his hands. The abbate went on to recount that the saint, having seen myriads of devils drag this impious soul to hell, had returned to a populated place and told of what he had seen, and a certain sea-captain, on returning to his own country, had it confirmed that on the very day and hour his sovereign had expired.

Amazing as this was, their astonishment was increased by finding on cross-examination that civility had prevented the good abbate from telling them in the first place that the hell-doomed tyrant was none other than their own reforming Henry VIII.[3]

On 6 May, having 'securely passed the poetical dangers of Scylla and Charybdis' they sailed into the harbour of Messina. As yet unaware of it being only a hollow facade, the travellers were struck with the beauty and magnificence of the city as the newly risen sun illuminated the splendid theatre of palaces which extended along one side of the bason of clear and unruffled water'.[4]

A boat came out to inform them that until they had passed a proper examination they could not enter the city and they were directed to a deserted spot on the shore where they waited for three hours before the officers of health came to question them and to submit them to rigorous tests of fitness. There was some merriment over Burton's 'corpulent unwieldiness' when they were required to leap a three feet bar, but at last after several trials 'and some oaths' his efforts were crowned with success and they were free to enter the city.[5]

What they saw excused the caution of the officers. The palaces were for the most part empty shells; the streets were almost deserted and grass covered the pavements; shops were closed and a few miserable stalls provided bare necessities. Six years before, this now silent and desolate city had been devastated by plague.

Charlemont, undoubtedly shocked but as a traveller of curiosity and in the interest of science, and perhaps with the idea of putting Thucydides to the test, was moved to make a full enquiry. Taking statements from the survivors, the merchants of the English factory, a Capuchin monk and the Governor himself, Don Giuseppe de Corbera 'a venerable old man', Charlemont gathered his data on symptoms, behaviour, spread of infection and disposal of the bodies.

The plague, raging in Morea, had been brought directly from

Patras by a Genoese vessel, showing false papers, whose captain pretended to have come from Brindisi. When, after being ordered into quarantine, the captain and some of his sailors had died in the Lazaretto, dreadful suspicion entered the minds of the harbour officers and they had had the vessel burnt. But this measure, extreme though it was, proved useless because the infected merchandise, corn, bale goods and wool, had already been smuggled into the port and distributed. When those who handled it died also, the alarm greatly increased, but the Messinese were unwillingly to admit to plague in the city and the local physicians aggravated the acutely dangerous situation by diagnosing an epidemical fever. The Viceroy at Palermo, Don Bartolomeo Corsini, sent a team of three doctors to make an independent enquiry and they, having no doubts, declared the plague and departed immediately. Troops were brought in, with orders to fire on any who tried to pass the barriers.

'The English factory, a numerous and respectable body of merchants, took alarm at the start and shut themselves in their houses' with 'no intercourse with the citizens' and supplied themselves from their warehouses. Not one of them died, but a Sicilian boy they had with them, bored with the lengthy imprisonment and home-sick for his own people, escaped from their fortress and succumbed the following day.

When the proportions of the disaster reached magnitude, it was estimated that in one day five thousand had died. Doctors withdrew and refused to tend the afflicted. As the medicines they administered only prolonged the torments of the dying, Charlemont judged the doctors 'not entirely immoral'. A loathsome stench permeated the whole city and the dead lay everywhere in heaps. To bury them, galley slaves and convicts were, with promises of pardon, released. Wearing frightful masks with long proboscises, they attempted to carry out their gruesome task, grappling the bodies with poles and iron hooks and trampling them down under a sparse covering of earth. But the masks through which it was 'foolishly thought the infected air might be breathed with less danger' proved hopelessly ineffectual and the galley slaves and convicts died also.

The Governor then came out of his palace and headed his soldiers in burning the bodies. In one day, he told Charlemont, they committed no fewer than twenty thousand to the flames. That some were alive and others threw themselves in a frenzy into the fire, scarcely increased the horror. While the soldiers were taken up with this ghastly duty, bands of ruffians roamed the streets, pillaging houses, the dead and the dying until they too succumbed. Within the space of three months, out of a population of sixty thousand, by Charlemont's reckoning, forty seven thousand must have died.[6]

While the merchants watched from their vantage point near the harbour, hideous sights were played out before their eyes. Pestilence-infected demoniacs 'rushed violently through the streets in frenzy' turning their 'ungoverned fury' on all they met as they ran to the water's edge and threw themselves into the sea. 'This extraordinary fact was authenticated' to Charlemont 'beyond all possibility of doubt by the testimony of the English merchants, who from their windows, which looked to the harbour, had seen daily numbers of instances', and Thucydides, observing the same at Athens, had put it down to the burning heat by which the affected were inwardly tormented.

Virgins were ravished in the streets, 'inordinate concupiscence' being another fatal symptom, and 'speedily revenged' by the instant death of the ravishers.

At the beginning of August for the first time some of the infected recovered. Soon there were no fresh cases and by the end of that month it was over, but nothing remained for the Messinese except famine. Trade and economy were shattered and endless squabbles and litigation resulted, hopelessly involved since whole families had been wiped out, and almost impossible to disentangle.

Charlemont talked with an old Capuchin, who, unlike so many other pastors, had not fled his duty and had administered to the dying throughout. He told Charlemont that he would not presume to think himself worthy of the 'immediate interposition of Heaven' and 'attributed his safety principally to his having always chewed tobacco and to his keeping leaves of that herb constantly in his nostrils'. But at one time he thought 'he had caught the infection, having perceived some extraordinary symptoms, which could only be accounted for by the usual operation of the distemper, that though an old man of near eighty, he had felt with amusement certain desires, accompanied by proofs of ability, to which he had long been a stranger'.[7]

It is perhaps not so surprising that, following a lengthy essay upon Messina and the pestilence, Charlemont wrote no account of the journey south along the east coast of Sicily; travels in Sicily, though scarcely a commonplace, were within the range of other British archaeologists and topographers. When they reached Catania they met two English gentlemen with their artist engaged upon the antiquities, and the voyage gained a draughtsman.

Before they sailed from Messina, Charlemont made one excursion which he thought worthy of mention, maybe because it was so directly in contrast to the horror of the history of the pestilence or more simply, an enjoyable outing.

At six o'clock on the morning of 8 May they set out in a felucca for the Calabrian coast. Hugging at first the Sicilian shore, where Indian fig trees grew down to the water's edge, their boatmen pulled up the Straits. Questioned by Charlemont, with his thoughts on Charybdis, they were talkative and told him of a cave where no man dare enter, and which they contended was inhabited by devils. They also gave him some account of the currents and the methods of the Sicilian fishermen, whose boats all round them crowded the Straits. A look-out from the top of the rock of Scylla called out the movements of the sword-fish in modern Greek, the familiar tongue of the Greek Islands adopted so as not to alarm the catch, while the fishermen closed in with barbed darts and played them until they could be drawn ashore.[8]

The head of a freshly caught sword-fish, dressed in the kitchens of the Prince of Scylla was 'luscious and palatable' and with cold meat and wine from the village at a penny farthing a bottle, provided an excellent picnic on the summit of the rock. They flung the bones to Scylla's dogs beneath! All Charlemont tells us of the Prince's palace is that the cannons on the ramparts bore the royal arms of the King of Naples, who had lately laid claim to the Sovereignty of Scylla.[9]

It was at Catania that they met Roger Kynaston and John Frederick with Richard Dalton and joined forces. We know from Dalton's account (Charlemont makes no mention of it) that they continued on to Syracuse and from there, with the Englishmen's felucca following in the wake of *L'Aimable Vainqueur*, they sailed to Malta.[10] It was agreed that Dalton should join Charlemont; if Charlemont had any misgivings about Dalton, whom he may already have met in Rome, at this late stage any draughtsman was preferable to none. Moreover he had an Irish connection in his favour and is said to have studied at the Dublin Society schools.

Dalton had come to Rome on this, his second visit, with Thomas Patch, travelling mostly on foot. His purpose had been to make drawings from the tapestries in the Vatican worked after Raphael's twelve lost cartoons, a performance, which by his own estimation, he had completed with the 'greatest care and exactness'. He then intended to engrave them in the hope that they would be 'not entirely unacceptable to the public'.[11]

Charlemont's first stay at Malta was brief, but it laid the foundations for a second visit on the return journey and a lengthy essay on the subject, and to such time we may leave it. However, to this visit belong the stories of British valour in the recent war, 'so generously undertaken and so vigourously carried on by England in defense of the ungrateful House of Austria'. Every exploit was sure of a mixed reception among the Knights, Austrian and Piedmontese on the one hand, French and Spanish on the other.

Among the stories which appealed to Charlemont was that of the English privateer, who achieved happy notoriety by 'falling upon any French ship that fell in his way and daily sending into the port of Malta prizes of considerable value'. Loss of trade and the taunts of British sympathisers drove the French Knights to demand retaliatory action from Marseilles. A vessel, splendidly equipped and commanded by an officer of the highest character for courage and naval knowledge, was speedily despatched. When she sailed out to hunt down the Englishman, the French partisans crowded the ramparts confidently while the English dreaded the outcome of so uneven a contest. But coming in boldly under French colours, the Englishman then hauled them down and engaged. After a long conflict, and with his ship totally disabled, he at length prevailed and, boarding the Frenchman, he towed his own 'impaired conqueror' into port.[12]

NOTES

1. RIA 12.R.5, p. 14.
2. W.B. Stanford & E.J. Finopoulos, ed. *The Travels of Lord Charlemont in Greece & Turkey 1749*, London 1984 pp. 225-6. F. Haskell, *Patrons and Painters*, London 1963, p. 200.
3. RIA 12.R.7, p. 147.
4. Ibid, p. 463.
5. Ibid, p. 465.
6. Ibid, pp. 467-474. Horace Mann estimated 30,000 but 40,000 is the figure generally accepted.
7. Ibid, pp. 483-5.
8. Ibid, pp. 464-466.
9. Ibid, p. 468.
10. R. Dalton, *Antiquities and Views in Greece & Egypt*, London, 1791, n. to p. 12.
11. Advertisement for subscription to the public for *Musaeum Graecum et Aegyptiacum*, London 1751.
12. RIA 12.R.7, pp. 555 & 557.

4

CONSTANTINOPLE

Sailing by way of Smyrna, Tenedos, the Troad and the Dardenelles, they reached Constantinople in late June and as they entered the harbour Charlemont was inspired to think 'the Golden Age had been restored'; myriads of sea-birds flocked around the boats, 'fearless of hurt and danger' and were pushed aside gently by the boatsmen's oars.[1] Ashore droves of dogs followed them and at first they found the incessant barking disconcerting and alarming, but then they saw that passers-by threw them food and all the dogs looked for and received was their daily pittance from those whom Charlemont had been led to believe were heartless in their treatment of animals.

They were made welcome by the British Ambassador and the entire party was comfortably installed at the Embassy as his guests. James Porter, the Ambassador, was an Irishman and kept up his Irish connections. He had been born James Le Roche, but his father, after the Battle of the Boyne when the cause to which he had allied himself was irretrievably lost, had changed his name to Porter. The then young man, who had a gift for languages and mathematics, had made a successful career in commerce, which had brought him, through the influence of Lord Carteret, to his present prestigious post.

Porter had nothing but good to say of Charlemont, 'the worthiest youth I ever knew, as full of good sense as of virtue, abounding with amiable qualities',[2] but must have on occasion found Charlemont, as 'a traveller of curiosity' a remarkably wearisome guest with his constant demands and enquiries about their enigmatic hosts, the Turks.

Charlemont on the other hand was openly critical of Porter following the publication of *Observations on the Religion, Law, Government and Manners of the Turks* by Porter in 1768, which might be regarded as arrogant in view of Charlemont's one month's stay, had he not, by the time he came to write his Essay on Constantinople, read widely on Porter's subject.[3]

Unwilling to give official sanction to what might be construed by the 'haughty' Turk as impertinent intrusion, Porter passed on Charlemont to the official dragoman* to the English, Signor Pisani, who was game enough to be a party to Charlemont's adventurous intention to penetrate the Porte itself.

On ceremonious visits Charlemont was obliged to dress and powder his hair and was stopped in the streets by Turks, who asked him 'why, in the name of wonder, he chose to put such a quantity of flour into his head'.[4] This time he would go happily in disguise as a mere sub-dragoman in Pisani's train and thus 'travestied ... *à la Greque'* he entered one early morning 'the Whitehall of the East'.

Pisani's business took them first to the offices of the Reis Efendi. It was here from a window in one of the secretary's chambers that Charlemont had a discreet but excellent view of the Divan already in progress. At the upper end of the room, which was to Charlemont's surprise but an ordinary one, was a sort of alcove or semi-circular recess, raised by three steps above the floor, where, upon a throne, was seated the Grand Vizir. Behind him stood an officer holding a large plume or whisk of feathers, which he waved about the Vizir's head; the flies at this season were exceedingly troublesome. On either side of the Vizir stood the Tezkereci Efendi, whose business it was to receive and read aloud the petitions. Beyond, at a distance of about four paces and nearly on a line with the throne, sat, at the head of two benches on either side, the judges who were to assist the Grand Vizir as council.

The method of justice seemed to Charlemont summary indeed. Here were 'no pleadings, no oratory, no demurrers, no writs of error'. The Grand Vizir after a little consideration or in a difficult case with a short consultation with the judges, gave his decree, 'signified by tearing to pieces and throwing behind him the petition which he rejects, or by delivering to one of the secretaries those of which he approves'. The client had not here the satisfaction of paying to have his cause ably defended, but then the loser lost nothing but his cause and success came unattended by ruin.[5]

Either Charlemont's new acquaintance, the secretary in whose chamber he watched, or his own awkwardness in Greek clothes, betrayed him, and on the rumour of Pisani having in his train a stranger of rank, messages came commanding Charlemont's presence. Obediently Pisani conducted him to the Reis Efendi, who

* Interpreter and guide

received him with 'most cordial, easy and unaffected politeness' and after enquiring his name and rank, desired him to sit down beside him. Pisani was kept standing. Charlemont, whose object was to question, was himself questioned as to where he came from and where he went and how he liked Constantinople.

Meanwhile servants came with a silver vessel filled with a sort of perfumed marmalade with a large gold or silver gilt spoon, which was presented to Charlemont and coffee was brought in and served. With the help of signs from Pisani, Charlemont had so far acquitted himself well. But, as he rose to leave, his host begged him to remain seated and servants in postures of the deepest respect, crouched upon their heels, offered iced sherbet and sprinkled from the long narrow neck of a silver bottle, rose water on his hands and dress. Charlemont was confused and when another servant came forward with a silver urn, resembling the incense pots that he had seen in Catholic churches, he unluckily laid his hands upon it and burnt his fingers. To his astonishment since he had been told Turks were incapable of laughter, the Reis Efendi laughed heartily and with great good humour told him he was happy to see him accommodating himself to their customs.[6]

Leaving the Reis Efendi, they were no sooner outside the door than the servants crowded round for a distribution of piastres. This was not such a surprise to Charlemont as might be expected. In Ireland at the time one was compelled to tip the servants at the houses where one dined and indeed as Charlemont complained, paid as dearly for hospitality as at an inn and sometimes for very mediocre fare. Here but a few piastres satisfied.[7]

After instruction by Pisani as to the proper method of perfuming, 'by holding the urn between my two hands and putting it into my bosom under my gown or pellice', the audiences continued. He was received most politely by the Mektupchu, private secretary to the Grand Vizir, who after questioning him about his travels, asked whether he was acquainted with the late Ambassador, Sir Everard Fawkener and for news of him.

Charlemont may not have known Sir Everard personally, but he had been much in the public eye. Friend of the Duke of Cumberland, host to Voltaire, he had surprised society by marrying a very young woman. It had caused amusement at Lord Lovat's trial for treason two years before when Lovat, facing death by beheading, had calmly declined to question Sir Everard's opposing testimony and had instead, with exaggerated civility, wished him joy of his young wife. The Mektupchu, on hearing of the marriage, expressed his concern and charged Charlemont not to fail when he should see his old acquaintance 'to present his compliments to him and to tell him that he pitied him greatly for having been weak enough to take a young wife in his decline of years'.[8]

All the ministers had offices adjoining their chambers and Charlemont, looking into half a dozen, was astonished by the multitude of clerks. It was claimed that the filing was so accurate that any reference could be traced within an half hour. There were no desks. The scribes used their knees, 'apparently in a most uneasy and inconvenient posture' and which differed little from that 'in which Raphael has placed the beautiful figure of the young disciple in the *School of Athens*'.[9]

Apart from this reference to Raphael, there is in the lengthy Constantinople Essay (most of it written in retrospect and in the light of later knowledge), but one hint of his developing connoisseurship and this in his description of the private apartments of the Grand Vizir in the Porte.

'I, now, for a few piastres, was admitted into the Grand Vizir's private apartments, which are truly magnificent. The rooms are large, lofty, and well proportioned. The ceilings are elegantly carved after the manner we style arabesque, and richly gilt. The walls of some rooms are covered with large china tiles, which have a very pretty effect. The furniture is, after the Turkish fashion, superb. The sofas are extremely rich, some covered with the finest silk Persian carpeting, others with silks embroidered. The pier glasses, of which there are a great number, are large and fine, most of them I believe from France. But that which seemed to me the most singular piece of magnificence was the number of clocks, all of them English, with which the chambers are crowded. In one large room I counted no less than six standard clocks, such as usually stand in our halls, only rather more elegant.'[10]

So far in his slight dealings with the Turks they had shown 'such amazing and much more than Christian politeness among a people whom I had been taught to believe little less than barbarous', but on another and more ceremonious occasion, Charlemont saw the other side of the coin. We cannot but suspect that Charlemont, some thirty years later, employed a trick he had learned then from the Turks to out-wit his arch-enemy, the Earl Bishop of Derry, when protocol dictated he should receive him at Charlemont House.

Following in the train of the Austria internuncio to an audience with the Grand Vizir, Charlemont and his party were ushered into a room in the palace of the Captain Pasha or High Admiral. The palace was not magnificent, but beautifully situated overlooking the harbour. The chamber in which they found themselves was poorly furnished, a sofa arranged in a corner for the Grand Vizir and opposite a stool for the Austrian envoy. It was already crowded with the Grand Vizir's attendants, but as yet without any sign of the Grand Vizir himself.

The Austrian envoy was left unceremoniously standing while they waited and all were aware that the late arrival of the Sultan's first minister was intended to ensure he would not have to rise to receive a foreign ambassador, a compliment the Austrian could not expect and which Turkish dignity would not permit. The Porte sent no envoys to foreign countries and had for those sent to them the sort of contempt with which they regarded merchants, or at the best honourable spies. At last, preceded by the Reis Efendi flanked by two officers and the cry of Long Live the Sultan and his Grand Vizir, the Vizir arrived and finally sat down, with the Austrian on the stool opposite him. Compliments were exchanged and the Vizir explained that he had chosen to receive him there rather than at his own palace because of the cooler air by the harbour.[11]

The Austrians had lately made a peace treaty with the piratical States of Barbary, but until now there had been no ratification of the agreement by the Turks; letters received two months before from the Emperor and Empress had remained until this moment unanswered. The Sultan's reply delivered to the Austrian and the ceremony completed, caftans were distributed to all the attendants. The ambassador informed the Grand Vizir that he had brought with him a nobleman from England 'whose curiosity had led him to Constantinople', and Charlemont was desired to come forward and was presented with an embroidered handkerchief, which although in itself of little value, he esteemed as a mark of distinction and favour.[12]

The audience at an end, the Austrian retired with obsequious bows, acknowledged by the Grand Vizir with a slight inclination of the head, and Charlemont, with his party immediately followed. But not quickly enough for the Turkish attendants, who with much rudeness fairly turned them out with cries of 'hush, hush, hush'. Nevertheless, at the gate outside, presents from the Sultan awaited the

Austrian envoy: a fine Arabian horse with 'magnificent furniture richly embroidered' and several dishes of fruit, sweetmeats and flowers.[13]

As it appeared that the Sultan would not be holding any audiences during their stay, Charlemont and Burton decided that they would take their chance along with the humblest of Mahmoud's subjects and try to get a glimpse of him in the streets. Every Friday at this season he came from the summer palace to attend mosque in the city, not to Santa Sophia but to the conveniently situated Zelie Ali Pasha close to the basin. It was his custom to ride from Beshiktash and return by barge.

Two lines of janissaries marked the route on either side of a track of fresh earth, sprinkled with water to settle the dust. The crowd around Charlemont and Burton were good-humoured and friendly during the long wait. First to appear were the turban bearers, who dismounted and posted themselves at either side to the entrance of the mosque, one carrying the diamond-encrusted turban of state and the other a footstool of rich brocade, which he set down for the Sultan to alight upon near the door.

A half hour passed and then a sudden silence signified the approach as the main body of the procession came into sight. They could discern detachments from the various bodies of troops which formed the Life Guard, but the lofty ostrich plumes rising from the Solak's helmets almost completely obscured any view of the Sultan's person. He seemed to be plainly dressed and without ornament. The trappings of his horse, an animal of the most perfect beauty, were on the other hand, splendid beyond description and shone with a profusion of jewels.

Immediately after came the Kizlaragasi, Chief of the Black Eunuchs, superbly mounted and followed by attendants. Charlemont believed he had never seen so ugly a human being and was struck with horror. At that moment the Sultan alighted, a royal salute was fired and all the people shouted in a deafening roar, Long Live Sultan Mahmoud.

While the Sultan, the Kizlaragasi and the principal officers were at prayer, the grooms walked the horses about. They were very beautiful, 'all Arabians but of that kind which we seldom import, and which are better fitted for war than for the course, high crested, light shouldered, but broad behind, and the furnitures, which, according to the Turkish fashion, covered a great part of the horse's body, were of a magnificence difficult to describe. Embroidery made the smallest part of their splendour and seemed to serve only as a ground upon which jewels of every sort were set in the greatest profusion. That by which I was more particularly struck was the horse on which the Kislar Aga rode. His trappings were of blue velvet embroidered with silver and powdered over with a multitude of pearls. The bosses of the bridle were of gold enriched with precious stones; but the most splendid of all was the breast-plate set with various jewels of great value, and in its centre or front an emerald of the most enormous size.'[14]

The Sultan reappeared and, remounting, rode to the waterside, where a magnificent barge with twenty-four oars, awaited him. At the first stroke of the oars a royal salute was fired and all the people shouted as before.

Quite overcome by the length, the solemnity and whimsicalities of the occasion, it was at this moment that Burton collapsed into uncontrollable laughter. Had not the crowd mistaken his convulsive heaving for a fit and drawn back to give him air and Charlemont taken the 'lucky hint' and showed the greatest concern, it seemed likely they would both have been torn to pieces by the mob before Charlemont could lead him to a safe distance, and out of hearing, where this most risible of God's creatures could laugh his fill.[15]

One evening driving out towards Belgrade with Mr Porter, Charlemont had the opportunity to study more closely the monstrous Kizlaragasi of the blackened teeth and hideous countenance as he passed their carriage, riding with a great train of attendants. Hardly had he gone by when one of his train returned and desired of the Ambassador that he would send his master a pinch of snuff. Mr Porter, having with him a very handsome gold box, concealed it and borrowed from one of the party a travelling leather one to send back. The request Porter assured them was for no other object than to gain possession of the coveted box, which would never be restored to him, but seized upon as a present, a trick now stale from use since it had been played upon other foreign ministers.[16]

Charlemont had it 'on good authority' that the loathsome Kislaragasi, this 'emasculated negro' with his few remaining teeth blacker than his skin, this obscene slave, who was first favourite of the Sultan and guardian of his wives, kept himself a harem of virgin beauties 'doomed to attend the odious call of his impotent lust'. Mahmoud I was said to be as high-minded, as magnanimous and merciful as the eunuch was rapacious and treacherous.[17]

Mahmoud is known to us today as the builder of numerous kiosks used by him and his boon companions for their nocturnal orgies. Charlemont's version of the tale is more bizarre. The Sultan would have been the happiest of men and princes had he been blessed with children, the lack of which embittered all his pleasures and overcast the glories of his reign. The tragedy through its publicity was made absurd. Women of all complexions, of all types and regions, had been put to the test and physicians, astrologers and quacks consulted. Dr McKenzie, a learned sensible man, who was physician to the English merchants told Charlemont, he too had been asked for his opinion, which he had given openly and frankly. If the Sultan slept well, ate well and performed the functions of nature normally and the external marks, signs and exertions of virility were as other men, the case was beyond his skill.

One aspect of the tale Charlemont thought more 'strikingly whimsical and absurd' than all the rest. Years before astrologers, casting the Sultan's horoscope, had pronounced he was not fated to beget a child on land. Therefore it was decided to try 'what could be done upon the water', the physicians concurring in the expectation that the motion of waves might happily contribute to facilitate conception. A magnificent yacht was built and moored opposite the Seraglio. Later, persevering with this notion, a kiosk was constructed upon floats and anchored in the channel at the most turbulent point. Having himself seen the kiosk, Charlemont gave credence to 'so wonderful an absurdity'.[18]

Charlemont's sources of information having so far been only European, he determined upon an interview with a 'sensible Turk, unprejudiced and well-informed'. In vain he pestered Mr Porter and he was beginning to think the British Ambassador's acquaintance was very limited when at last, one Mustafa Efendi arrived in Constantinople. He was the Turkish secretary to the English and he was highly rated for his honesty for having refused a bribe from the Russian minister to reveal the contents of a memorial he was translating and for telling the Russian he could not betray the country whose bread he had eaten. Once he had been in running for office at the Seraglio, but wearied by intrigue he had put ambition aside for his present post, which gave him time for study. A rare accomplishment for a Turk, he had 'no small proficiency' in Latin, and Charlemont had high hopes of a successful interview.[19]

Unfortunately the interview was short and with Porter and Dr McKenzie present and Pisani translating, a respectful reserve inhibited it throughout. Charlemont expressed his desire to ask a few questions if he might do so without giving offence. The reply came he might ask as pleased and take what licence he chose. Did he believe in astrology? 'I do not but think it a foolish science. For whilst a man pretends to foretell events, he does not know what his own wife is doing'. Questions and answers on the law and sexual morality followed and then Charlemont turned to religion. 'There are in all religions many things which should be understood metaphorically. Do you believe literally those relations in the Koran, of Mahomet's ascent into heaven?' etc. and the Turk countered with another question and a smile. 'Do you believe that Christ came from heaven and is gone thither again?' and then 'I am obliged to believe what is written in the Koran. I believe the world was created because, when I see smoke, I am sure there is fire. I have read a translation of the New Testament and believe the miracles of Christ, such as his restoring sight to the blind, his curing the diseased ...'

Then Charlemont tried to find out, as was the dream of Western scholars, whether the missing parts of Tacitus and the lost decade of Livy existed still in the Sultan's library. 'If there be any, they are in the Treasury, and impossible to come at because they are sealed with the Sultan's own seal ... the Caliphs in Egypt found a book in which there was nothing written against the Law, but on the contrary, where many good rules of conduct were to be found. They asked their prophet Omar if they might keep this book. But he desired them to burn it and ordered them to destroy whatever Greek or Latin manuscripts they should for the future meet with.' Charlemont wondered if this book could have been a copy or even the original manuscript of the Septuagint.[20]

This 'sensible' Turk left Constantinople the next day to Charlemont's chagrin; he felt he had failed to make the best of the opportunity.

Turning his attention to the business methods of the British merchants, he quickly formed the opinion that they were 'generally impatient to make their fortunes and return home quickly'. One Mr Barker, 'whose principal business was to supply the Seraglio with set jewels' admitted to selling his stock at a hundred per cent over its true value because his dealings were conducted through the office of the Kizlaragasi, a most precarious tenure, and upon the dismissal of that officer, or more likely his death, he stood in a hazardous way of not being paid. His over-charging might be a hedge against such a disaster, but Charlemont considered it 'must undoubtedly produce frequent disputes and consequent animosity.'[21]

Merchants and ministers alike had their villas at Pera, and here Charlemont found the pleasures of the table were well understood and there was scarcely an evening 'without balls, concerts and assemblies'. The women were remarkably handsome and well-dressed, their manners most pleasing and, so pleasant was society at Pera, that Mr Fawkener, a nephew of Sir Everard's, regarded a recall to England as little short of a sentence of banishment.[22]

It was Fawkener who accompanied Burton and Charlemont on an expedition to a brothel or, as Charlemont more delicately put it, to 'one of those modern temples of Venus' which are to be found in every metropolis. Burton of course was the instigator, his 'activity and curiosity with regard to some certain points of natural knowledge was as great as traveller ever possessed' but the proposal was by both Fawkener and Charlemont 'cheerfully accepted'. A Greek guide was hired and at midnight they stole out of the Embassy.

Having been only a short time in a country of whose inhabitants their Western prejudices had taught them to form 'terrible notions' and conscious that their purpose was licentious and for all they knew illegal, 'the dead silence', 'the pitchy darkness' of the streets made them susceptible to alarm, so that when without warning the silence was shattered by a great clamour, the darkness broken by a great blaze of light and they found themselves surrounded by men striking the ground with heavy clubs at their feet, they were terrified. Not understanding one word, thoughts of immediate destruction at the hands of Turkish barbarity, chased frantically through their minds. Then Fawkener laughed. It was only the Night Watch. Their Greek guide assured the Captain that they were merely English strangers walking out for recreation and to enjoy the night air. The Captain wished them goodnight, the lanterns were extinguished, and the patrol departed as silently as it had come.[23]

The matron of the house to which their Greek guide led them was an elderly Greek gentlewoman, who received them in a large room furnished with convenient sofas. On being whispered to by Fawkener she retired and presently they were surrounded by 'eight or ten goddesses' who with a liberality they found all the more pleasing since it 'so perfectly contrasted the cloud-envelopped apparitions' to which their contemplation had been confined since their arrival in the city, 'disclosed the full blaze of their heavenly charms', much as those who had disputed the prize of Beauty upon Mount Ida and revealed themselves to the Trojan shepherd. The ladies, none of them Turkish, although Turks frequented the brothel, were Greek, Jewish, Armenian and Christian, all of them extremely beautiful and 'well skilled in all the necessary arts and allurements of their calling'.[24]

The encounter with the Night Watch opened Charlemont's eyes to the effectiveness of Turkish policing methods. The stealth with which the patrols moved could well be applied in European cities where house-breaking and robbery by assault were the commonest of crimes, where felons had warning of the approach of the watch and could time the intervals between patrols. Neither did he underestimate the effectiveness of the heavy clubs he had seen, which he was told, could be thrown with the utmost dexterity between the legs of fleeing miscreants to bring them down.[25]

On the other hand, the administration of justice in the courts, if Pisani was to be believed, was unaccountable. Judges were open to bribes, but some of their decisions seemed incalculable more than corrupt. In one case a sea-captain was sued by the owners of a ship for a cargo, which he had jettisoned in a storm. The judge held the plaintiffs were entitled to its value – to be estimated at the moment before it had been thrown overboard to save the ship.

Stranger still was the case of a horse deal involving the sum of 200 piastres. The horse was not dear but the purchaser had found it unsuitable and recollecting he had spent more than he could afford, he went to the judge with half the sum to find in his favour. The vendor too went to bribe the judge with a similar sum. The affair was settled by the judge handing over the money to divide between the plaintiff and the defendant while he kept the horse.[26]

But these matters were by report and Charlemont, as a traveller, had to see things for himself and could not in conscience leave Constantinople without witnessing the dance of the Dervishes. Every Tuesday and Friday afternoon the order known as the Mevlevis, monks who had taken vows of poverty and austerity, held a public service in a spacious hall in front of a large congregation. They wore distinctive garb, whitish cloth gowns fastened at the waist by leathern belts, jackets and petticoats and caps of camel-hair stiffened into sugar-loaf shapes.

The service lasted two hours and began with a sort of hymn, its purport, Charlemont was told, a recommendation of charity and good works. An unintelligible sermon followed and then prayers by the Superior without book. Next there was a long hymn of which

Charlemont obtained a translation from one of the French residents (who also gave Charlemont translations of Turkish love lyrics), the gist being, '*Ne t'imagine point que celui qui trouve des riches trouve du Bonheur! Celui qui trouve le Bonheur n'est autre que celui qui trouve Dieu!*' The hymn was accompanied by a tabor and a sort of flute or hautboy and performed 'with great vociferation', shouted rather than sung. The music changed and the dance began. The monks revolved and revolved with astonishing velocity and Charlemont trying to count the revolutions thought he estimated sixty a minute, but nobody seemed to know whether they revolved in an expurgation of sin or in remembrance of their founder, who had fasted and turned in this manner until he had fallen into ecstacy with resulting revelations.[27]

More bizarre was the service of the Santons, an order named by the Franks (Europeans), Hough Houghs from the sound they emitted in the frenzy of their devotions. Although prepared for a strange and frantic scene, and aware that no women would be present as they had been at the former ceremony, the travellers had not supposed the monks would be so unkempt, their beards 'uncombed and nasty', their legs and feet bare and dirty, their persons 'squalid and nauseous'. As with the Mevlevis there were prayers and a long hymn, which the monks 'roared out all together as loud as they could bawl' and with 'a wildness of enthusiasm that had something shocking in it and seemed to promise the scene which followed'. The hymn ended and the dance began. The monks formed a close-knit circle leaving their superior to continue to sing alone, which he did with 'amazing vociferation', while they jumped as high 'as their strength and agility could raise them' and accompanied their violent activity with the most 'hideous howling' and a continual reiteration of what sounded like 'hough, hough', their features so distorted by the effort as to appear hardly human. Some 'overcome by the violence of the exercise, giddy with turning' fell inside the circle and lay there in ecstasy, howling and barking like men in a fit. Those still upright closed in and entwined their arms and continued to shout and jump 'like one great body, a furious monster with many heads, with many legs, jumping with all its feet, yelling with all its mouths' until their superior gave the signal by ending his song. Silence followed and then the performance was repeated until all lay gasping on the floor.[28]

These visits had Mr Porter's sanction, but Charlemont and Burton kept to themselves their determination to experience an 'unadulteratedly Turkish' bath with 'no foreign refinement' and in the depth of the city away from the English quarter, with only their janissary as a guide.

Subsequently they found themselves at a bagnio in a neat and convenient room heated by vapour, from which they were led to another, and then another, progressively hotter but not disagreeably so, and much as they had been led to expect, until they came to a room that was excessively heated, where the attendants indicated they should undress and assisted them to do so. When they were quite naked, the Turks tied about their middles a short apron, which served the same purpose as 'Adam's fig-leaf' and led them to a final chamber, which was intensely hot.

Here they were left, the doors closed upon them and the only light coming from small glazed cupolas overhead. At the centre was a large sunken bath with mats laid out on the marble floor for them to sit on. Soon they were sweating copiously and wishing the ceremony at an end. They called out but the attendants did not, or chose not, to hear, probably because they were not prepared to indulge them in the singularity of curtailing the stated time. As their cries continued to go unheeded, they began to feel faint and also seriously alarmed that they were going to pay dearly for their curiosity.

At length the door opened and two gigantic Turks appeared naked except for their aprons and each carrying a tub full of suds. They were seized by the Turks, laid out on the mats and covered all over with 'unsavoury lather', which got into their eyes and mouths. Disagreeable as this was, it was mere discomfort to what followed. The giant Turks drew over their hands a sort of mitten of hair-cloth and started rubbing them with such activity that Charlemont feared for his skin, but he resigned himself to the torture. Burton, on the other hand, 'roared like a bull'. His tormentors remained unmoved, 'without either pity or laughter' and continued in perfect and 'dignified gravity', to pull and draw their limbs until the joints cracked and then to sit upon their chests and press their shoulders.

That ended the torment and they were led to the bath and soused in lukewarm water before being conducted from one cooler room to another until at last at a normal temperature they lay upon beds and were served with the most excellent coffee. When they rose and dressed themselves, they felt wonderfully well and full of strength and alacrity, although they were somewhat subdued on their return to the embassy by the Ambassador's 'indifferent reception' and a severe chiding for venturing into a part of the city never free from plague.[29]

NOTES

1. RIA 12.R.5, pp. 103-4.
2. HMC Rept. 10 App. pt. 1, p. 303.
3. Stanford & Finopoulos, p. 6.
4. RIA, 12.R.5, no. to p. 7.
5. Stanford & Finopoulos, pp. 163-5.
6. Ibid, pp. 166-7.
7. RIA, 12.R.5. pp. 8-9.
8. Stanford & Finopoulos, pp. 167-8.
9. Ibid, p. 170.
10. Ibid.
11. Ibid, pp. 172-4.
12. Ibid.
13. Ibid.
14. Ibid, p. 182.
15. Ibid, pp. 184-5.
16. Ibid, p. 192.
17. Ibid, p. 193. (RIA, 12.R.5 p. 90.)
18. Ibid, pp. 189-90. H. Ganem, *Les Sultans Ottomans*, Paris 1902-3, Vol. 2, pp. 79-107.
19. Stanford & Finopoulos, pp. 176-9.
20. Ibid.
21. RIA, 12.5.5, n. to p. 2.
22. Stanford & Finopoulos, p. 205.
23. Ibid, p. 210.
24. Ibid, p. 206.
25. Ibid, pp. 211-2.
26. Ibid, pp. 213-8.
27. Ibid, pp. 219-223; RIA, 12.R.5 p.90.
28. Ibid, pp. 224-235.
29. Ibid, p. 231.

5

THE GREEK ISLANDS

Leaving Constantinople, in July, the travellers reached the first of the Greek Islands, Metelin (Lesbos), the islands where the 'parching heat of summer is never felt'. 'The thick shade of trees, and thousands of crystal springs, which everywhere arise, and form themselves into numberless rivulets, joined to the refreshing sea-breeze, qualify the burning air, and render the year a never-ending May.' ... Nature here reigns triumphant ... The mountains whose rugged tops exhibit a pleasing interspersion of rock and pine-groves, have their sides, for many miles along the coast, covered with olives, whose less agreeable verdure is corrected, embellished, and brightened by a lovely mixture of bays and of laurels aspiring to the height of forest trees, of mulberries growing wild, and laden with fruit, and of every other tree of noblest kind for sight, smell, taste! While the luxuriant vine, climbing wild and unrestrained even to their topmost branches, adorns and enriches them with its vivid green, and with its clustering fruit.'[1]

Thus wrote Charlemont, the essayist, years after in transposing the journal he kept at the time into literary form. Though on occasions we might prefer to hear more from Charlemont, the diarist, and of those observations made on the spot, in this particular instance the rhetoric is not inappropriate since it is used to describe 'nature triumphant' and has bearing on Charlemont's precept for the poetic, romantic landscaping of Marino, his villa outside Dublin. Moreover he was probably writing while he was engaged upon those improvements.

Charlemont's investigations, as at Messina and at Constantinople, continued to be as thorough as time and his inexperience allowed. The sense of adventure, the feeling of wonder and curiosity survived to the end, but throughout the Greek travels, as one would expect from a classical scholar, his studies had prepared him for identification and recognition of the ancient scene rather than the surprises that came with contemporary life and Turkish domination.

Charlemont was a product of the age, an amateur and a dilettante before such terms had lost their meaning and respectability. He travelled with a library of books of classical reference, a notebook in which to copy any ancient inscriptions he came across and an array of measuring instruments for the proper and approved examination of antique monuments and edifices.

The island of Metelin was 'full of broken basso relievos, mutilated inscriptions, marble columns, and capitals of different orders, wrought in the best taste", some of the columns fluted and others worked spirally. In the court of the Bishop's palace they saw an antique chair with fine bas reliefs, which bore an inscription stating it was the throne of Potamon; perhaps the same Potamon listed by Strabo* as one of the island's eminent men. But their principal discovery was a marble aqueduct at an hour and a half's ride from the town and this, because Charlemont could not find any reference to it by other travellers, they measured in all its particulars, with great industry and we must suppose accuracy, as he recorded their findings precisely.[2]

The modern buildings had a peculiarity of construction which enabled the islanders to enjoy fully the prospect over their enchanting island. 'Each house is a square tower, neatly built of hewn stone, so high as to overtop the trees'[3] an exterior staircase led to the apartments at the top and beneath were granaries and storehouses. Another singularity was the way the Metelines propagated their vines from shoots buried in dung heaps.[4] The wine, although good, did not come up to Charlemont's idea of its ancient fame, but the fruits of the island, particularly the figs, were incomparable. He also made notes on the island's trade in sponges and olive oil.

But the chief peculiarity of Metelin was the behaviour of the women, and years later Charlemont read a paper on the subject to the Royal Irish Academy in Dublin. On their perambulations, the travellers found themselves the focus of the undisguised curiosity of the female islanders, who boldly stopped them, immodestly examined their clothes and their persons and pointed and laughed in their faces. The girls were very handsome in spite of their complexions being masked by make-up, their eyebrows shaved and a line of gummed hair subsitututed. Their figures were scarcely concealed by a transparent shift to the waist and a handkerchief covering the breasts, a

* Stabo (*c.* B.C. 63 - A.D. 24) widely travelled Greek geographer.

small sop to modesty imposed by the Turks, and a matter of patriotic grievance since any departure from old custom was regarded as a betrayal of national identity.

A French resident explained the odd behaviour. This was an Amazonian society. The women wore the breeches. On marriage the man took his wife's name and dared not interfere with management of house, garden or estate, which was hers. The eldest daughter inherited her mother's possessions. Her brothers were apportioned small dowries or turned out penniless to seek their fortunes. Her younger sisters, 'condemned to perpetual celibacy', might think themselves lucky to wait on her and wore home-spun clothes, while she was dressed magnificently and her clothes were embroidered with pearls and gold sequins. It was a society in which men rode side-saddle and women astride. These women were content with absolute sway, without endeavouring in any other particular to change the course of nature, and it would seem that Sappho's manly inclinations merely conformed to the 'whimsical manners of her countrywomen'.[5]

It was Burton's contention that there was every reason to think that, in spite of their haughtiness, they would have been the 'kindest ladies on earth' had they not been strictly watched by the Turks, whose 'ungallant laws' were enforced through the threat of arbitrary fines. The closest they came to a Meteline was to persuade one to sit to Dalton for her portrait.

The full implications of Turkish domination did not strike the travellers at Metelin, but became apparent at Chios,[6] where outside the harbour were two very large men o' war. Inside a number of Turkish galleys, flying pennants, flags and colours made a pretty sight. The harbour however was badly neglected and silted up. The island, accounted the richest in the Archipelago, paid dearly for the Captain Pasha's protection, ostensibly against the corsairs who infected the seas. Besides the annual dues of sixty purses, there was the cost of entertaining him and his entourage ashore during the visit.

The Turkish presence had a depressing effect on the islanders. Fear of the levantis*, who, like other seamen coming ashore were inclined to be 'troublesome, expensive and dangerous', restrained the women from appearing in anything but the poorest apparel and behaving in a very reserved manner. Charlemont was not entirely sure that the fears and complaints were justified. The Levantis offered neither insult nor riot while he was there. Many Turks, 'allured by the

* Turkish sailors

wealth of the island' made Chios their place of residence and seemed to live with the inhabitants on a friendly footing. Religious tolerance was evident; there were six mosques, numerous Greek churches and convents and the 'Latins' had five churches and monasteries besides.

Rambling around the island and visiting the mastic villages,7 the source of much of the island's wealth*, they came across a convent of nuns, 'the jolliest girls of the kind I ever yet met with', who for the reward of a sequin chanted their whole service 'most angelically'. Their church was small and pretty and, like many of the churches, in a good style of architecture, 'the Genoese and Venetians having left behind them many obvious traces of their taste'.

The country houses too were well built, 'neat, elegant, and designed with taste', each with its paved court and fountain and trim garden.

Charlemont's account of their visit to Néa Moné is one of the rare extracts from the missing journal. Saturday August 2nd 'We set out on mules for a Greek monastery the principal in the island, called Néa Moné, i.e. new retreat. In about two hours we travelled little more than three miles through mountains of solid rock ... the road was execrable. Here one may observe with pleasure the indefatigable industry of this people, for wherever there is half a foot deep of soil ... it is cultivated to the utmost. At length we arrived at the monastery, which is a large, but ugly building resembling an old castle, such as with us are frequently seen. The church is pretty enough for the age in which it was built. Its plafond, which, according to the fashion of architecture during the Greek Empire, consists of several small circular domes, is covered with tolerable mosaics. The monks informed us that it was built in the year 1045, and showed us an old painting of the Emperor and Empress who founded and endowed it.' Charlemont copied the inscriptions above the portraits and added a note that they were of Constantine IX and the unfortunate and wicked Zoë. 'The history of this imperial dame makes Messalina appear a prude.'

'The body of the church is made out of pieces of most precious marbles, collected from more ancient buildings, but these fragments are ill put together, and wretchedly jointed ... They [the monks] showed us many relics, dirty and ill preserved – among others an old piece of board, with scarce an atom of colouring upon it, which they

* Chios was the almost exclusive producer of mastic or gum resin obtained from the bark of the lentisk, an evergreen shrub.

call a portrait of the Virgin by St Luke. Nothing can be more ridiculous than the paintings in the porch of the church. The Virgin is represented on the top of Jacob's ladder – in the burning bush of Moses, and in the little stone which broke Nebuchadnezzar's image. They have a sort of library with many manuscripts lying in dust and rubbish. We spent an hour in looking them over, hoping to have discovered some ancient treasure, but found nothing but some manuscripts of the Greek Fathers. There are also many printed books, and, among others, a St Chrysostom printed at Eton, 1612 ...'[8]

Another visit was to an exiled prince of Tartary, who resided in the palace of a Pasha of Rhodes, whose acquaintance they had made at Malta. Sending up word that 'some English gentlemen, travellers from curiosity, were desirous of the honour of paying their respects', they were shown into his apartments, where he received them. He was surrounded by his guard of Tartars, who had followed him into exile after his unsuccessful revolt against the reigning Cham, all dressed in Tartarian fashion, fur caps and green gowns. The prince, a very handsome man, who combined good sense with a graceful manner and polite condescension, asked them many questions about their travels and particularly about England and the circumstances of the war with France.[9]

So far little or no contact had been made with the Turks. On first arriving at Chios Charlemont had openly expressed his wish to call upon the Captain Pasha, but a deputation of Greeks had come aboard *L'Aimable Vainqueur* to warn him that the Admiral was unlikely to receive him kindly. He had shown 'a strong inclination to order the bastinado to be inflicted' on the Consul's dragoman, who had been lax about laying their firman* before him immediately on their arrival. But an Aga, in command of the garrison of janissaries on the island, paid a courtesy call. He was forbidden by his religion to taste wine, but 'he was greatly delighted with what he called our *English sherbet, viz.* arrack punch' and on leaving, withdrew from his girdle a sabre and presented it to Charlemont, remarking that it had already killed two men and he was sure it would not lie idle in his service either. Charlemont reciprocated with a pair of English pistols and tells us that at the time of writing, the sabre was still in his possession, ever since 'perfectly at rest'.[10]

On the last evening before their intended departure, they gathered together 'a parcel of pretty country girls' and danced with them on

* Passport

the shore close to the spot known as the school of Homer, a small amphitheatre cut out of the solid rock with a square seat like a pulpit at the centre, flanked by defaced lions. The girls were handsome, plump and had lovely complexions, 'the large eyes of Juno' and 'the true Grecian nose', but their dress unbecoming and their petticoats 'so short as to show a great part of the leg', which Charlemont would not have complained of had they not rendered it a disadvantage by 'a whimsical predilection for thick legs', which he thought they must esteem a beauty for they wore several pairs of stockings![11]

Sleeping aboard that night with intention of sailing for Myconos at the first change of wind, they wakened early and discovered a barge of twenty-four oars drawn up alongside. This turned out to be the barge of the Captain Pasha's second-in-command, who had come to enquire for their health and, supposing they would be pleased to inspect a Turkish man o' war, invited them to accompany him. Greatly obliged they dressed in clothes kept in readiness for such occasions, and sent for an interpreter.

Met on the quarter deck of the man o' war by the son of the Commodore, they were conducted to his cabin, where he was sitting on a sofa surrounded by a number of handsome boys, perhaps not there for any honourable purpose. He excused himself from rising because of an attack of gout, but he entertained them very politely with the usual coffee, sherbet and perfumes and presented them with gold and silver-bordered muslin handkerchieves.

His son was their guide and led them over the entire ship. Named, as it would seem all commanding ships were, the *Capitano*, she mounted seventy-four guns. Her enormous breadth in proportion to her length, the height of her stern, and the heaviness and confusion of her rigging, made Charlemont think her unwieldy and clumsy. He did not believe their young conductor when he told them the guns on the lower deck carried a ball of no less than a cantar, 110 lbs., and he noted with some national pride that the sailors, compared to British seamen, went awkwardly and slovenly about their duties.

Then a strange thing happened. Noticing four seamen who eyed them wistfully, Charlemont asked who they were and was told they were Christian slaves, who did duty aboard. He went forward and spoke with them. Each bore his fate according to his country; there was an Italian who was peevish and impatient, a Spaniard who was 'grave and sullen' and a lively talkative Frenchman, who laughed at the lubbardly seamanship of the Turks, paid the travellers a thousand compliments and appeared as full of spirits as if 'in the most prosperous situation' at home. The last was an Englishman, who was philosophical and seemed glad to meet his countrymen, but made no show of it. He declared his situation by no means a bad one. He had been captured at Oran and was better treated as a slave than as a mercenary of the Spaniards. It being 'the peculiar property of every Englishman to love Liberty', it was no surprise that he had written to Mr Porter at Constantinople, but he seemed unconcerned about the outcome of his appeal. All four agreed that the Turks were lenient masters and showed, after an initial attempt to convert them to the True Faith, the greatest religious tolerance. They had made over a cabin to them for a chapel, which Charlemont asked to see. Astonishingly, considering Muslim detestation of image and picture worship, the little chapel contained a sort of altar on which were images in baked clay and prints of the Crucifixion and the Virgin and Child.

Before leaving, Charlemont distributed some money among the crew and 'a particular bounty' to their Christian brethren. A salute of three guns was, on Charlemont's previous instruction, returned by the firing from *L'Aimable Vainqueur* of the Royal Salute.

Their Christian friends hung on the shrouds cheering and the Frenchman called out, '*Milord, oserois je vous demander si vous avez été en France?*' and Charlemont shouted back, '*Oui, j'y été*'. The Frenchman called again, '*Avez vous vû Fontainebleau?*' '*Non, je n'ai pas vû,*' Charlemont replied. '*Ah, Milord si jamais vous retournez en France pour l'amour de Dieu voyez Fontainebleau. C'est bien le plus bel endroit du monde.*'[12]

Gifts in compliance with Turkish custom and also as a testament of gratitude were despatched, a silver *étui*,* made in Birmingham, for the Commodore and a silver snuff box for the Captain. The wind being favourable they set sail. As they passed the enormous and stately man o' war they fired nine guns. The salute was acknowledged, one, two and then three guns, as great a compliment as the haughty Turk allowed himself.

In contrast to Chios, where Charlemont had dwelt on the beauties and richness of the island, the wealth of the mastic groves of the evergreen Lenticus and the industry of the inhabitants, his observations on Myconos were summary. The idleness of the Mycones was extreme and 'except for a few cotton stockings, and an abundance of cuckolds, nothing is made in this island'. The men were sailors with

* A small case fitted with useful articles.

large caiques carrying commodities between the islands while the women, expensively dressed and with chains of gold and strings of pearls about their necks, had the impudence to beg in the streets.[13]

Here, on the report of Dr Askew, a physician and classical scholar, that no women on earth were as 'fair and all-accomplished' as those of this barren and rocky island, they contacted a pimp, (Charlemont chose to call him their 'obliging Mercury'). Because of a Turkish squadron in the harbour and the town full of *levantis*, he arranged an assignation at the ruin of a castle in the distant countryside, in the dark and rain and at the dead of night. After a long and most uncomfortable wait, the pimp returned in great state of agitation and begged them, if they valued their lives, to flee. A band of Levantis had snatched the 'maiden', beaten him cruelly and only by the aid of darkness and his superior knowledge of the country had he escaped to warn them.

Charlemont and Burton, requiring no second bidding or further explanation, instantly followed the pimp, who ran full speed ahead of them. 'Poor Frank especially, whose body, any more than his soul, was never formed for flight, exhibited the most exact and the most humorous representation of Sir John Falstaff's precipitate retreat from Gadshill. Out of breath with running, and scarcely able to keep up, he damn'd the *levantis*, the Pimp, the Whore, the Greeks and the Turks'– 'Is it not better to have one's throat cut than to burst one's wind? I cannot stir an inch farther. Let them come and be damn'd. Zounds, I'm in a Ditch – up to the Neck, by Jove! What the devil brought me awhoring in this unchristian Country? Stay for me. Let me recover breath. Zounds, man, stay!'"[14]

A few days later, having regained their courage and being vexed by the disappointment, they persuaded their Mercury to arrange another assignment, this time in the town, but, alas, as Charlemont had to admit, the damsel was more fit for the arms of the levantis than their 'more refined and sentimental passion'.

After Myconos, they parted with the ship and hired a felucca for the shallow waters and inadequate harbourage of Delos, Naxos and Tinos, and arranged for a rendezvous at Paros.

Delos, the sacred island, was uninhabited except for rats, rabbits and a singular kind of lizard, which agreed with the Koscordili of Tournefort's drawing. For three days they toiled among the ruins and found nothing other than what had been described by Tournefort*.

* J.P. Tournefort *Relation d'un Voyage de Levant* 2 Vob. Paris 1717.

Delos, 'the Mecca of the heathen world, enriched with gifts from the greatest monarchs', decorated by 'the most exquisite sculptors' had become 'a quarry for the neighbouring islanders,' who found stone here for their meanest purposes. The fountain of Inopus, so famous to the ancients, yielded little better than mud and they had been well advised to put a supply of fresh water aboard the felucca. For want of food they had to send one of their Greek boatmen to the neighbouring isle of Rhenea for mutton and for want of lodging they improvised a bed of dry seaweed on the shore and covered this with 'a homely tent' of awning, where they slept for three nights.[15]

On 15 August they rowed across to the island known as the greater Delos and here Charlemont, quoting from his journal, lists at length the antiquities, all 'extremely ill-treated by time'. They took the measurements of the colossal body of a headless lion, of which Strabo, usually so accurate, made no mention.

Returning late one evening from their 'toilsome researches', they were agreeably surprised by 'a singularly pleasing night scene', and here the essay reverts again to Charlemont's later literary style, with a description that pays homage to Edmund Burke's *Of the Sublime and Beautiful.*

'Three musicians, two lyres and a guitar, passing from Tinos, had spied our boat, and in the hopes of employment, had landed here. Our crew, who were all Greeks, had willingly received them, and were dancing their country gambols by the light of a parcel of dry sticks (for we had no candles), burning in an iron pot. The view of Mount Cynthus, at the foot of which our homely tent was pitched. The contemplation of those venerable ruins, which raised in our minds the most awful and painfully pleasing ideas. The sprightly whimsical music, not a little improved and dignified to our fancy by the respected and consecrated name of *lyre*, and accompanied by the solemn buzz of the still sea, which served as a sullen base. The grotesque dancing and the strange illumination, which looked as if prepared for enchantment. All these circumstances joined to the genial feel [?] of this delightful climate, and a night beyond expression serene and beautiful, contributed to render as agreeable as it was picturesque and singular this unexpected scene.'[16]

Naxos was hilly and finely wooded with little torrents dashing down the mountain sides through trees to form the small rivulets that watered the valleys below. 'The veneration of antiquity' conspired to 'sanctify the region' and added 'its awful charms, its reverential ideas to the romantic beauties of these enchanting scenes' among which oranges, pomegranates, mulberries and figs grew in abundance. Here they climbed to the top of Zia, the mountain of Jupiter and were rewarded for their toil with a prospect over all the Cyclades, island after island as far as the eye could see. About half way up they came upon a vast rock of marble with an inscription, which Charlemont copied and, close by, a romantic and spacious cave. An amazing vine grew nearby, its vast size and apparent age suggesting to their imagination that it was planted by Bacchus himself, the cave being traditionally the scene of Bacchanalian orgies.

Throughout their stay at Naxos they were the guests of a Gascon nobleman, Baron François de Lastio de Vigouroux, who invited them to his house, 'a large and handsome habitation' on a hill above the town. The Baron was eighty years old, tall, robust and of 'a plumpness' that went with health and good humour. He had as a child been page to Louis XIV and in all the wars of 'that restless Prince' had served with credit until, risen to the rank of Lieutenant-General, he had at length grown tired of the pursuit of pleasure and ambition and of the trifling intrigues of court life, and retired with his wife and his young son to Naxos. His wife had long since died, his son had grown up and was married to 'one of the principal women of the island' and it was she, 'handsome, lively and affable', who acted as their hostess.

Every day the travellers were entertained to 'a splendid repast', and every evening there was a ball in their honour, to which the handsomest youth and the prettiest women were bidden. Many were Catholics, descendants of the Venetian occupation. Under the Baron's roof the natural aversion between Greek and Latin was forgotten. All were equally his friends and he was the equal friend of all, his good humour and keen but kindly comment delighting the company.

Charlemont believed him the happiest of men, spending the remaining years of an honourable life, the father, the protector, the friend of his people and doing more good in his country than all the potentates of Europe could boast of in a century. He was idolized by the populace, as Charlemont saw when on one of their perambulations through the town in the excessive heat of the August sun, the Baron suffered a fainting fit. The consternation was general; the whole town was in tears. These expressions of love and sorrow touched Charlemont and even more, the transports of joy and emotion when at length the Baron recovered and the people kissed his hands and embraced his knees and then, making a lane for him, allowed Charlemont and his party to lead him back to the house.[17]

When in the last years of Charlemont's life Dr Halliday, in a letter to Charlemont, enquired for his family, he made it clear that it was to the whole Irish nation that he referred. There can be little doubt that Charlemont's self-adopted role, the father of his people, was inspired by this model of benevolent rule.

Thousands stood on the shore at Naxos and expressed their goodwill in acclamation as the travellers departed. The last kindness of their host, the Baron, was to have the felucca filled with every sort of provision, sheep, bread, wine and fruit.

Tinos,[18] the next island, was also free of visits from the Captain Pasha. Formerly under the dominion of the Venetians, the island had surrendered only by treaty, a treaty strictly observed by the Turks, who received a tax of forty purses paid in Constantinople and had but one deputy, the only Turk, residing on the island. Such had been the spirit of liberty that a tyrannical Voivode* having been torn to pieces and an armed galley sent by the Turks to demand the murderers, the whole people had assembled themselves on the shore and openly and unanimously declared their guilt, if to destroy a tyrant was culpable. Even the Turks were awed by this unity of front and retired.

The island struck Charlemont as beautiful with its hills and dales and the inhabitants 'industrious, well clothed, happy and lively'. The resident Venetian consul was candid enough to say that though the silk trade had decreased and the Tiniotes paid higher taxes, he was convinced that under the Turks they fared better.

At a ball given by the British consul, all the belles of the island were present and Charlemont was struck by their beauty. They danced until midnight, not only Greek dances but the minuet; and their dresses, unlike those of the other islands, resembled the Venetian contadine, retaining something of the superior elegance of the former influence.

In contrast there was little to be said in favour of Syros,[19] the last island to be visited before the rendezvous with *L'Aimiable Vainqueur* arranged for Paros. Two things impressed Charlemont about this island: the 'so whimsically built' capital around 'a steep and pyramidical rock, every tier of houses forming a step, so as that the flat roof of the lower house serves as a courtyard to the upper, only a little incommodated by the chimney', and that the town was more like

* Voivode, or Vaivode, local govenor.

'a pigsty than an inhabitation for Christians of any sect. Pigs and Capuchins are indeed in such abundance here that one can scarcely walk through the streets without stumbling over one or the other ...' There was only one Greek church and the Latins completely predominated. The people were hospitable and good-natured and they put on board the felucca a parting gift of excellent figs and honey.

The travellers were not particularly dismayed to find no sign of *L'Aimable Vainqueur* at Paros and sailed on happily enough to Antiparos to view 'with astonishment the famous grotto, which, both in magnificence and difficulty of descent' exceeded all their expectations and here Dalton recorded their presence in a drawing of the cave lit by their flares. Charlemont felt it unnecessary to give any further account, except of one curiosity discovered since Tournefort's day, a small chamber in the rock with two springs of water, only nine feet apart, one fresh, cold and sweet, the other not distinguishable from the saltiest sea-water.

It remained only to settle their small accounts and re-embark for Paros. 'Upon an exact inspection into each man's purse', they were shocked to find they had between them a mere three sequins or the equivalent to a guinea and a half, all that was left of the money they had brought from *L'Aimable Vainqueur* or thought necessary for their expedition in the felucca. A council was called and it was agreed they should avoid immediate discovery of their poverty by 'gallantly paying' what was owed at Antiparos and return at once to Paros, where they might rely on the good-nature of the Voivode and his wife, whose son they had met at Myconos.[20]

In 'sad trim' they arrived at Parechia. Charlemont's huzzar jacket was all in rags from climbing rocks and creeping into caves; 'Burton's long plaid banian, at best the worst of nightgowns, was torn and greasy'. But the most wretched figure of all was Dalton, who, having the ill-luck to spill on his coat a lampful of 'stinking oil', was reduced to a waistcoat, which had once been laced with gold, but now had its back pieced together with remnants of an old canvas with some mutilated figures painted upon it, which gave it the appearance of 'a sign hung out to testify the poverty of the miserable inhabitant'.[21]

Notwithstanding, they were received by the Greek Voivode and his wife with the utmost cordiality and cheerfulness and their 'dear fat landlady' provided a most hospitable board and saw to it that the anxious days of waiting for the ship were filled with sight-seeing and festivity and their evenings spent in the best company.

But the wind continued to blow steadily and unfavourably. Every day brought fresh anxieties, which they could scarcely conceal from their amiable host and hostess. They blushed in company when the everlasting topic, the amazing wealth of England, was brought up, and cursed the importune females, who, on their walks about the town, teased them, as rich strangers, to buy from them the cotton stockings manufactured on the island. 'Fears of the most serious kind began to intrude'; there was an amount of money on board *L'Aimable Vainqueur* and the stores were valuable. The ship was well manned and in some sort armed. They knew little of their captain's character and what they did know was not of the most comfortable kind; they had heard and read of seamen turning pirate.[22]

From such melancholy thoughts they turned gratefully to every distraction. They were bidden to a Greek christening and were much entertained by 'the odd behaviour' of the priest, who was as careless and relaxed, as if he was 'employed in the most trifling affair, talking to the bystanders of indifferent matters during the most sacred parts of the ceremony, and handling the poor little animal in so rough and awkward a manner' that the travellers feared 'at every instant some fatal accident'.[23]

They visited a number of churches, most of which were in a pretty style of architecture. A priest informed them that the Madonna, accounted the largest and most magnificent of the archipelago, was built by a student of the architect of Santa Sofia. Charlemont considered that, if this were the case, the pupil had outdone even his master in bad taste.

The visit to the famous quarries provided another distraction. The entrance to the great quarry was dignified by a basso relievo cut in the solid rock, representing Bacchus and the Bacchanals and dedicated in an inscription to the nymphs of the country. The workmanship seemed careless to Charlemont suggesting some statuary (sculptor) waiting to load and amusing himself in an exercise of his talent. Another quarry had recently been discovered and the entrance only partly cleared. The cavern was deep and dark and confirmed to Charlemont Pliny's assertion that the quarries were worked by lamplight. There was evidence of ancient chiselling and the practice of squaring and smoothing the marble before cutting.

That from this womb had issued all the fine sculpture of Greece and from this island the Arundel* marbles, was a thought that gave

* Collected by Thomas Howard, 2nd Earl of Arundel (*c.* 1585-1646) on his travels and through agents. Given to the University of Oxford, 1667. Including the Parian Chronicle, a marble slab recording events of Greek history between B.C. 1582 and B.C. 354.

Charlemont infinite delight. Parechia, in ancient times the most splendid of cities, had everywhere evidence of its past glories, the walls of the town, the houses and the little chapels were all built from ruined edifices; 'not a cottage but has its doorcase of the finest marble, the remains of ancient architraves and friezes.'

Their stay, prolonged by the non-appearance of their ship, coincided happily with a visit to the island of none less than the Archbishop of Naxos, who was waited on by the Voivode, and whom Charlemont and his party most willingly accompanied. They were entertained to a dinner, the company consisting of the Archbishop with his chaplain, the Voivode, their own ragged fraternity and a bard. The repast was composed almost entirely of kid, which was considered in the islands the first of delicacies, roasted and dressed in savoury sauces, and followed by fruit, principally grapes and figs, the whole accompanied by incomparable wine. The kid, as Charlemont afterwards discovered, had been raised from the time it could leave its dam in a dry well or narrow pit (and there were plenty of these on the island), and fed with the milk of two cows until after six months of inaction, it had grown to a great size and was deemed fit for the table.

The jolliest feature of the Archbishop's banquet were the toasts, which, with the extempore stanzas sung by the bard, the emptying of full goblets and the choruses, made for a truly classical scene. Charlemont was extolled for his nobility and the extent of his travels, Burton for his extraordinary size, Dalton for his skill in painting and the two tutors for their faithful attachment, Murphy the Achates of Charlemont, Scott a Patroclus to Burton's Achilles.[24]

They would have been very happy but for their predicament and when at last the wind changed and their ship appeared on the horizon, they imagined 'the Argo freighted with the Golden Fleece, was not more acceptable to the Greeks'. There was firing of guns and every mark of 'nautical joy', and Charlemont was at last able to settle their accounts and distribute gifts to their so many benefactors.

Taking leave of their 'dear fat landlady', who for eight days had succoured them with an excellent table of mutton, game and the best partridges, and of all their other friends, they sailed away for Egypt.

At sea somewhere between the isles of Crete and Cos, Charlemont celebrated in the old style of dating his twenty-first birthday with a feast and much dutiful firing of cannon. No kind bard being there to write his birthday ode, he was obliged to write his own.[25]

NOTES

1. Stanford & Finopoulos, p. 19.
2. Ibid, p. 26.
3. Ibid, p. 19.
4. Ibid, p. 27.
5. Ibid, pp. 20-4.
6. Ibid, p. 29.
7. Ibid, p. 34.
8. Ibid, pp. 41-2.
9. Ibid, p. 33.
10. Ibid, p. 44.
11. Ibid, pp. 35-6.
12. Ibid, pp. 36-40.
13. Ibid, pp. 46-51.
14. Ibid, also Craig, App. II, pp. 260-3.
15. Stanford & Finopoulos, p. 52.
16. Ibid, p. 54. The indecipherable word in the Ms may be 'feel'.
17. Ibid, pp. 56-9.
18. Ibid, pp. 61-2.
19. Ibid, p. 63-4.
20. Ibid, p. 65.
21. Ibid, p. 66.
22. Ibid, p. 69.
23. Ibid, p. 68-9.
24. Ibid, pp. 67-8.
25. Hardy, p. 15. The Birthday Ode is also given in full in Craig, pp. 57-8. Craig repeats Hardy's mistake that Charlemont came of age in Constantinople. See Charlemont's letter to Marlay from Alexandria.

6

EGYPT: THE LAND OF WONDERS

Of Charlemont's sojourn in 'that astonishing country' we are told by him only a part; the essay he planned either was never written or the manuscript was lost. The few marginal notes relating to Egypt which are incorporated with his accounts of the Turks are barely chronological and for any sequence of events we must turn to Dalton's publications: *Musaeum Graecum et Aegyptiacum* or *Antiquities of Greece and Egypt*, illustrated by prints, engraved from drawings 'taken on the spot by Mr Richard Dalton, in a late voyage to the Levant, in the company of the Right Honourable Lord Viscount Charlemont, and Francis Pierpont Burton Esq. *Ann. Dom.* 1749 and 1751 (1752)'. Another edition with seventy-five prints followed in 1791.

Dr Johnson was discussing with Boswell how little does travelling supply to the conversation of any man who has travelled. Boswell: 'What say you to Lord Charlemont?' Charlemont had a high reputation for the ease and charm of his conversation. Johnson: 'I never heard him but once talk of what he had seen and that was of a large serpent in one of the pyramids of Egypt.'[1]

In the first week of September *L'Aimable Vainqueur* docked at Alexandria, and the party going ashore was welcomed by Mr Browne, the British Vice-Consul, who led them to the Consulate, where there was lodging for the party and what proved to be very hospitable entertainment for the length of their stay. For protection, and as a guide, one Mahomet, a janissary in the service of the Consulate, was detailed to accompany them wherever they went. If Charlemont expected the kind of civility shown to travellers of curiosity in Constantinople, he was quickly disillusioned. Ostensibly under Turkish dominion, the Egyptians showed none of the courtesy of their masters, and it was not safe to walk the streets in European clothes. When Scott was struck by a stone thrown by an unfriendly native, they proceeded with greater caution, changing their tricorn hats, their jackets and knee breeches for the less conspicuous garb of Greeks and Armenians.

On 6 September there being a ship about to depart for Leghorn, Charlemont wrote to Richard Marlay and sent him his Birthday Ode. It was the first opportunity in three months for getting a letter away. 'As we are but just arrived you can expect no account of anything here; all I can say is that everything we meet strikes us with wonder. In a day or two when we shall have well examined this port, we propose to set out for Grand Cairo, for which purpose we are now busied in getting ready our Turkish masquerades, for 'tis necessary in that voyage to go travestied *à la Turque*. How many times I wished that you could but have seen us in some of the droll equipages we have been in during our abode in the islands, mounted on asses, and glad to get them, pack saddles, without either bridle or stirrups; seven or eight days without a bed to lie on, encamped on desert islands ... I have been very busy measuring a column above one hundred feet high, which is of one stone, a most beautiful granite, seventy feet long. The women here are most droll animals! those of the Greek islands are deities compared to these gypsies.'[2]

The column was of course Pompey's Pillar, of which Dalton made a drawing, with two spectators, unidentifiable but presumed to be Charlemont and Burton. Unusually Charlemont's measurements, as reported to Marlay, are less than exact.

There were but two obelisks; one remained standing though half-buried in surrounding ruins and rubble; the other was fallen down and broken. Neither bore comparison with those in Rome, particularly with the one found in the Campus Martius.

Earnest attention was given to the catacombs. Murphy with the measuring rods, and Dalton with his sketch book, between them made a scale plan of the entrance and the temple, and one of the chambers was carefully examined. But the city where the immense library of the Ptolemies had fallen prey to devouring flames, where the ancient Pharos lay buried deep in the sea and without any certain indication of where it had stood, held nothing further to delay the travellers.

Charlemont, however, perceiving a Turkish galley in the harbour, could not resist a courtesy call upon her captain, and being now conversant with Turkish ceremony, was well received. He found the slaves, the majority of them Christians 'singing and conversing' with the utmost gaiety and good humour and again he was assured that the Christians were encouraged to observe their holy days, for which at Christmas, Easter and Whitsuntide their Muslim captain provided sumptuous feasts. He seemed to Charlemont a good man, who supplemented from his own pocket a Government allowance for their clothes and other necessities.[3]

On 25 August (O.S.) Mr Browne sent his report to the British Ambassador at Constantinople. Mr Porter was informed that Lord Charlemont had left Alexandria and was going well for Cairo.

Twenty-five miles of desert lay between Alexandria and Rosetta. The heat was intense, the sand deep and burning and stretching as far as the eye could see. Mounted on mules, the Christian travellers, with water to drink and water-melons to chew, could scarcely endure the extreme conditions. Because it was the season of Ramadan, their Arab guides, whom they pitied greatly, neither drank nor ate until the sun went down. Not that they suffered 'this horrid abstinence' with any sign of distress; on the contrary they ran beside the trotting mules, ankle-deep in the burning sand, jumping and shouting and diverting themselves 'with a thousand antic tricks'. Their janissary too observed the strictness of the fast; Mahomet, although nearly fainting, could not be prevailed upon to wet his lips.[4]

According to Dalton, for the first part of the journey, a Sheik and his son, with one of their men, mounted on fine Arabians, rode with them. At parting Charlemont thought a present was indicated and consequently the Sheik's attendant continued on with the little caravan after his master had ridden off. Further along the route two Arab horsemen approached, one riding the most beautiful Arabian, and after some palaver with their escort, went away. Seemingly they were reconnoitering, but had been discouraged by the Sheik's officer.

Bypassing a town they came presently to a ferry. On the far side was a khan or caravanserai, but this they were advised not to enter 'as infected persons had been there lately' and they took their refreshment in the open air.

About a mile out from the town of Rosetta they were met by Monsieur Chabère, who conducted them to his house and entertained them with great civility on the recommendation of Mr Browne.

From Rosetta they sailed up the Nile 'in a large commodious boat'. The first night they were tormented by gnats 'to the last degree'. Along the banks were miserable villages, clusters of bee-hive dwellings made of clay and the inhabitants mostly naked or barely covered with a few filthy rags. It amazed the travellers to see a great extent of fertile country and, in the midst of abundance, such poverty.

At Cairo, Charlemont and Burton were guests of the British Consul and his wife, Mr and Mrs Barton; the others lodged with a Mr Harris. Charlemont, it seems, was soon on very good terms with the Bartons, and especially Mrs Barton, who was his chief informant about the Turkish ladies, of whom Charlemont despaired of catching even the barest glimpse.

She conceded their good looks, if not great beauty, but was feminine enough, to Charlemont's amusement, to mention their most lavish use of medicated baths, drugs, cosmetics and perfumes. Mrs Barton was herself excessively thin and bore with entire equanamity this disadvantage in a society where embonpoint was an accepted standard of beauty. She was a victim of the undisguised ridicule of the Turkish ladies of her acquaintance, who were almost as forcibly fattened as pullets crammed for the table. She also told Charlemont that at the houses where she visited she was questioned with great curiosity about the freedom indulged to women in European countries. Far from being envious of Christian liberty, the ladies exclaimed with one accord against such unnatural licence and expressed horror, even disgust, at what seemed innocent enough to her.[5]

Mr Burton seems to have been less cheerful. Young gentlemen with too much curiosity were in his experience a potential source of trouble. Either a shrewd assessor of character or naturally cautious, he started off by informing Charlemont and Burton there was not a brothel in the whole of Cairo, and any intercourse between Franks, other than husband and wife, whatever the denomination, was forbidden by law, and the penalty an exorbitant fine. In the case of a Turkish woman being found with a Christian, death by drowning was her punishment, and the man likely to be beheaded. Charlemont was most indignant. These barbarians seemed to think they alone had right to the joys of love.

As a cautionary tale Barton cited the instance of his own nephew young Lethieullier, who had not long before on a visit to Cairo been misfortunate enough to 'inflame the passion of a Turkish lady'. One evening Lethieullier was lingering in a shop when the lady entered and shut the door. She was being followed and the young man had but a minute to escape by the back door. The woman was seized and, Mr Barton feared, put to death as she had not been heard of since. Information being lodged against Lethieullier that he was the object of the lady's unlawful desires, a strict search had been made for him, although they were but a minute alone together. Fortunately he had succeeded in hiding until the matter had been accommodated by his uncle, but at the cost of fifteen hundred sequins.[6]

Dalton also had his warnings of the aversion of the inhabitants to being depicted. This he discovered applied also to their animals when he went to make a sketch of a camel in the courtyard of the Consulate. The least accident to the camel would be imputed to a spell cast by the Christian artists.

Charlemont soon perceived that, even disguised in Greek dress to accommodate themselves to the superstition and unfriendliness of the people, they owed their freedom from insult entirely to the presence of the janissary, who went with them everywhere.

The strange dances of the Dervishes were but weak performances compared with those of the Santons here. These holy men, some of them truly mad, others counterfeiting madness, the attribute of saint and prophet, were a common spectacle of the streets. There was one whose claim to holiness rested literally on the hardness of his head, which was bald and uncovered, though otherwise he was clothed normally as a Turk. His performance was to approach a stone pillar, retire back a little and then, like a ram, run tilt against it with such impetuosity and force that must have fractured any reasonable skull. When they expected to see his brains dashed out from the violence and report of the blow, they perceived him 'perfectly unhurt and unconcerned'.[7]

Another ran stark naked in the streets. This struck Charlemont as incomprehensible in a country where the conduct of women was so strictly supervised. Yet they followed him in droves, believing it in his power to cure infertility. Such was the force of custom and superstition over every other consideration that 'happy was she who could contrive to kiss that part of him, which was likeliest, if properly applied, to perfect her cure.'[8]

In the evenings at the Consulate these strange and 'beastly' things were much discussed. A French physician, who supped often with the Bartons, recounted some of his experiences. Sometimes sent for to treat Turkish women, his patients were so muffled up as to be completely concealed from his view. Pulses he might feel only through the thickest of pieces of muslin. Generally such cases were venereal disease (that 'bane of love' was Charlemont's remark), in which the wives had been infected by their husbands. Before giving the physician any account of their symptoms, 'these innocent creatures' invariably prefaced their recital by declaring they 'got the disorder by a fright'.[9]

A discussion about Turkish disregard of the principle of quarantine in cases of infectious or contagious diseases recalled to Mr Barton an unnerving incident. One day, sitting upon a bench in front of his house, he was accosted by a Turk of his acquaintance whom he had not seen for months. The Turk sat down beside him and taking his hand, told him, with a melancholy countenance, he was the unhappiest of men. The plague was in his family. Two of his sons had died and the previous night he had lost his favourite wife. The consul edged off as fast as he could, endeavouring 'to put a speedy end to this dangerous conversation', but the poor Turk, thinking no harm, was not easily put off from persecuting him with his family complaints. Mr Barton regarded it as his extraordinary good fortune that no mischief ensued![10]

But what of the Egyptians themselves? In answer to Charlemont's plea to be allowed to talk with a sensible Egyptian, Mr Barton recommended one Hadgie Mahomet, a rich merchant of Cairo, who was 'esteemed a man of superior sanctity' for having made for many years the pilgrimage to Mecca annually. Charlemont prepared some notes on the Koran as a basis of discussion, and as Hadgie Mahomet was about to depart once again on the journey, which it transpired brought him gain in this world, Charlemont made a point of seeing him as often as was convenient during the few remaining days. The Egyptian emerged as one who very successfully reconciled service to God and to Mammon. He combined the annual course of devotion, which brought him esteem and respect, with a trading journey, and bought at the great fair at Mecca commodities to be sold on his return at considerable profit. Charlemont could not resist asking how he reconciled this *modus operandi* with his conscience. The merchant was blithely untroubled by any doubt; having made the first journey for devotional reasons only, he felt himself entitled thereafter to put his pilgrimage to profit. Charlemont privately considered him superstitious and bigoted and the information obtained from him scanty and uncertain; but he found him civil enough and the whole party were invited by the merchant to dine with him.[11]

Before the departure of the Grand Caravan, there was the customary procession through the streets to parade the coverings and embroideries to be sent in devout tribute to Mecca and Medina. This could only be watched through latticed windows from a house on the procession route and, at no small expense, Charlemont hired a secret viewing place in a principal street. Dalton was advised of the danger of being discovered with a sketch-book and had to content himself with meagre notes, perhaps to be worked up at his lodging afterwards. Mahomet and another janissary from the Consulate stood guard in the room. There was a long wait, but Charlemont, happening to glance towards another latticed window, flattered himself he had in that instant caught a glimpse of a Turkish lady looking out. Though he saw her but imperfectly, she appeared to him very handsome. When at last the procession came in sight, it was something of an anti-climax, merely twenty men bearing upon their shoulders embroidery worked with Koranic inscriptions and some asses carrying dark-coloured cloth laid upon their backs.

On the other hand nothing could be more worthy of a traveller's curiosity than the Grand Procession with the Emir Hadge, or Prince of the Pilgrims, sumptuously arrayed and mounted upon a beautiful Arabian with a thousand attendants and three thousand camels in his train and with an escort of troops to guard the Caravan on its journey.

Charlemont took 'much satisfaction' in the spectacle; the number and beauty of the horses with splendid trappings; the seemingly endless procession of camels carrying water and provisions, some with aged or infirm pilgrims in wicker chairs on top of the store hampers on their backs; the Emir Hadge's pages with their bows and arrows and the military escort, including the Horse Guards mounted on white Arabians and carrying long ceremonial lances. Above all in splendour was the Holy Camel, an animal forever freed from labour for having this once carried the sacred pavilion. Multi-coloured plumes crowned its head. The pavilion embroidered in gold upon green with Koranic texts, was mounted with gold vase-shaped finials. As it passed, handkerchiefs were thrown from the balconies, which on touching the tent became holy relics; and Charlemont noted that the percentage reaching the target was much higher than he would have expected.

In the wake of the procession came crowds of Santons, who brought to the scene an air of savagery. Some were naked. Others wore various and fantastic garb. The most numerous had monstrous serpents entwined about their bodies so that they were virtually clothed in snakes. That the venom of these dangerous animals had been extracted, as he knew, hardly lessened Charlemont's horror of their clinging presence. But when the counterfeit madmen, as he believed them, mingled with the crowd, none drew back or showed any fear.[12]

After the departure of the Caravan, Charlemont and his party set out for Saqqara. We learn from Dalton of their slow passage up the Nile, their boat getting stuck in the mud and the travellers being transported to land on the backs of porters. The incident necessitated a stay over night at the house of Sheik Solimen el Habiri.

Charlemont makes no mention of this episode or of the entertainment prepared in honour of a Christian nobleman and his retinue, but Dalton tells us something of the occasion. The room they found themselves in was surprisingly plain. Apart from a lantern of Moorish design hanging from the ceiling there was no furniture. They sat down in a row, cross-legged, on the floor opposite their host. Between them a simple board was set down, with no eating utensils nor any ornament, and with a ridge of small loaves around its edge, and yet the supper that followed was more than plenteous. Eight servants waited upon them and served thirty-eight different dishes.[13]

In the morning a breakfast of coffee and pancakes was brought to them before they set out again, this time in a boat provided by the Sheik's brother.

The river traffic presented a pageant of curious sights. Drifting down in rafts of small tree-boughs covered with palm leaves, were scantily-clad Ethiopians bringing stores to sell in Cairo. They were very poor and those that survived the journey would try to work their passage back by boat. Close to the city, where there was less danger from crocodiles, they saw a gardener swimming to market, drawing a load of melons and vegetables behind him.

Visits to the pyramids are not described by Charlemont. At Saqqara, according to Dalton, led by 'villainous wretches' calling themselves guides, they searched the mummy-pits and found only bones and skulls and nothing could be more disagreeable than the perpetual cries of the grinning savages as they led them from chamber to chamber creeping along the dismal passages. They had been told they might find feathers in the catacombs of the Ibis, but all they found was evidence of recent disturbance.

A more cheerful scene was a performance by some dancing girls, belly-dancers scantily clothed with large rings in their noses and ears. Dalton's sketch, drawn from memory, showed a circle of spectators, Arabs with muffled women and Mahomet smoking a pipe with a dispassionate air.[14]

From Saqqara they sailed up the Nile to Gizeh where they lodged at the house of a Mrs Vernon, noted by Dalton for its delightful situation. From here at four o'clock in the morning they set out for the pyramids, arriving only 'with difficulty' at eleven o'clock. From then until sunset they applied themselves to as thorough a survey as they could manage in the limited time. Dalton's weak drawings convey something of the amazement of their Lilliputian figures gazing at these wonders of the ancient world.

Following the scramble over the fallen masonry at the entrance of the Great Pyramid and the crawl downwards through the narrow shaft, Dalton recorded, by the light of one flare held high, their ascent of the Sloping Gallery and this drawing conveys, with its primitive perspective, the eeriness of the climb to the inner chambers, where, in another drawing, the apprehension of the party is suggested by the pistols they hold. But dutifully they measured the inner chambers. It was midnight before they were back safely at Mrs Vernon's house.

Mahomet's presence at moments like these and throughout the entire sojourn in Egypt, must have been a comfort to Dalton; not quick to praise and having no vested interest in feats of courage (and indeed there are innuendos of discontent with some of the hardships and discomforts), he spoke well of Mahomet, 'a most faithful janissary'. Charlemont too, to whom Mahomet attached himself with slavish devotion, questioned whether there was ever a more faithful and affectionate creature.

At first Charlemont had found Mahomet's broken English confusing and sometimes incomprehensible, as for instance his favourite phrase 'no force', which turned out to mean 'willingly' or 'without compulsion' and 'thinking it no hardship'. It amused him to hear Mahomet rattle on about his wife; between the couple Charlemont could detect no great refinement of love, but a good deal of practical benefit. 'My last wife no good wife. She not wash my shirt. She not make my broth. I sell her no force. Buy another. This wife very good wife. She wash my shirt well. She make my broth good. Very good wife.'

But when Charlemont asked to see this paragon, promising not to speak to her and if necessary to remain hidden, Mahomet was adamant. 'Ah, Master. Me fight for you. Me die for you. No force. But my wife no show. No good Turkman show his wife.'[15]

NOTES

1. Boswell, May 13th 1778.
2. H. Grattan, *Life and Times of Henry Grattan* by his son, London 1839, Vol. 2, p. 109-12. Dalton, but not Charlemont refers to Pococke as the authority on Pompey's Pillar.
3. Ibid, 12.R.6, p. 21.
4. Ibid, 12.R.5, p. 101.
5. Stanford & Finopoulos, pp. 203-4.
6. Ibid, p. 200.
7. Ibid, p. 228.
8. Ibid.
9. Ibid, pp. 198-9.
10. RIA, 12.R.5, n. to p. 107.
11. Ibid, p. 110.
12. Stanford & Finopoulos, p. 229.
13. R. Dalton, *Musaeum Graecum et Aegyptiacum*, London 1752, Pl. XVIII.
14. Ibid, p1. XII.
15. Stanford & Finopoulos, p. 198.

7

OFF COURSE: HALICARNASSUS

On 22 October they sailed from Alexandria, 'intending for Cyprus' and Rhodes in their passage to Athens. They came within sight of 'this isle of Venus', but contrary winds prevented their landing. The disappointment was attributed by Charlemont to the anger of the Paphian Goddess that 'during our abode in the inhospitable and ungallant regions of the Nile, few or no sacrifices had been by us offer'd to her divinity' and she had 'forbad our entrance into her sacred isle, and by her well known interest with Aeolus, and with her uncle Neptune, frustrated our anxious expectations'. This to our modern ears sounds a very indirect way of referring to a strong easterly gale and reminding us of Egypt's stringent sex laws![1]

The winds continued, alternating with calm and it was not until 30 October that they made harbour at Rhodes. Here painstakingly, they measured the distances and angles between the two rocks with their square towers erected by the Knights*. Even allowing the Colossus a height of 120 feet, they could not credit a straddle of 200 feet.

The town was smaller than anticipated. The principal street was still named the Street of the Knights, but was nearly uninhabited. The armorial bearings remained intact upon their different colleges or auberges and they thought those of England, like the others, 'not unhandsome, considering the early age in which they were erected'. St John's Church, the ancient cathedral, was now the principal mosque and not without 'a degree of magnificence'.[2]

The Palace of the Knights was, comparatively, a ruin, but with some apartments in tolerable repair. In one of these was confined a brother of Tahmasp II, Emperor of Persia; recalling that other princely detainee at Chios, Charlemont concluded this was Ottoman poli-

* Hospitallers of St John of Jerusalem, Rhodes 1310-1528 when they were expelled by the Turks and moved to Malta.

cy, but feared that in this case, the Turks and Persians being natural enemies, the prisoner was not well treated.

Over the ruined Church of the Virgin they identified the famous inscription of the Grand Master Pierre d'Aubusson, commemorating his victory over the Turks, and they made a tour of his fortifications. There were also excursions to other parts of the island and they visited the ruins of ancient Lindos.

Unfavourable winds made their stay rather longer than intended and this gave them time to contract 'some degree of intimacy' with the Archbishop of Rhodes, a very great dignitary of the Greek church, with whom they exchanged visits. They were also honoured with a visit on board from the Mazulheim or Deputy Governor, which was preceded as usual with a very acceptable present of sheep, wine and fruit, which had to be reciprocated 'with usury'.

Rhodes being the most Turkish of the islands, Greeks were not permitted to live within the town walls. Their houses, neat and well-built, were delightfully situated amidst groves of orange, lemon and pomegranate, the pomegranates of an amazing size. It was now November, yet everything here was fresh and verdant.[3]

However, for its house, its garden pavilions or 'Chiosks' and plantations, the Pasha's villa made the most favourable impression, 'being by far in the best Turkish taste of any we have yet seen. The taste indeed is rather formal, and somewhat in our old style of gardening; but perfection in any style is beautiful, and the novelty and extreme luxuriancy of the plantations far more than compensate for any deficiency in their arrangement.'[4]

This comment on Turkish taste made no claim to be a direct quote from his journal and therefore has to be taken as a considered opinion; perhaps rather more so than his enthusiastic description of the Grand Vizir's apartments in Constantinople, his only other reference to Turkish taste in his *Essays*. It may therefore have significance in the future improvements at Marino, the villa outside Dublin which he created on his return home. His villa, like Hadrian's, was to be an evocation of all his travels and not, as his contemporaries and later commentators would have us believe, a backward glance to the years in Italy and with only a passing reference to the voyage.

L'Aimable Vainqueur set sail for Athens, 'the final object' of the voyage on 7 November. Tacking all day between Rhodes and the mountainous coast of Caria, Charlemont noted, in a direct quotation from the journal, 'The tops of the mountains, which are extremely high, are covered with snow, and have a most wintry aspect forming a perfect contrast to the torrid plains of Egypt, the burning sands of the desert, and those scorching heats which fourteen short days have suddenly changed into winter.'[5]

The following day they were becalmed, but on the third day a breeze sprang up and, hugging the Carian coast, they sailed for Cos. They were about three miles short of the point of the promontory when they spotted, on the mountain side, considerable ruins, seemingly the remains of a great city. The situation agreeing with Cnidos and the wind being unfavourable to their intended course, they lowered a boat and rowed towards the shore. From the ship they had not seen any harbour but closer in they found the port, formed by a peninsula joined to the mainland by a very narrow isthmus.

On the side of the hill above the harbour 'a most noble theatre all in white marble' commanded the extensive and beautiful prospect. Going to work with rods and rules they recorded the measurements of a semi-circular amphitheatre of thirty-six seats or steps with entrances at the extremities of the curves and a dividing landing, used, as they supposed, to facilitate the audience's movements or as a demarcation between the ranks of the citizens. The seats were hollowed-in which made for more comfortable sitting, a feature that struck them as singular as they had not seen it in other ancient theatres.

Higher up the hill they came upon the remains of a magnificent temple of the Corinthian order with very finely wrought capitals and cornices and 'a pediment of excellent workmanship and exquisite taste, though somewhat impaired by time, clearly evinced that it had been built in the best age, and in the purest style of architecture'. Because of the order Charlemont reasoned this was perhaps the third and most modern of the three temples reckoned by Pausanias to have been dedicated to the Cnidian Venus and which Praxiteles had enriched with the most famous statue of the goddess. This seemed to be borne out by there being several other temples in a ruinous state, apparently of greater antiquity and pre-dating the establishment of proper orders.[6]

Still farther up the hill were great ruins, which seemed to be the remains of 'stately palaces'. Many terraces still survived supported by walls of white marble, strongly built and of excellent masonry. Door cases of simple but beautiful architecture remained standing and Doric columns, although many of them fallen, were still entire. They were puzzled by the number of subterraneous passages, the use of which it was not easy to explain.[7]

Finally, their ascent brought them to the walls of the city where one square tower still stood. Above them at the summit more ruins were visible, probably the remains of the citadel, inaccessible and strong against attack.

Descending to the harbour, they found more evidence of former grandeur: the immense thickness of the walls and the gate leading to the sea, still more or less intact, and its foundations cut into the solid rock; great walls and a round tower of a second port and town constructed of white marble, which confirmed this was the double city of Cnidos, described by Pausanias and Strabo. That night they returned to the ship, blessing the contrary winds that had brought them to a site which had afforded them 'the highest delight both as antiquarians and lovers of arts'.[9]

The next morning, Monday, 10 November, there being no wind for Athens, the decision was made to put into Cos. Here they found little worth a traveller's notice except the great and beautiful plantanus tree in the middle of the market place of the small and ill-built capital town. Stone pillars supported the extremities of the tree, which spread over fifty yards. Late as it was in the season, here in its native clime, the foliage was only tinged with autumnal hue. In northern regions, Charlemont remembered it as being one of the first to shed its leaves, and he recalled the many references to the tree's properties by ancient poets and naturalists and that the Persians credited it, by the number that grew about Isfahan, with saving the city from plague.[10]

Nothing else of singular interest presenting itself, they enquired of the inhabitants for marble remains thereabouts and were directed to Bodroumi (Bodrum) on the mainland where, they were told, were a great quantity of ruins. Immediately it occurred to them it could be the great and ancient city of Halicarnassus and they returned to the ship in a mood of high expectation.

Putting in to the little port of Patera on the evening of 10 November, they despatched their dragoman to the Governor at Bodrum to present their firman and then went ashore to ramble about the countryside. They came across some fishermen and bought from them *tapodi* which Charlemont took to be the *polypus* described by Lucian in the fourth of his *Marine Dialogues*. Boiled, it became firm and made a 'tolerably' good supper and they finished the evening in drinking the King's health, it being His Majesty's birthday.[11]

Their servant did not return until the next morning, which slightly alarmed them; but he arrived with horses and a favourable reply from the Musselim.

They set out at about 8 o'clock and, passing through a small, ill-built town, Pietromi, they came in three hours within sight of Bodrum, which, with its castle built upon a promontory, presented a most pleasing sight. About a mile out they were met by servants of the Aga with fresh horses for them, a polite attention which Charlemont found most gratifying, and were escorted into the town. They were received most politely by the Musselim, who immediately granted their request to enter and inspect the castle and assured them they were at liberty to make drawings of any antiquities they should find there.

But on quitting his apartment they were accosted by the Kadi, or chief officer of Justice, who with hardly any ceremony, forced them into his chamber and with a stern countenance demanded how they dare presume to enter the Castle without first obtaining his permission. Their protestations of having sent their firman to the Musselim and obtained his leave, were ill-received; the Musselim, he remarked, was an old man and easily imposed upon. The Kadi's insistence that he saw their firman presented a serious difficulty. It had been left on board following the dragoman's return. There was nothing for it but to send a messenger.[12]

While they waited for his return, they explored the environs of the town. A quarter of an hour's walk brought them, on the rise of a hill overlooking the sea, to the magnificent remains of a noble theatre. Again, as at Cnidus, the marble seats were hollowed out. Measurements were taken and recorded, a front of 300 feet, 64 feet the depth of the arena and the height of the whole 115 feet with 36 steps or seats. What particularly struck Charlement was, 'the walls of this structure are singularly built with great blocks of marble, not all of equal size, nor laid in level lines, the upper ashlar being for the most part dovetailed or let into the lower, a manner of building which, though it may be deemed deficient in point of beauty, adds, as I should conceive, greatly to the strength of the edifice, and was probably for this cause preferred'.[13] Dalton made a drawing of this on the spot.

The view, as from almost all ancient theatres, was extensive and beautiful, overlooking the semi-circular harbour 'bounded by hills romantic in their shape and beautiful from their verdure'; the castle on its lofty peninsula and the town, which though not large or well-built, had its share in the prospect by adding 'the idea of population to this romantic scene'.

Above the theatre the hill was cut into several 'grots or caves', their use not apparent to the travellers, except perhaps as places of burial.

In a field below they found an altar, large and enriched with figures in *basso relievo* in the finest taste, of exquisite workmanship and which Charlemont thought belonged to the best age for sculpture. Not far away were the remains of some very ancient building of which a part of a Doric portico still stood, and here too they found inscriptions, which they copied.

Returning to the village, they found their messenger had arrived back with their firman which had been shown to the Kadi and a bargain struck for a permit to view the castle. This they immediately ratified and attempted once more the seemingly impregnable citadel. For a further fee to the porter the gates were at length thrown open.

They recognized from the crosses and coats of arms over the gates and the planning and construction that this was a former stronghold of the Knights of Rhodes, and might have been disappointed had not their eyes been at once attracted to several *basso relievos* set in the inner walls. In both taste and execution they were the finest they had ever beheld and their imagination prompted them to suppose they were a part of the renowned Mausoleum, which had ennobled the city of Halicarnassus and was ranked among the seven Wonders of the World.

This 'pleasing supposition was still farther fortified by a more attentive investigation of their astonishing beauty'.[14] The subject was a battle with the Amazons. They immediately set about making drawings, but hardly had their work begun when all their delight was shattered, by the adjutant of the Kadi telling them time was up and fairly turning them out and shutting the gates against them.

'Provoked at this disappointment' and tantalized by a bare glance of these masterpieces of art, they applied again to the friendly Musselim. Their desire was to investigate fully these 'beauties' and by copying them exactly make them in some sort their own. The good old man pronounced the Kadi a rogue and the adjutant an impertinent fellow, but more practically suggested leaving their measuring rods, the cause of the alarm, behind and entering the fortifications one by one. If they would stay over night, he would send his secretary in the morning to sit by Dalton until he had completed his work. 'This discourse he concluded by a gentle hint that a little coffee would not be disagreeable to him.'[15]

The next problem was a shortage of beds in the village. It was decided that Charlemont and Burton being 'less delicate in point of accommodation' should remain with Dalton, and Murphy and Scott return to the ship.

That evening they spent rambling about the environs and finding extensive substructures, great walls, pieces of columns and cornices and other indications of ancient magnificence. Charlemont had by then little doubt from what they had seen, that they had discovered the site of the lost city of Halicarnassus, described by the ancients but unknown to modern travellers.

In the morning with the Musselim's secretary for watchdog, Dalton returned to the Castle and Charlemont, infected with thoughts of the magnitude of their discovery, wandered about the hills tracing the circuit of the ancient walls built with very large blocks of stone and constructed by the same method already observed in their investigation of the theatre.

The little town itself was a wretched place and the inhabitants, Turks and Greeks, very poor, but Charlemont had noticed how good the fruit was, and for the first time since they left Constantinople he had tasted well-flavoured apples. He was told that beyond the hills were fertile valleys and upon their cultivation the people depended for a living. There was no wine and the travellers were obliged to drink water until the captain of a French ship in the harbour sent them a little bad wine, which in these circumstances was acceptable. Even then Charlemont's British distrust of the French brought forth the comment, 'The French send a few ships hither – indeed where do they not send them? – to be laden with timber and pitch'.[16]

Bodrum was the scene of yet another major discovery of which Charlemont, as an amateur, disdained all public recognition, although as with the discovery of the friezes from the Mausoleum, he was fully aware of the importance of his finding. The following from the *Essays* is his account of his copying an inscription on a stone in Bodrum.

'Having observed a very long inscription upon a stone, which formed the upright of the door belonging to a small house in the village, I set myself down to copy it, but was presently interrupted by a cobbler, the owner of the hut, who told me peremptorily that I must not sit there, for that his harem was near that door. I could not help smiling at the *cobbler's harem*, but the matter was of a nature too serious to admit of joking, and I found myself obliged, after much altercation, to pay a sequin in order to induce the jealous Turk to evacuate his house, which was accordingly done, the wife being brought out muffled and veiled from head to foot, and deposited in the harem of one of the cobbler's friends and neighbours.'[17]

We know from his essay that Charlemont regarded the inscription as a very curious one indeed, the characters excellent, though in some parts defective, and the language very obscure, 'yet still I hope to be able to make out its meaning, so far as to render it one of the principal curiosities we have met with in our voyage'. This hope Charlemont was able to realise and he later made a translation in Latin of the inscription, which he had from the first recognized as the recording of an ancient law of Halicarnassus.

Nearly a hundred years later, in 1846, the friezes were removed from the Castle by Charles Thomas Newton, who claimed their discovery and that of the inscription as his own. The friezes and the stone were brought back to England and are now in the British Museum. Newton, as keeper of Greek and Roman antiquities, published the inscription in *Essays on Art and Archaeology*, 1880. 'This inscription, which I found built into a house at Bodrum ... contains a law, the exactment of which must have been the result of some kind of political convention between Lygdamis (a tyrant exiled about B.C. 455) and the people of Halikarnassus on the other. The object of this law is to secure certain persons in the possession of lands and houses by assigning a term after which their titles could not be disturbed.'

But between 1877 and 1893, Gustav Hirschfeld, working on *The Collection of Ancient Greek Inscriptions in the British Museum*, gave Charlemont the credit. Hirschfeld had access at that time to what he called Charlemont's MS. diary, which could have been either the missing journal or the missing inscription book kept by Charlemont or merely the relevant page from either. Charlemont's original copy was in lead pencil; it became somewhat obscured by time and rubbing, as he notes in his *Essays* and he made two more. We know from Hirschfeld's facsimile copy of the transcription that it was the original and that it was used in the restoration of the stone, which by the time of Newton's rediscovery had been cut into two pieces to form the jambs of a window and the text defaced.[18]

What is so particularly intriguing about this is that Hirschfeld quotes from the journal or inscription book essay with Charlemont's first spontaneous reactions. For 'much altercation' we have 'after a good deal of difficulty and scolding, at length by force of paying I got leave to set at a door to take a long ins[cription] in very old and as yet unintelligible Greek ...'[19]

Charlemont could have chosen, had he wished, to publish his remarkable find. Richard Chandler, who was sent by the Society of Dilettanti with Nicholas Revett and William Pars to explore the antiquities of Ionia, with Charlemont on the committee organizing the expedition, wrote twice to Charlemont for a copy of his transcription for his *Inscriptiones Antiquae pleraeque nondum editae* of 1774 and received no reply.[20]

NOTES

1. Stanford & Finopoulos, p. 75.
2. Ibid, p. 77.
3. Ibid, p. 80.
4. Ibid.
5. Ibid, p. 83.
6. Ibid, pp. 82-6.
7. Ibid, p. 85.
8. Ibid.
9. Ibid, p. 86.
10. RIA, 12.R.6, p. 79.
11. Stanford & Finopoulos, p. 89.
12. Ibid, p. 90.
13. Ibid, p. 92.
14. Ibid, p. 93.
15. Ibid.
16. Ibid, p. 97.
17. Ibid, p. 98.
18. G. Hirschfeld, *The Collection of Ancient Greek Inscriptions in the British Museum*, 1916, pp. 49-54. I remain indebted to the late Professor Stanford, who first drew my attention to Hirschfeld's report.
19. Ibid.
20. HMC Rept. 12, App. pt X, p. 317.

8

ATHENS AT LAST

Charlemont reached Athens a year ahead of James Stuart and Nicholas Revett, which chronologically made his first view of the Acropolis an historic event; but as a link in the chain leading up to the Greek Revival and the Neo-Classical movement, its importance is difficult to assess. Having come so far to see the famous edifices and so painstakingly to measure them, he chose on his return to Ireland to build in the Roman-Doric style and appointed, in William Chambers, an architect whose dislike of the *Gusto Graeco* was proverbial.

Caught up as Charlemont must have been in the Graeco-Roman controversy during his years in Rome, it is remarkable that he so successfully evaded the issue in his *Essay on Athens*, that we are left without a hint of his considered opinion. The *Essay*, like the others, was of course written in retrospect, but in this case he was writing after he had made his decision to build, and while the actual building of his Roman-Doric masterpiece, the Casino of Marino, was in progress. His claim that so much had been written about the antiquities of Athens that it would be superfluous to dwell upon them, reads like an ill-disguised feint. More especially since he does mention the monuments, but mostly in such rhetorical terms that nothing is revealed, as for instance 'the awful antiquity of the Temple of Theseus, the massive magnificence and towering majesty of the Parthenon and the other wonders of the Acropolis, the ornamented purity, and the graceful elegance of the Fane of Erectheus, the rich and elegant singularity of the Choragic Monument ...'[1]

Back in Rome Charlemont could not have avoided the close questioning of those who had not themselves seen the monuments and were the most concerned, Abbé Winckelmann[2] on the side of Greek superiority and Piranesi, the champion of Rome. There is no account of any of the discussions which must have taken place. However Dalton told Piranesi 'the caryatides were the work of a mediocre mason' and that 'some of the remains of the reliefs on the tympanum of the Temple of Minerva [the Parthenon] were beautiful, but that if everything else described by Le Roy were to vanish, lovers of the fine arts would suffer no loss at all'.[3] There is no reason to suppose this reflected Charlemont's opinion, any more than Dalton's; Dalton saw in Stuart and Revett's expedition to Athens, a threat to the success of his own intended publication of Charlemont's voyage.

We know from the engravings after Dalton's drawings that the Parthenon and the Erechtheum were the subject of at least nine and four drawings respectively, made on the spot, and that there were besides sketches done of the Tower of the Winds and the Choragic monument of Lysicrates, both of which are given prominence in Stuart and Revett's *Athens*. Presumably the choice of Dalton's subjects was under direction from Charlemont and there is some evidence, which will be considered later, that Charlemont thought of the Choragic monument for Marino.

Much of the *Essay* is taken up with reflections on past glories. Charlemont tells us 'I find in my note book the following fantastical flight on my first contemplating the ruins of Athens, which, with the assistance of a little superstition, might be exalted into *something prophetic*, and therefore only I have copied it: "Is this the renowned Athens? How melancholy would be the reflection should we suppose, what certainly must come to pass, that in a few ages hence, London, the Carthage, the Memphis, the Athens of the present world, shall be reduced to a state like this, and travellers shall come, *perhaps from America*, to view its ruins."'[4]

In eight closely written pages he traces 'the lamentable history of Athens since the fatal period of its downfall', finding Hadrian of all the emperors its greatest friend and in contrast the Venetian occupation 'a complication of Gothicism and cruelty' in having presumed to profane by one single Gothic shell the Acropolis ... 'that favoured seat of Minerva, that Nursery of the Arts, that Treasury of the Muses'. He concludes: 'Such is the precarious and transitory tenure of sublunary grandeur! Cities, kingdoms, empires ... finally perish and fall to decay'.[5]

Panegyrics, so much a feature of this particular *Essay*, fall uneasily on modern ears, and we had rather hear the blunt acclamation of a Richard Wilson standing before the falls of Terni and crying out 'Well done, water, by God' than a eulogy which might be designed to cast a veil over a feeling of inadequate response.

However, one small but interesting point arises from these melancholy reflections on the past glories of Greece, when in the *Essay*

Charlemont relates them to a decline of the British Empire from the year of William Pitt the elder's enforced resignation in 1761. 'What was the British Empire under the administration of William Pitt? Alas, what is it now? Dying – dying – dying ... Britain! the Greece, the Italy of latter Times! The illustrious daughter of the Ocean – the Queen of Commerce! The Patroness of Science – the Mother of Philosophy! Invincible in war – unrivalled in the arts of peace! The Arbitress of Europe! ... She is fallen!' The same sentiments we shall find summarised in the dedicatory plaque purported to have been laid with the foundation stone of the Casino at Marino.[6]

Charlemont's final decision for Rome as evinced in the Roman-Doric style of the Casino, although with some backward glances towards Greece, came after nearly five years spent in Italy; his sojourn in Athens lasted only a week or two. To come down on the side of Greece might have seemed to him a betrayal of the chief source of his connoisseurship and the development of his taste.

On the morning of 23 November 1749, the wind failing after a hazardous and very stormy passage which had forced them to seek shelter at Syros and again at Cythnos, in a dead calm they entered the Piraeus on tow. 'Hymettus, and Pentelicus, and Parnes, appeared in full view' and over a great plain of corn stubble and olive trees 'Anchesmus showed itself, and the Acropolis reared its venerable head, crowned with the lofty Parthenon, whose massive columns, even from this distance were clearly visible by our glasses'.[7]

Having sent their dragoman ahead with their firman, they rowed ashore, rejoicing in setting their feet at last on Attic soil. They spent the evening investigating the remains of the towers, platforms and wharfs of the harbour.

The following morning they set out eagerly to cross the plain, making their way along the sheep-walks. They were particularly struck by 'the pastoral elegance of the shepherds and of their sheep. Each flock was preceded by its *vir gregis* with his horns richly gilded and adorned with ribands; and the shepherds were neatly dressed, each having his crook and pipe'.[8]

Later having committed himself to Rome and an architect who was uncompromisingly Roman, in one of the most endearing of Charlemont's sneaking backward glances, we find him introducing the motif of a ram's head with the unusual gilded horns and the ribbons, in the decoration of the Casino.

The modern city, as they drew nearer through the olive groves, appeared more considerable than they had expected, with perhaps two thousand houses, scattered and most of them with a garden, and, allowing five persons to each house, they reckoned the population at ten thousand.

The Voivode received them with the greatest civility. He placed their firman on the back of his hands, bowed his head to touch it with his forehead and read it with great solemnity. Its order being to protect the bearer from 'every species of insult', the Voivode assured them that, exclusive to his master's sacred command, he would be glad to do them any service that lay in his power. He was as good as his word. Rather more valuable gifts than usual, a chased silver *étui*, some yards of English cloth and a case of pistols, were presented to him and he looked for nothing more throughout their stay and continued to help them as much as he could.[9]

As at Bodrum, their experience with the military governor was less happy. His permission to enter the walls of the Castle to measure and draw, was obtained at the cost of a considerable present of cloth, pistols and coffee. But when they launched themselves onto the Acropolis, with what appeared to the Turks as too great an apparatus of rods, rules and lines, they were fairly turned out and had to enter into fresh negotiations with the Disdar Aga at further cost. The Turks were apt to entertain a notion that engineers had come to make plans of the fortifications or, worse still, with their strange instruments they were conjurors looking for hidden treasure.[10] At last with one ten foot rod and a foot ruler they were allowed in.

Murphy, their chief measurer 'and the most minutely accurate that ever carried rule'[11] found that the intercolumnations of the Parthenon were by no means equidistant, though never more than by two inches and not apparent to the eye. Charlemont thought this served to show 'the inutility of those measurements to a hair's breadth on which Stewart [Stuart] piques himself'.[12]

Charlemont was struck by the amazing exactness and contiguity of the joints. They were so perfectly wrought that he could not pass the edge of a knife between them. Robert Wood, when he came with James Dawkins, was to be similarly impressed and to make an experiment similar to Charlemont's. Taking a jointed stone, a broken-off piece from the temple, he tried to separate it in order to find out whether any kind of cement had been used. Unable to get the stone asunder by any other method, he resorted to a hammer. To his amazement the stone broke beyond the joint, leaving the joint unshaken. The only explanation that occurred to him was that so exact a contiguity produced an attraction and was further strengthened by an exudation from the marble itself.

The experiment strikes us today as an act of vandalism and yet we find Charlemont was not regardless of what we term conservation. Observing that 'this admirable masonry ... was also assisted, particularly in the Minerva, by cramps of copper, with which the ashlars were bound and tied together' he noted 'from the use of these cramps a very disagreeable consequence has ensued, as the superficial stones of the building have in many places been broken in order to get at and purloin the metal. Had it not been for this circumstance the surface of the Parthenon, where not destroyed by the infernal bomb, would probably to this day have remained perfectly entire.'[13]

But even with these ravages, injuries and breaks, 'these wonderful edifices' had an air of newness and freshness that was astonishing and yet, as we know, not unexpected, although it was sixteen hundred years since Plutarch had written that as soon as they were finished they had an air of venerable antiquity and when old the freshness of a modern building with the bloom of perpetual youth and unfading elegance.[14]

Some time was spent tracing the contours of the Themistoclean walls and the ports of Piraeus. In examining the walls surrounding the Munychian port Charlemont made what he believed was a discovery. Finding that for the most part they were composed of previously used stone with all the appearance of great age, it occurred to him Themistocles in fortifying the city would not have neglected its port when the city's strength depended upon her navy. Somehow historical records had neglected to mention this. Making a more thorough search, the party found ancient columns, split or sawn lengthways and forming what seemed to be a part of a dry dock, where ships drawn up from the water could be held erect. Although delighted with this observation, Charlemont had to retract an earlier conclusion that he had identified the three ports of the Piraeus and accept that this was the actual third.

Wandering along the promontory of the Munychia, the English party as usual attracted a following of natives, friendly and curious Athenians, who impeded research, but were, within their limits, informative. They appeared to Charlemont extraordinarily ignorant. However, conscious that his proper business was with mankind, he gave them his full attention.

Drawing his attention to a passing boat, they told him it carried two prostitutes on their way to banishment on the island of Salamis, the punishment it seemed for 'common strumpets'. The incident led to discussion and the Greeks were bitter about injustice imposed upon them by Turkish governors. The women in the boat were prostitutes, but they complained that the most innocent maidens, daughters of wealthy Athenians, were not safe from the same criminal charges. By the most wily and unscrupulous methods and to the odious end, which was to fill the coffers of the Voivoide, the victims were ensnared. A creature of the Voivode was introduced into the household with the vile purpose that, acting on his false information, the Voivode's officers could search the house and seize the girl. In vain she would protest her innocence, but the evidence was too strong; the wretch suborned to bring about her ruin, would confess his own guilt, thereby including hers, and nothing was left to her but to claim inspection in order to prove virginity and all to no avail, since the matrons would be bribed to declare her guilty. To save her from the penalty of being sold as a slave, her father would purchase her pardon by a liberal gift to the magistrates, procuring her release at the cost of his fortune and her good name.[15]

The Athenians, Charlemont thought, were more unfortunate than the rest of the Greeks, in as much that they retained a stronger idea of their ancient splendour and in consequence repined more at their present degradation. When they were told such stories and asked 'in the most pathetic manner whether there were not, in our more powerful and flourishing parts of Europe, some prince or people, who, reflecting on the ancient renown of Athens, and on its present wretched prostration, might be induced to seek by force of arms their deliverance from Turkish bondage,' their pleading brought tears to Charlemont's eyes.[16]

But although he was greatly moved, he heard too their boasts of intrigue at the Porte, whereby they claimed that playing on the avarice and pride of the Kislar Aga, they had it in their power to drive away his Voivodes and even to have them imprisoned. From James Stuart's later account of Voivodes removed during his time at Athens, Charlemont concluded their boasts were not without foundation. He concluded that these, 'by far the most ingenious people of Greece' had degenerated, through their sad dereliction, 'into low cunning and knavery' and were 'generally addicted to the most refined species of cheating, and the countrymen of Aristides are now perhaps the keenest and the most accomplished rogues upon the face of the earth.'[17]

The Athenians, looking to the West for their delivery were politically instinctive, but like Charlemont's flight of fantasy about the ruins of London, there was an element of prophecy. It was, of course, not some prince, but an English peer, who was to ally himself with their cause, and die at Missolonghi.

Despite Greek intrigue at the Porte, the crushing effect of Turkish rule was more evident here than anywhere among the Islands and went deeper than the usual injustices. New churches built by the Athenians were locked up until the people agreed to pay twenty purses for the privilege of using them, and there were but two free schools in a city, which was once 'the seminary of the whole world'. These schools were badly attended and the teachers seemed to Charlemont 'profoundly ignorant'. While allowing for an allegiance to ancient manners, the reserve of the women seemed extraordinary; they seldom appeared in the streets and young girls were never seen at church until after they were married. There was 'a very great and sad difference' between here and the Islands, where conversation with the ladies had been a great part of their 'happiness and entertainment'.

The Latins were few and were left more or less undisturbed by the Turks. Charlemont mentions the one Catholic monastery belonging to the Capuchins, but not that the Lysicrates monument was a part of it and that the monks used it for their library. Perhaps he felt he had already fully expressed his poor opinion of the Capuchins in his account of the island of Syros.

However, in this cultural wilderness Charlemont found a paragon who, we cannot help noticing, was more than a match for our learned young milord. The monastery of St Cyrianee (Kaisariani), of which Father Paeseus was abbot, was not far from the caves on Mount Hymettus from which since ancient times had come the famous honey. The hives, Charlemont was satisfied, lived up to their classical reputation, since he who never before had tasted honey without disgust, could relish it daily. An excursion to the caves led to the good fortune of their becoming acquainted with the Abbot.

Father Paeseus was singular among those Charlemont met in Greece. He was erudite, 'well-skilled in Latin learning and a perfect master of the ancient Greek'. Desiring to render his talents useful to his country, he had converted his monastery into a sort of college, where he educated several Athenian youths 'in the most proper manner'.

In conversation with 'this sage' Charlemont happened to remark upon the veneration in which Homer was held among the learned in all parts of Europe. The effect of the remark was unexpected; Father Paeseus went into raptures. While he expressed no surprise that such a poet should fill with astonishment those who could barely pick out his meaning without being sensible of a thousandth part of his beauties, he denied that anybody other than a native Greek could understand the niceties of his language nor feel Homer and enter into his true spirit.

Charlemont was piqued at not being allowed to understand a poet he had studied so painstakingly and argued that Homer's renown as well as the curiosity and pleasure with which he was read, was surely tolerable proof of foreign perception, but the Abbot would have none of it. He scorned the feelings of a cold scholar labouring through his author in a dead language and with this, he took from his pocket a copy of Homer and opening it at random, read a page or two. The effect was astonishing. 'He seemed in ecstasy – totally enraptured. His eyes rolled, his features were changed and in every particular he appeared like Virgil's Sibyl, full of God.'

Then closing the book and endeavouring to compose himself he said, 'You may judge of the cause by its effects, and if you feel in reading Homer as I do, you may pretend to perceive his beauties like me'.[18]

Whether or not there was some affectation in the Abbot's transports, Charlemont could not determine. They appeared genuine, and taking into account the affinity between ancient and modern Greek and 'a delicacy and sensibility' of temperament which Northern climes could never produce, he concluded the rapture was real and natural.

Once Charlemont had toured the hinterland and observed in the modern Greek so many of the characteristics of his ancient counterparts, he was convinced the affinity went closer than language. The Athenians had the natural gift of their forefathers for oratory, utmost fluency and precision and a grace and manner peculiar to themselves. James Stuart was also to notice a fondness for congregation and dissertation. At Thebes too Charlemont found the moderns lived up to their old reputation. They remained good-natured, honest, undesigning, but heavy and dull and immoderately addicted to drink.

The proposed tour of Corinth, Thebes and Chalchis brought warnings from their Athenian friends. The perils of the road were many, chiefly the danger from robbers, and when the party set out at the end of the first week in December, they were accompanied by a janissary and two Albanian guards and carried with them letters from the Vaivode to magistrates along the route, recommending the travellers to their protection. That the letters were unsolicited and given free, was unusual politeness, and they proved useful too.

The Albanian guards attracted Charlemont's curiosity; their dress was shorter than the Greek and 'upon the side of their head' they wore 'a whimsical kind of small hat, fastened round the hinder part of the head with a strap or riband, wrought with wire, and sometimes plated with brass'. Though hard, it covered so small a part of their head, it hardly seemed useful. Neither man showed the slightest awe of the janissary normally 'feared and honoured like a sort of demi-deity' and treated him as an equal. They were in every respect formed to make good soldiers, well-made, strong and sinewy, light and alert and accounted of 'undaunted bravery'.[19]

One of the striking things about this journey is the evident hardiness of the travellers. It was winter. They rode all day and at night their accommodation was, for the most part, 'as bad as possible'. At Eleusis the only lodging was 'an old, waste, uninhabited castle', where they passed the night lying on the ground shivering with cold. The following night at Megara their shelter was 'a sort of oven', perhaps an old kiln, because there was a chimney, and a fire was lit. Burton laid his bed down on one side and Charlemont, proud that he made no use of bedding, wrapped himself as usual in his cloak, and lay down on the other side. During the night Burton, 'the most chilly of mortals', got up and threw a long piece of green wood on the fire carelessly, not noticing how close the end of the log came to Charlemont's face, until it burnt, spitting scorching sap and caused him to bounce out of his sleep in terror.[20]

At Corinth they were received by the Bey, 'a very great personage', and entertained with the usual ceremony of coffee and perfumes, and they obtained leave not only to visit the Castle, but to travel by an unauthorised route to Thebes. That night they were well lodged and looked after by the British consul, a Greek of a Venetian family.

The beauty of Corinth's situation is well-known and, as Charlemont remarks in his *Essay*, there was perhaps never any city, 'so perfectly placed in point of healthfulness, strength, pleasure, and commercial convenience', but the city was now reduced to villages within the circuit of the ancient walls and some of the villages consisted of only a few houses. But they were well and neatly built, Charlemont noticed, and the space between them beautifully planted with orange, lemon and cypress trees.

All that remained of this proud city were the ruins of a Doric portico, of which there were eleven columns still standing. Today there are only seven, but what is of even more interest is that Charlemont, hitherto indirect in his comments on Greek architecture, is explicit here. 'Nothing can be in a worse style than this portico ... There are eleven columns yet standing, fluted and shaped in the same manner as those of the Parthenon, but much shorter in their proportions, being, exclusive of the capitals, not more than eighteen feet high, by six feet across at the bottom of the shaft, which gives them an altitude of three diameters only, whereas those of the Minerva are somewhat more than six diameters in height. Their capitals are out of measure clumsy and unprofiled, and the whole of their composition and workmanship would induce me to suppose that they were of very high antiquity, and previous to the birth of true taste ... These columns are not of marble, but of a hard free-stone, each of them being made out of one stone. Pillars nearly of this sort are to be seen at Syracuse, and at Paestum in Calabria."[21] Thus Charlemont describes the Temple of Apollo, VII century B.C., and although we know of his visit to Syracuse, there is no evidence of his having seen Paestum. Nevertheless the description, apart from the last comparison, reads as if straight from the missing journal, without the adulterations of the Athenian essay and is therefore a rare example of first response.

Visiting the Castle, the ancient citadel, the Acropolis of Corinth with its Venetian fortifications, Charlemont looked out from this lofty and almost pyramidal rock over the wonderfully extensive and beautifully romantic prospect: the richly cultivated plain of Corinth, the isthmus with its two seas and beyond Cithaeron, Helicon and Parnassus covered with snow; to the east Athens; and to the south the endless mountains of the Peloponnesus. He pondered upon the history of the city and its destruction by the Romans in 146 B.C. and referred to the descriptions of Pausanias.[22]

His imagination fired by thoughts of the fountain of Pirene, sacred to the Muses, and which in all its history had remained unexhausted, even in the driest summer, and had supported the Venetians in the seige by the Turks, Charlemont made the difficult and dangerous descent by candlelight of a steep passage in the rock and copied some almost certainly indecipherable inscriptions upon the rough stones of the wall. However he felt himself amply repaid for his toil by the venerable appearance of the sacred spring, surrounded by ancient walls of excellent masonry and the sight of 'two Doric pilasters supporting a well-constructed pediment'.[23]

From Corinth the travellers made excursions to survey the remains of the Isthmian Wall, the Stadium and to Sicyon. On 8 December they set out on the journey to Thebes, by way of the unauthorized road for which they had a permit from the Bey, back to Megara, which they reached after nine hours' ride. In describing the ride, Charlemont in his *Essay* reverts to the journal, which records their satisfaction at finding marks of the road's antiquity and the giddiness and terror at passing over precipices where the ancient substructure had given way.[24]

On 9 December, mounting before day-break, they rode across the plain of Megara and arrived at the mountain pass of Cundora. It was wild, rocky and steep but the path was good and it was here, notwithstanding the presence of the janissary, that the Albanians fired their muskets and raised a song of triumph, which they followed with a mournful ditty commemorating a bloody action in which a hundred Albanians had ambushed and cut to pieces a thousand Turks, the rearguard of a Turkish army marching through the pass to Morea against the Venetians.[25]

Another mountain pass, higher than the first brought the travellers to the descent into the plains of Boeotia, 'watered by a thousand rivulets, which descend from the mountains, and covered, excepting only where cornfields and vineyards are beautifully interspersed, with innumerable herds of cattle whose size and condition speak the fertility of the soil'.[26]

They crossed the Asopos and in nine and a half hours after leaving Megara, reached Thebes. Numerous ancient marbles, broken columns and capitals were to be seen, but only a part of the walls and two gates, one arched and of considerable size, and the other, smaller but of excellent workmanship, its style resembling the more ancient architecture of Delos. There was no English consul and as usual they went to the house of the French consul, whose dragoman entertained them hospitably in his master's absence. The Thebans had a fund of traditional stories, most of which Charlemont dismissed as historically inaccurate and one of Alexander burning vanquished villagers alive, he thought 'silly'. But they were kindly people, if 'the least sprightly among the Greeks' and very hospitable and rather drunken on wine which Charlemont thought might have been excellent but for the quantity of resin in it.[27]

Quitting Thebes they rode away across the Theban plain, 'fertile, luxuriant, watered by innumerable rivulets, and covered with numerous herds of large and pampered cattle', and after six hours in the saddle arrived at the bridge which crosses the Euripus. Alighting here they spent some minutes gazing with astonishment at the rapidity of the famous current.

Here they were met by the French Consul's servants with 'a train of fine and well-accoutred horses' on which they made a triumphal entry into Chalcis (known to Charlemont as Negripont). The ships in the harbour saluted them as they passed and they were met at the gate of the city by the French Consul, his family and servants 'in their best attire', with the whole factory of French merchants, and escorted to the Consul's house. It was insisted they take up their quarters there.[28]

Their entertainment at the Consulate was 'sumptuous and elegant' and in every respect the Consul endeavoured to do honour to his country in his treatment of his English guests. He accompanied them on all their excursions, as did the principal merchants of the factory; but there were no ruins to see except those remains which marked the site of ancient Eretria and which Charlemont noted as 'inconsiderable'.

He observed that the Turkish fortifications were in poor repair and were daubed with white-wash, which gave them a singularly 'unwarlike' appearance, while the Greeks complained much of oppression. Charlemont seems, with one exception, to have made no contacts with the Turks, who lived within the walls of the city, where none other than a few Jews were also permitted to dwell. The Greeks with a few Franks, most of them French, lived in the better-built and more populous suburb.

When Charlemont returned to spend some hours studying the variations and changes of the currents of the Euripus, a Turkish officer of the bridge fort supplied him with information which did not agree with the observations of the ancients. Watching the gentle motion of the waters begin to increase in rapidity until it began to rush with all the impetuosity of the most rapid mill-race, and continuing thus for the space of two and a half hours until it gradually subsided, became motionless, changed and started up again, Charlemont was not certain that he could depend on the officer's observations, as there were but four changes on that day and the officer claimed that on occasion the change occurred as many times in an hour.[29]

On 13 December the travellers began the journey back to Athens by boat. Carried along rapidly, with their boatman pulling across towards the Boeotian shore, they gained the famous Bay of Aulis, 'the renowned rendez-vous of the Grecian fleet destined to revenge the rape of Helen'. But they saw no ruins, and with the wind and current in their favour, they glided swiftly to Vathy, where the Consul and his friends parted from them with the most polite and friendly regrets. The consular horses and servants were waiting to convey them the rest of the journey.

The politeness of the Consul well nigh cost Charlemont his life. Having insisted on lending them horses, Charlemont was mounted on a beautiful young stallion, which turned out to be vicious and ill-broken . When night came on and it was imperative they kept to the beaten road, the horse suddenly took fright and Charlemont was run away with into the open country until, stopping suddenly at the edge of a steep fall of ground, it plunged and kicked so violently that Charlemont could scarcely sit him and yet feared to alight. His companions searched for him, but one of the foot guides was the first to find him. 'This wise Euboean thought at first to coax the horse by calling him fondly by his name, but finding that fruitless, he took the much more dangerous measure of throwing stones at him', many of which hit Charlemont, who entreated him to desist. At length one of their company rode up, and at no small hazard, put a switch into Charlemont's hand and he was able eventually to bring the horse to reason.[30]

Lingering at some ancient though inconsiderable ruins, which they took to be the remains of Delium, they reached Athens that night and the next morning were visited by their Athenian friends, who congratulated them on having escaped the many perils of the road.

Since Charlemont in his *Essay on Constantinople* made such a point of regretting his youth and his inexperience at the time of his travels, and his 'avocations in search of antiquities, which were then my principal objects', it is perhaps not so surprising that we are told nothing of the circumstances in which he acquired an Attic stele of the mid fourth century B.C., presumably during this Athenian visit. No mention of the stele is found in any of his papers and its existence would not have been known had it not been discovered in the undergrowth in the grounds of Marino near the Gothic Room and at no great distance from the Casino in 1980, more than two hundred and thirty years later.[31]

NOTES

1. Stanford & Finopoulos, p. 108.
2. Winckelmann's acquaintance with Charlemont is confirmed in a letter from him to Baron Stosch. J.J. Winckelmann, Briefe 1952, Vol. 1, p. 311.
3. Jonathan Scott, *Piranesi*, London 1925, pp. 156-7.
4. Stanford & Finopoulos, p. 135.
5. Ibid, p. 134.
6. Ibid, pp. 134-135.
7. Ibid., p. 106.
8. Ibid., p. 119.
9. Ibid., pp. 129-130.
10. Ibid.
11. Ibid., p. 130.
12. Ibid., p. 132. He is referring to James Stuart.
13. Ibid.
14. Ibid., pp. 132-4.
15. Ibid., p. 128.
16. Ibid., p. 128.
17. Ibid., p. 114.
18. Ibid., pp. 122-6.
19. Ibid., pp. 136-7.
20. Ibid., p. 138.
21. Ibid., p. 139.
22. Ibid., p. 140.
23. Ibid.
24. Ibid., pp. 144-5.
25. Ibid., p. 145.
26. Ibid., p. 146.
27. Ibid., p. 147-149.
28. Ibid., pp.150-1.
29. Ibid., p. 155.
30. Ibid., pp. 156-7.
31. C. O'Connor & B.F. Cook, 'A Greek Stele in Dublin', pp. 29-34. *Journal of the Society of Antiquaries of London*, Vol. LXI, 1981.

9

RETURN FROM THE VOYAGE

With three weeks unaccounted for, we next hear of *L'Aimable Vainqueur* on 20 January 1750 in a passage between Rhodes and Malta with the weather dark and threatening and the Captain, unable to navigate accurately in these conditions, ignorant of their position. A great storm blew up and Charlemont, braced in the gangway, watched as night came on and the tempest increased its fury. 'The gloom of the night was unnaturally horrid. The scudding clouds at times divided, affording faint and transient gleams of brassy light ... the waves rose mountain high ... the whole ocean appeared in flames, through which the vessel ploughed her desperate way. Sometimes perched on the giddy brow of the stupendous accumulation, and again plunging precipitate into the flaming abyss'. Unable to support the violent motion, he was preparing to go below when a sudden squall laid the ship down almost on her side and broke three of her five main shrouds. The cannon broke loose together with their loading and the great part of the ballast rushed to the lee-side with a crash, so that it seemed the vessel would burst in pieces, and even after the immediate shock was over, the consequences were not less terrible. The ship weighed down was unable to right herself and lay 'gunwale under water, at the mercy of the billows'.[1]

The captain, calling for a volunteer to make fast the buoy rope to the main-head to serve as a false shroud and possibly preserve the mast, was interrupted by one Tom Sillers, who taking the plug of tobacco from his cheek cried out, 'By G..., master, if we must die, tis better to die doing something,' and this truly brave British sailor (Charlemont would never forget his name) was soon aloft and the danger at least postponed.

Charlemont retired to the cabin to wait with his party in horrid uncertainty, but not without hope, when the captain entered and told them that the ship might possibly ride it out, but they should prepare for the worst. Breaking the dead silence that followed, Frank Burton suddenly burst out with an oath and exclaimed, 'Well, this is fine indeed! Here have I been pampering this great body of mine, for more than twenty years, and all to be a prey to some cursed shark, and be damned to him!'

So odd and unexpected a remark at such a profoundly serious moment was irresistible and they burst out laughing. Their merriment was of short duration; the ship's carpenter, a favourite with the party, entered the cabin, evidently with the intention of reassuring them that the ship was a tight one, strong and good but added there was 'one *rotten plank*, and that a principal one – let that hold, and we are all safe'.

With their minds running on the soundness of the ship and that one rotten plank, they passed the tedious night, 'shut up in a noisome and agitated dungeon, the gloom of which was made visible by the dim twinkling of a swinging lamp, and which had but too much the semblance of a tomb already prepared' for them. Soaked by sea-water, 'which dashed in through every crevice', bruised in every part of their bodies from being thrown by the violent agitation, they still hoped '... the principle of religion was active' in their souls and they prayed.[2]

The storm abated, but the shattered vessel still lay with her gunwale close to the water's edge and they were still utterly ignorant of their whereabouts and knew not what course to steer. At length, one of the men sent aloft sighted land and the land was their very destination, the end and purpose of their voyage, Malta.

A few hours brought them safely into harbour. They were surrounded by a multitude of boats, laden with fresh fruit and vegetables and they had not eaten for two days. Everything concurred to delight them; past misery was present comfort and all nature smiled on them. When they found they were condemned by the port authorities to a quarantine of forty days, it seemed no hardship, and they chose to stay with the ship to avoid the trouble of moving and for fear of infection in the Lazaretto. Also they felt a sentimental affection for the brave little vessel. The seamen had much to do to put the ship aright and they themselves were busy putting their papers and journals in order. Permission was given for them to stretch their legs daily in a small space of ground from which they could speak with their acquaintances at some distance, separated from them by a double row of railings.[3]

After ten days they began weary of their situation and, following a petition to the Grand Master with sound bills of health, they were granted a shortened confinement. On the twenty-third day they went ashore with much rejoicing and took up residence at the British Consul's house, where they were received with the most hospitality and 'the most cordial affection' among their acquaintance of their previous visit.

Now began such a round of festivity, every day great dinners and in the evening, revelry, dancing and drinking that Charlemont began to fear that their constitutions would not stand up to this Circean riot. In the mornings, for the good of their health, they rode out on horses provided from the Grand Master's own stables.[4]

They had constant access to the Grand Master's villa, La Boschetta, which in this torrid region with its orange groves, its fir trees and cool streams appeared 'like a rich jewel in an Ethiop's Ear'. There were lawns, which covered about a hundred acres; verdure too common in the British Isles to be properly esteemed, but in this climate ravishing; shade from orange trees, which grew to an exceptional height, their golden fruit and their flowers breathing a 'celestial fragrance'.

The Grand Master, Don Emmanuel Pinto de Fonçeca was an old and very respectable Portuguese nobleman. Charlemont's introduction to him was the scene of a curious and long-standing ceremony. All grandees of Spain and peers of France and Britain were required to be presented with their heads covered and consequently Charlemont was wearing a hat when he entered the chamber and was received by the Grand Master likewise. After the first compliments had passed hats were removed and the remainder of the company was then presented, heads bared.[5]

The Grand Master invited the party to dine at his palace and, though etiquette forbade his eating in their company, he joined them after and spent the evening with them. His civility went so far as to re-introduce masked balls in their honour, which had previously been banned due to some 'unlucky riots'.

Nobody could doubt the great respectability of the Grand Master, and Charlemont was impressed by the tender care of the knights for the sick, who administered in rotation to the patients in a most kind and affectionate manner. The hospital was magnificent. Every culinary vessel was made of solid silver. But Charlemont was shocked, if not entirely surprised, to find, considering that such a multitude of gentlemen in the prime and vigour of life were cooped up together on one small island, that the holy knights were thoroughly debauched. 'Obliged by their vows to celibacy, they made no scruple to take, without bounds, illicitly, that which is denied them in a lawful way'.[6]

La Valette with its broad long streets, its large houses of hewn stone and the lanes which intersected the streets with their flights of stone steps, was a beautiful city, but it was one vast brothel. In the principal street, at a signal, every window displayed a cap with all its appendages*. 'Hither flock as to an establish'd Mart for Beauty, the Female Votaries of Venus from every distant region – Armenians, Jewesses, Greeks, Italians, all such as, either from accident or from too great Notoriety have lost their price at home, touching on this happy coast instantly recover their Value and every distress'd Damsel is here certain to find an adventurous Knight, who will bravely redress their Grievances.'[7]

Every woman in the town was a knight's mistress, the respectable women having taken themselves off to live in Medina. Sodomy, too, was rife. Charlemont met one French knight, who not only impudently professed himself for what he was, but 'gloried in his enormity', even attempting to justify it by argument. Mechanics and labourers were fit to toil for the continuation of the species, but men of birth, of sense, of breeding should quit the vulgar paths of pleasure. What, he asked, was to be learned from intercourse with a woman? How to dress or talk nonsense? Whereas in male society instruction of every kind was to be found and friends might mutually improve each other. The Chevalier was not, Charlemont admitted, without genius. He had a taste for poetry but most of his poems were 'too odious' to relate.[8]

While Charlemont was conducting this enquiry into 'a detestable vice', that other 'accurate' traveller was pursuing an independent investigation. The irrepressibly earthy Burton had discovered on the island a conjuror with unusual powers and in the interests of scientific research he was taking lessons from him and called Charlemont to be a witness to the honesty of the magician's performance. 'By the exertion of an astonishing Talent of venting wind backwards Ad Liberium' this man got his livelihood. 'He began by charging himself with air, which he took in at his Mouth, and which pass'd thro' him as an eel does thro' the Cormorant, only with this difference that our Adept had his Bowels under perfect Command. As soon as He was charged, He laid himself down on his Belly and let out the wind, at what Intervals, and in what proportion seem'd most fitted to surprise his Audience. Neither could there be any Deceit as plainly appeared by his Breeches being puff'd out at every explosion, and all this perform'd without any noisome smell.'[9]

To Burton's annoyance and disappointment, he failed in his lessons. Charlemont consoled him. He told him he believed the

* presumably the Maltese version of a red light.

science incommunicable. After ten months of voyage, and in spite of being cooped up with him in a small cabin often for days at a time, Charlemont could still regard 'the dear companion' of his travels with amusement and affection.

The parting was now close. After their disembarkation at Naples, Charlemont was not to see Burton again for nearly five years, but there was news of him. Richard Marlay wrote from Dublin that reports had reached him that Burton and Scott were on their way home. He expected to find Burton much improved. 'Though he had always a good deal of good humour and good nature, he was in many things very childish and ignorant, but if he has tolerable good sense and has lived with you for a year, he [may] be altered for the better.'[10]

By 12 March Adderley had the favour of seeing Burton and Scott; the latter, whom he had not met before, seemed 'a very sensible genteel man and if I do not make mistake, well-tempered'. Burton was soon to be married to Miss Clements, the eldest daughter of Mr Clements of the Treasury, and there had been some mention of his paying his debt to Charlemont, but no money was so far forthcoming. Burton had given to Scott a lease worth about a hundred and twenty pounds a year for three church livings and thrown in a fourth for the consideration of twenty shillings a year. This, Adderley thought, reflected great honour on Burton and he was almost as pleased on his account as on Scott's. It is evident that Adderley knew nothing of the Borra affair nor Charlemont's resentment. Marlay may have been better informed. Later he was to write to Charlemont that news of Scott which Charlemont could only have been delighted to hear: Scott was to be married to 'a girl in England with two hundred a year for life, very ugly and disagreeable'.[11]

NOTES

1. Hardy, pp. 18-22, for a full account of the storm.
2. Ibid.
3. Ibid.
4. Ibid
5 Ibid p. 23.
6. Ibid p. 24.
7. RIA, 12.R.7, p. 548.
8. Ibid pp. 551-3.
9. Ibid, p. 550.
10. Ibid, 12.R.21, no. 10.
11. Ibid, 12.R.9, no. 12.

PART TWO

Italy

10

THE TRAMMELLED PATH OF THE TOURIST

The adventures, dangers and the discoveries of the voyage behind them, Charlemont and Murphy, Dalton with them, returned to Rome and the tranquil routine, or comparatively so, of a young milord abroad with his bear-leader.

Rome, usually so empty, was filled with visitors, among them a great number of English, who had come for the Jubilee Year celebrations under the mistaken notion, as Horace Mann* observed from Florence, that it would be a time of 'great mirth and diversions of all kinds',[1] only to find there was to be no carnival, no opera and that all social activity was curtailed. Nevertheless they were not too bored. They had themselves for company and there was no shortage of spectacle – even a rhinoceros was on exhibition.

Charlemont's *Essay* on his years in Italy has never been traced; perhaps it was never written. A few footnotes to the other essays are all that we have of a first-hand account of his experiences. It is in relation to the scenes that he had witnessed in Constantinople with the dervishes that he describes an adventure, which probably dates to the Holy Year of 1750, and immediately after his return from the voyage.

'The horrid masquerades' of the flogging processions of Good Friday in Rome had often been described, but still the habits of the voyage persisted, and it was as a traveller of curiosity that he went out one Friday evening and joined the throng entering a large and magnificent church of an order of flagellant friars.

A long sermon recommending 'mortification and above all things self-discipline as the sure means of washing away every trace of sin' was followed by an 'excellent concert' during which servitors, carrying large silver plates, distributed scourges of twisted and knotted whipcord like cats o' nine tails to the entire congregation. The music ceased and the lights, which had illuminated the scene with 'the

* Best known of the British diplomats in Italy. There was no British representative in Rome.

utmost brilliance' were extinguished and 'at the same instant all the doors were clapped and secured with a noise like thunder'.

What followed, in total darkness, was 'sufficient to dismay the firmest mind' and Charlemont came close to hysterical laughter. The sounds began quietly with a rustle of disrobing and then rising to a crescendo, the cutting of whips, the clank of chains (for some had brought their own more cruel instruments) and the groans and shrieks of the penitents. This was Charlemont's idea of 'the infernal regions'.[2]

When at last the church was relit and the doors again opened, he escaped and thereafter there were no more of these investigations and Charlemont's life abroad took on the more conventional tenor of the Grand Tourist in Rome.

Hardy, writing of this time, makes much of Charlemont's connections with some of the most eminent men of the age (of whom more hereafter), and we cannot discount the effect of Charlemont's contacts with the Duc de Nivernois, Marchese Scipione Maffei and later the great Montesquieu in France and even with the Pope himself (Benedict XIV), if only because such connections were not the lot of any average Grand Tourist. But in attempting to analyse and weigh the influences which moulded Charlemont's career, due regard must be given to a group of less famous names, the fashionable young Englishmen on the Grand Tour with whom he formed friendships for life.

Rome was the finishing school and its playing grounds – or more precisely its antiquarian sites, galleries, museums and palaces – were the pitches where the battles of taste were lost or won. Out of boredom or from common interests and propinquity, grew a camaraderie and a bond, which was never to be severed and would continue to play an influential part in the patterns of connoisseurship, collecting, patronage and the architectural projects of the Grand Tourists, Charlemont and his friends, on their return home.

Lord Malton was in Rome and also Charlemont's old acquaintances from The Hague, John Ward and Sir Thomas Kennedy. Soon Philip Stanhope and a contingent of Irish visitors arrived, some of whom Charlemont already knew from early days.

Broadly speaking, the Tourists were divided into two groups. The young Englishmen who came from a tradition of Grand Tourism, with the background of England's architectural renaissance, were already well versed in Italian cultural influences and the vocabulary, however superficial, of taste and style. The Irish, on the other hand, came almost as pioneers and from a climate of newly-acquired prosperity (a lull in the troubled history of their country), and were in Rome to gather up, perhaps rather too obviously, the trappings of their new-found wealth and power.

Charlemont, without undue snobbery, inclined towards the English group and was totally accepted as one of theirs. At the same time he was on amicable terms with his compatriots or at least with the younger members, who moved under the redoubtable leadership of Joseph Leeson, future 1st Earl of Milltown, a Dublin brewer and banker.

Leeson, a man of considerable drive and self-importance, was, at the age of forty-nine, the doyen of all the Grand Tourists and on his second visit to Italy. He had already shown he had good judgement and a considerable flair for fashion. His portrait by Pompeo Batoni, painted on his earlier visit in 1744, was one of the first of that long series of Grand Tourist portraits by the artist in Rome. At the same time Leeson had patronized Giovanni Paolo Panini and Claude Joseph Vernet. Leeson had built Russborough, an imposing Palladian house in Co. Wicklow, to the designs of Richard Castle. It was the loss of many statues, pictures, etc., intended for Russborough, when the merchant ship carrying them had been taken by the French, that had precipitated the second visit to Italy in search of replacements of further works of art.

Russborough was one of a limited number of palatial and truly great houses which had begun to grow up in a country, which for so long had been restricted to fortified or semi-fortified building and where landowners of previous generations, more concerned with securing their property against the native Irish, had few architectural aspirations and consequently little interest in the fine arts.

Leeson's portrait by Batoni and Vernet's full-scale copy of Salvator Rosa's *Atilius Regulus* had survived shipment and now Leeson was once again back with Vernet and with Batoni, from whom this time he commissioned a portrait of his son, Joseph Leeson junior, who accompanied him in Rome.[3]

Leeson had taken a house, rather than the usual rooms or apartments, in the English quarter around the Piazza di Spagna, and here he was joined not only by his son, but his nephew, Joseph Henry, the son of yet another Dublin banker.

Joseph Leeson, junior, a chinless youth and much over-shadowed by his father, had spent a year at the Academy at Turin and he and Charlemont had this at least in common. He had a talent for mimicry which made him a not unamusing companion.

His cousin, Joseph Henry, the son of Joseph Leeson senior's sister, was a very different character. He had already been wandering around Europe on his own for two years and was to continue to do so for eight or nine years more. He was a collector and a bibliophile. According to Robert Adam, who met him at Pisa in 1755 and Florence in 1757, he had taste and a considerable estate, the two most desirable attributes of a prospective patron, although there is no evidence of his having employed Adam.

It is to be wondered why he and Charlemont were not closer friends. As usual it is that indefatigable gossip and the most faithful of Charlemont's irregular correspondents, Richard Marlay, who throws light on the matter in one of his waspish letters to Charlemont from Dublin.

Marlay enquired, 'Is Jo: Henry at Rome now, is he as fine a gentleman as ever, as conceited and full of himself as he was in his native country, or is he more affected since he trod classic ground, seen every court, heard every king declare his royal sense of operas or the fair? What an unaccountable thing it is that a person, who does not want sense should make himself ridiculous by his vanity or how can vanity and good sense meet in the same person; and yet we find they often do. I believe it is owing to self-love which intoxicates the brain and gets the better of understanding, and makes men say or do things which they imagine will raise them in the esteem and opinion of the world, but in reality makes them despicable and come (as Pope says in his character of the Duke of Wharton) most contemptible to shun contempt.'[4]

Whether or not this was a just criticism, Marlay knew his audience and he hardly would have risked expressing such an opinion if he was not sure of a sympathetic hearing.

Neither would Marlay have dared, however much confidence he placed in Charlemont's sense of humour, to have been so explicit about the exploits of Charlemont's erstwhile friend, Jack St Leger, as related by St Leger's mother, had he not been sure of Charlemont's change of heart.

Marlay wrote, 'I am told Mr St Leger is a great favourite with the Pope, My Lady St Leger says they often drink a jolly bottle together, toast c--t to the Church, beat the watch and bugger the Cardinals, but there are many here rude enough to doubt the Lady's veracity!'[5]

To the relief of all concerned, St Leger was no longer in Rome. Although far from shunning his compatriots, Charlemont understandably spent more of his time with Malton, his friends from The Hague, and a newcomer, Lord Bruce of Tottenham,[6] who was to become the closest friend of all.

Leeson's progress was enough to flutter the entire Roman art market with painters, sculptors and antiquarians vying for his commissions. Malton, formerly a sought-after patron, was now obliged, under instructions from home, to retrench. His father was complaining of expense and of the monies advanced for sculpture intended for Wentworth Woodhouse. Malton had done his best to explain to his father that the people were so poor that without an advance the greatest sculptor would starve before the work was finished, but no sooner than the first cases being delivered, word came to Malton that no more money was forthcoming. He was very disappointed, and particularly so because he had just discovered 'a most surprising genius', an English abbé, who had invented a harpsicord. Two had been made, one for Cardinal York, which, left in for some adjustment, the abbé had played for Malton. Malton could not conceal his pleasure; whereupon he was shown the other, which the inventor insisted on completing as a present to him, a present he could not gracefully refuse although he knew it was going to cost him a pretty penny in a reciprocal gift.[7]

It can hardly be seen as a coincidence that for the second time Charlemont took his lead from Malton, the first in support of James Stuart and now in employing the sculptors which Malton had been forced to abandon. Charlemont's commissions for copies after the antique were given to Joseph Wilton, Simon Vierpyle and Giovanni Battista Maini. All three had done work for Wentworth Woodhouse.[8]

Charlemont's other life-long friendship, with Lord Bruce, was based rather more simply on compatibility and a shared sense of humour. It was not a common interest in architecture which first brought them together in Rome in 1750, but the lack of occupation, as Charlemont would recall to Bruce some twenty-five years later, which made them believe themselves in love and with the same young woman, Eugenia Peters.

As Charlemont recalled, Eugenia was plain, almost to ugliness, but endowed with all the choicest accomplishments of her sex. She sang well and was a perfect mistress of the harpsicord. In striking contrast to her mother (an ill-bred and vulgar woman), who accompanied her, it was evident that Eugenia had received a most careful education. The disparity made for some talk at the time but was soon forgotten, and only revived when Eugenia, as the widow of Philip Stanhope, had the temerity to publish Lord Chesterfield's famous letters to his natural son. Gossip then related that she was the illegitimate daughter of Mr Domville, an Irish gentleman.[9]

In Rome, at the time, Charlemont and Bruce could see that Philip was also smitten, but it had never occurred to them he would marry her. The marriage was kept secret from Lord Chesterfield and only became known to him after his son's death, adding bitterness to his grief. All the worldly advice and devotion he had lavished upon Philip was, by this marriage, rejected.

The letters, published after Chesterfield's death, have been castigated by later generations as immoral, due to a lack of principle acquired on the Grand Tour and the time Chesterfield had spent at foreign courts. But as Charlemont pointed out to Lord Bruce (by then 3rd Earl of Ailesbury) the letters were never meant for publication; they were 'unjustifiably forced into the world by the poverty and resentment' of their old acquaintance Eugenia. 'If a physician should write upon a particular case, it would seem hard and unfair to criticize his work under the idea that he intended it for a complete system of physic' when, as in this case, it was no more than 'the anxious efforts of a paternal physician to effect a cure in an incurable disease'.

Stanhope, as Lord Bruce would recall, had 'good parts and a great deal of clumsy liveliness' and might have gone well enough through life had not his father insisted on trying to make him a fine gentleman. Philip was not unhandsome, but 'Dutch-built, thick, short and clumsy', and what struck Charlemont as so surprising in the son of 'the punctiliously well-bred' Lord Chesterfield, he had 'an ungraceful demeanour and total lack of breeding'. Sir William Stanhope, on first hearing of his brother's chagrin, had remarked, 'Why, what could Chesterfield expect of him? His mother was a Dutch woman, he sent him to Leipzig to learn manners, and that under the direction of an Oxford pedant'. This Charlemont thought rather hard on Mr Harte, elegance in tutors being rare and Harte 'a good man of considerable erudition'.

Charlemont had a fund of stories about Philip Stanhope – most of them gleaned from a fellow traveller, Mr Eliot (later Lord Eliot), who had shared his studies with Stanhope at Lausanne – all of which combined to form a picture of a veritable Tony Lumpkin.

One of his failings was gluttony and on an occasion at dinner at Chesterfield House, he had seen a dish of gooseberries and cream, a rare delicacy then, being removed from the table unfinished and demanded that 'his darling food' be brought back, but so as not to interrupt the courses, he had placed the serving dish under his chin and begun to lap it up in a hurry. Lord Chesterfield, 'choking with rage', called out to the valet, 'John, why do you not fetch the strop and the razors? You see your master is going to shave himself'.

Another of Stanhope's failings was 'an insatiable curiosity'. 'Again at dinner with his father, in front of a select company, while voraciously indulging his appetite for good things, another of his appetites was aroused by an unusual noise in the courtyard. Up he bounced with the intention of going to the window, but unfortunately forgetting that he had with admirable grace stuck the table cloth into his button hole, by the effort he exerted in rising, the dishes were displaced and the soup overturned to the amazement and annoyance of the guests, and to the utter consternation of his distressed father.'[10]

But to return to Rome and the events of 1750, Charlemont's and Bruce's brief dalliance with the future Mrs Philip Stanhope was brought to an end by their leaving for Turin to attend the wedding of the Duke of Savoy, Charlemont's erstwhile fellow student, to Princess Marie Antoinette of Spain. By the time they were back in Rome, the amiable Eugenia had departed; with Philip Stanhope, it was said, travelling in the same direction.

Hardy implies that Charlemont's invitation to the wedding was a singular honour. Charlemont may have been a privileged guest, but Horace Mann complained of the crowds of English coming from the wedding at Turin, too many looking for attention.[11] We are told nothing by Charlemont of the pomp of the royal occasion, the ceremonious arrival of the Princess at Oulx on 31 May and the marriage at Turin, where, incidentally, the Turin Shroud was on rare view. There is no mention of a reunion with old friends, but very possibly, it was here that he had his first meeting with Guiseppe Baretti, whose dramatic dialogue commemorating the wedding had received official recognition.

Even at the moment of success and the publication of a slim volume, *Piacevoli Poesie*, Baretti was typically in trouble. A satirical piece ridiculing Don Guiseppe Bartoli, professor of literature at the

University, was the cause of his being shortly forced to leave. This gave rise to the story that Baretti was brought to England by Charlemont, which Charlemont himself later denied, claiming he had known him well in Italy but had not known about his coming to England until he met Baretti again in London.[12] It was then that Charlemont stood by him when Baretti was charged with murder.

Baretti's accident ('accident' being a contemporaneous expression applied to any setback, whether trivial or the greatest misfortune), was satisfactorily resolved and he was acquitted. But as with his other protégés, the path of Charlemont's patronage was strewn with accidents as we very soon begin to find. This was far from unique or necessarily Charlemont's fault. It was rather more often his unlucky choice of the lame dogs he tried to help over stiles.

When Charlemont left Rome for the royal wedding, he and Dalton were apparently still on equable terms. But Charlemont seems to have shown no disposition to back Dalton's intended publication of his engravings; these were to include drawings made after the Raphael cartoons, work done in Sicily before Charlemont invited him to join him, with engravings from sketches made on the voyage. This would suggest Charlemont had no monopoly of interest and therefore no say in the publication's presentation. The outcome was a book, said by Robert Adam, to be 'so infamously stupid and ill-done that it quite knock'd him in the head & entitled him to that name of Dulton which is generally given him.'[13]

No doubt much of the cause of Dalton's failure was undue haste because of his jealousy of Stuart and Revett, who had been given Charlemont's financial backing, and his anticipation of the success of their venture.

A further threat loomed with the preparations being made by James Dawkins, John Bouverie and Robert Wood for their expedition to Palmyra, carrying with them the architectural draughtsman Dalton had merely by chance superseded, Giovanni Battista Borra.

By the time Charlemont was back in Rome from the wedding, Dalton had left for London to start work on the engravings. He took with him a letter from Joshua Reynolds, who had arrived in Rome in April, to his friend Miss Weston, in the hope that she and Dalton might become acquainted so that when he, Reynolds, returned from Italy, they might all three have 'many agreeable jaunts together'. In a rare recommendation of Dalton, Reynolds wrote, 'a worthy man is he'.[14]

Dalton's first publication appeared in 1751. It was followed by Robert Wood's *Ruins of Palmyra* in 1753. The first volume of Stuart and Revett's *Antiquities of Athens* did not appear until 1762.

Early in 1753 Charlemont received a most disagreeable communication. Adderley wrote, 'I must now mention Mr Dalton (ye painter) in order to obviate anything wch. he may advance agt. paying every honour & respect to yr. Lordship's recommendation of him. As soon as I recd. yr Ldship's letter abt. him, not knowing where he may be directed to, I commission'd Mr Burton to subscribe for ten setts of the Grecian antiquities for me, wch. he did ... Mr Dalton has been paid for them. When I was at Bath I had the favour of a visit from Mr Dalton, who came there in order to solicit subscription, when I told him I was, from the recommendation I received, willing & ready to do him every service in my power & accordingly desired him to put me down for 5 setts I believe of the cartoons. Indeed I paid him no money at that time for that I intended to have paid him the whole subscription when I got to London.'

Adderley, having missed Dalton in London when he had called on him twice, wrote to Dalton to apologise for it and confirm that he desired the sets to be made up and would direct payment to him. Dalton had replied in a letter, which Adderley obviously thought was impertinent, that the sets were ready to be delivered to any person who was empowered to pay him. Adderley had discussed Dalton's attitude with Mr Scott, who assured him that he had been treated ill also.

The sting came in the tail of Adderley's letter. He wrote, 'I have lately heard that he intends to publish something against the authenticity of Palmyra & proposes to call upon yr. Lordship to support him in the charge. Should he do this without yr. Lordship's knowledge, he must be strongly fortified with impudence.'[15]

By this time Charlemont and Wood had become intimate friends and we can imagine Charlemont's embarrassment, if not fury.

We now have to return to Rome in 1750, before Charlemont had left for the royal wedding, or Wood with Dawkins, John Bouverie and Borra had departed for Palmyra. Here began another of Charlemont's essays into patronage, which considering his protégé's character, was liable to run into accident.

Charlemont probably first met Thomas Patch through Dalton. They had come to Rome together from England, making most of their way on foot. Patch, a Devon man, came from a family of surgeons; his father had held an appointment to the Old Pretender and Patch, intending for medicine also, had been apprenticed to an apothecary in Exeter. Here his talent for caricature had given offence to patients and he had soon abandoned a career in medicine for art. He was not without education and Charlemont may have recognised in the impoverished artist, who eked out a precarious living in Vernet's studio copying the works of his master, the kind of judgement and perception which gave Patch an understanding of the Old Masters, and later was to enable him to see Masaccio as a great painter while, as yet, the world did not. That Patch was difficult and quarrelsome, Charlemont could not have failed to be aware, but his civilising influence and Patch's gratitude for his encouragement promised a good effect. A growing concern for under-privileged British artists studying in Rome was partly the incentive and before Charlemont left for Turin, he commissioned from Patch a set of views of Tivoli. It was agreed Patch should find his own way there and remain at Tivoli for the summer.[16]

NOTES

1. PRO, London, SP. 98.56 p. 185. See Ed. W.S. Lewis, W.H. Smith, G.L.Lam, *Horace Walpole's Correspondence* with Sir Horace Mann, Newhaven, 1960 Vol. 4, pp. 83, 165, 127-8.
2. Stanford & Finopoulos, pp. 226-7.
3. M. Wynne, 'The Milltowns as Patrons' *Apollo*, Feb. 1974, pp. 104-6.
4. RIA, 12.R.21, no. 101, Pope, 'Epistle to Cobham', line 195.
5. Ibid.
6. Thomas Brudenell, Lord Bruce of Tottenham, afterwards 4th Earl of Ailesbury (1730-1814). Courtier and Gentleman of the Bedchamber, Tottenham Park, his seat in Wilts. was designed and built for Lord Bruce's father by Lord Burlington, his brother-in-law.
7. Gutteridge, pp. 1-9.
8. H. Honour, 'English Patrons and Italian Sculptors', *Connoisseur*, May 1958, p. 224.
9. HMC, Rept. 12, App. pt. X, pp. 325-9.
10. Ibid.
11. Walpole, Mann Correspondence, Vol. IV p. 159.
12. RIA 12.R.15, no. 16.
13. J. Fleming, *Robert Adam and his Circle*, London 19?2, p. 223.
14. E.W. Hilles, *Letters of Sir Joshua Reynolds*, Cambridge 1929, p. 19.
15. HMC, Rept. 12, App. pt. X, p. 201.
16. F.J.B. Watson 'Thomas Patch', *Walpole Society* Vol. XXVIII (1939-40), pp. 15-50.

11

THE CONNOISSEURS, THE CARNIVAL AND THE CARICATURES

The winter of 1750-51 was a period of unusual activity for the Grand Tourists in Rome, leading up to the Carnival which was expected to be more splendid than ever since there had not been one in Holy Year. Some of these activities are described in a letter from Richard Phelps to Mr Cornewall in England. The letter is of considerable interest since it gives us an account of Charlemont and the Musical Society from which he went on to found, in 1752, an Academy for British artists studying in Rome.

Phelps[1], a Welshman, had first come to Rome as travelling tutor to John Bouverie. Bouverie, with his friend James Dawkins, had fallen under suspicion from Horace Mann for having 'behaved himself so indiscreetly in contacting frequently the Pretender's people' and Phelps likewise when, during the war, he had procured passports for Naples for himself, Bouverie and Dawkins from Lord Dunbar at the Jacobite court. With friends in England never doubting his loyalty, Phelps had out-lived the inconvenience and now enjoyed considerable popularity with the English set in Rome.[2]

Phelps' letter of 30 March has no year date but can safely be ascribed to 1751 the day before the death of Frederick, Prince of Wales, on 31 March; sometime after the news of Bouverie's tragic death at Guzal Hissar, in Turkey, on his way to Palmyra with Dawkins and Wood, had reached Rome. Bouverie had died on 20 September 1750. Phelps wrote that he had not sufficient philosophy 'to dissipate the gloom the death of my dear Friend occasion'd' and had been ill, but now, perfectly recovered, was able to write once again.

He describes the activities of the winter. 'The greatest part of us form'd a Society & raised a Fund for the better carrying on the important and necessary Business of Musick & masquing. I had the honour of being appointed Manager, I need not say that merit had no share in this promotion, but as I have had no small Experience in the ways of this blessed Country, I was look'd upon as one that had forgot so much of the plain dealing of my own Country as to render me in some small degree a Match for the more refin'd honesty of this. We hir'd the first Apartment of a Palace towards the center of the Town & having furnish'd most of the Rooms in the usual manner we reserv'd our Sala where we made our musical Academy twice every week to be adorn'd by the English Students in Sculpture & paintings who were invited to send in the best of their Works. Our Room was soon fill'd greatly to the Credit of the several Artists, some of whom in Time I think cannot fail to do honour to their Country in both these Arts.'[3]

Unfortunately Phelps does not tell who the artists were nor of what the twice-weekly meeting consisted. Almost certainly Vierpyle and Patch exhibited works in the music room, where there were concerts for which professional musicians were engaged, but as Phelps himself sang 'like an angel' and Charlemont and Sir Thomas Kennedy and John Ward were all amateur musicians, one suspects that the meetings were often informal and the recitals unprofessional.

Phelps goes on, 'But we had design'd our grand Coup d'Eclat for those days of the Carnival when Masquing in the streets is carried by the Nobility here to a great degree of Magnificence. It was resolv'd that we ought to briller* for the honour of our Country, & a Triumph of British Liberty was agreed upon for the subject. I have taken the Liberty to enclose our Scheme of it as it came out of the hands of our Committee & which was never executed, I am asham'd to say some of our Brethren deserting us and others, tho' every Man was strictly engag'd to keep it secret having very soon blar'd it abroad. This last Circumstance would have been sufficient of itself to have put an end to all our Measures it being necessary to obtain leave for introducing into the streets a Vehicle with four Horses abreast which ours must have had, & the Government here would have invented many excuses for putting a stop to any Spectacle which they had heard was to do honour to our Government under the present Royal Family. If you meet with anything in this plan that may please you, the honour of it belongs to Lord Charlemont, for tho' we both sat down together to assist one another, I soon found myself sufficiently employ'd in being his Lordship's Amanuensis.'

'I do not know if you have heard of that young Nobleman's

* to shine, to sparkle

Character but amongst all the Men of fashion that I have had the honour of being acquainted with abroad, I know few who have made so great & indeed universal use of their Travels as he has done.'

The scheme, which Phelps described at length and accompanied with a rough sketch showing the placing of the figures, provided for nineteen figures to be staged upon three decks of a Triumphal Car drawn after the manner of the old Roman chariots, by four horses abreast. The decks were raised about two feet, one above the other, and slightly sloped so that 'the view of no single figure be intercepted'. The sides of the car were to have been painted with antique trophies and arms representing the British navy and military, at the front a shield charged with the Union Cross and at the back a white horse at full gallop and the device and motto of the House of Hanover.

For each of the nineteen figures appropriate attributes, mottoes and details of dress had been designed. On the highest stage at the back under a canopy of festoons of flowers and palms was to be Lord Bruce as Liberty in a 'flowing Grecian Robe of bright green, a Garland on her head', Genius Britannia and Monarchy on either side of him. Phelps was assigned the honour of representing Genius Britannia because as he wrote, 'I looked the jolliest of the company'. He was to wear a helmet and a coat of mail with an azure mantle over his shoulders, bearing in his left hand a standard with the British crosses in union surmounted by three imperial crowns, and in his right the Magna Carta with the motto *Reges in ipsos Imperium est*, his arm resting on a column decorated with military and naval trophies.

The plan for the middle deck divided nine figures into three groups. Patriotism flanked by Virtue and Truth, Industry with Plenty, and Victory and Prudence with Justice and Mercy. Lord Middleton was to have taken the role of Patriotism in the character of the Prince of Wales with ensigns and plumes of feathers, Sir Thomas Kennedy at his right hand as Virtue wearing a helmet and a close-fitting taffeta vest and, to his left, John Ward representing Truth in a transparent robe with 'her Hair flowing negligently over her shoulders'.

Presiding over the lowest deck with Theology, Philosophy and Poetry on the one hand and Mathematicks, Physick and Commerce on the other, was to be Minerva – Charlemont in 'her usual dress when she is represented as the Protectress of the Arts, a Helmet upon her Head with the Owls upon it, a flowing robe of azure with the

Gorgon upon her breast, the Olive branch in her hands with this motto *Victrix Sapientia*.'[4]

This extraordinary exercise with such attention to detail was not destined to come to fruition, which was perhaps just as well in a city where the Old Pretender held court and the nearest British Resident, Horace Mann, was as far away as Florence. But if there was temerity and a great deal of robust national zeal, there was also symbolism, iconography and humour. The object would seem to have been, not so much a tilt for the House of Hanover, but a cheeky attempt to compete with the French. The students of the French Academy every year excelled in the masque and never more than in 1746 when they had staged for the Carnival an unforgettable departure for Mecca, with the Marchesa Gabrielli, the most beautiful woman in Rome, playing the part of an odalisque and throwing down her handkerchief to the Sultan.

Significantly, Charlemont had chosen the role of Minerva presiding over the Arts. In Rome, British artists struggled to survive while the French had every advantage. Rich Englishmen, potential patrons who might yet provide gainful employment in the future, did little to encourage those studying in Rome. For example Reynolds, to whom the Grand Tourists would flock on his return to England, was without employment in Rome and his only commissions were for the caricatures. A part of the problem seems to have been the prevailing winds of fashion. Richard Wilson, arguably England's greatest landscape painter of that era, could hardly sell his landscapes because they did not conform to the classical ideal of Claude.

Charlemont was sympathetic to the impecunious students, but primarily he regarded it as a slur on British prestige that the sons of the most powerful and richest nation on earth should be under a disadvantage in a city where their late enemies thrived under the auspices of the French Academy.

At the same time he was becoming increasingly aware, as he fell more and more under the spell of Italy, and studied her language, her history and literature, of the country's decline. This was due, he began to think, to her being overrun by foreigners, bent too often upon a refined form of pillage and whom he had discovered were so regarded by Italians of learning who emphatically styled them Barbarians. Indeed Britons too, who had long resided in Rome, while making exception for those of their compatriots with knowledge and taste, had come to compare the hordes of Grand Tourists to an invasion of Goths.[5]

The early spring had brought a fresh flux of Grand Tourists, visitors from England come for the Carnival, and a fresh flutter in the art world since among them was Sir William Lowther,[6] who was young, amiable and extremely rich and who was known to be on the look out for Old Masters; his list of *desiderata* included a work by Claude.

Sir Matthew Fetherstonhaugh's party accounted for nine. He was about thirty-five years old, learned, and also very rich. He had inherited a fortune from a cousin, the conditions of the will being that he purchase himself a baronetcy and a place. Having settled upon Uppark in Sussex, he had married Sarah Lethieullier and was now travelling with his bride, her brother Benjamin Lethieullier, her half-brother Raymond Lascelles Iremonger and five other relations. The entire party sat to Batoni for their portraits, which were to be hung at Uppark and with them landscapes by Vernet and paintings by Old Masters that Sir Matthew had come to Italy to acquire.[7]

From Staffordshire came a neighbour of John Ward's, William Bagot,[8] and from Ireland Thomas Dawson,[9] the son of yet another banker, with estates in Co. Monaghan and travelling with a neighbour, Mr Maxwell, a connection of Lord Farnham's.

In this atmosphere of weighty opulence and expansive patronage, Vernet's book of *commandes* expanded; Richard Wilson was commissioned by Joseph Henry to paint a pair of views of Tivoli; Vierpyle began for Edward Murphy to copy the entire series of the seventy-eight heads of the Roman Emperors, a commission which it was to take him four years to fulfil, 'standing in the chilling Capitoline Museum to model so many busts' and Joseph Leeson startled the art world with a bid for the Furietti centaurs.

A visitor to Rome described in a letter to the antiquarian Dr Jeremiah Milles, the pair of black (*bigio morata*) centaurs, celebrated since they had first been dug up at Hadrian's villa in 1736 in the excavation carried out by Monsignor Furietti. 'The finest things in ye world of ye kind,' he wrote; and he had feasted his eyes on them for a full hour, while 'Mr Leeson, an Irish gentleman who was with me offered 2000 sterling for them, which proposal was received with indignation.'[10]

Had Leeson's offer been accepted, which was most improbable, a licence would have certainly been refused; Benedict XIV had set his heart on the centaurs for the Capitoline Museum and had shown his displeasure at Furietti's refusal to donate them by for some time passing him over for a cardinal's hat. Since Leeson could hardly have smuggled them out, one concludes the bid was an act of bravado. Nevertheless the centaurs did have their price and after the death of Benedict XIV, Clement XIII acquired them finally for the Museum against huge sums offered to Furietti's heirs by English negotiators in Rome.[11]

The stage was now set and all the characters present for *The Parody of the School of Athens.* This was the caricature painted by Reynolds for Joseph Henry, of the connoisseurs in Rome in 1751. In the past, while it was as yet unsuspected it had been commissioned by Henry, Reynolds came in for criticism for being so tasteless as to parody Raphael's sacrosanct masterpiece.

Joseph Henry had already demonstrated some independence of his uncle, not merely in his patronage of Wilson. He had discovered for himself the celebrated caricaturist Pier Leoni Ghezzi, who until then had been quite neglected by the Tourists. Whether it was that kind of vanity, attributed to him by Marlay, which found in ridicule an inverted form of flattery, or for some other cause, Henry had had himself caricatured by Ghezzi with the inscription "*Guiseppe henry Inglese, huomo assai erudite nella antichita e en Lettera.*"[12]

A series of caricatures by Ghezzi followed: Charlemont seated with the younger Leeson taking coffee, and groups in which Joseph Henry appeared variously with Lord Bruce, Lord Middleton and John Martin junior of Overbury among others.[13]

It does not seem to have occurred to Joseph Henry to make use of Patch's talents; perhaps he did not find him sufficiently biddable and indeed it was not supposed until recently that Patch painted any caricatures while in Rome. But a letter from Lord Bruce (by then Earl of Ailesbury) to Charlemont in 1792 refers to 'our caricature painted by Patch', a caricature which could only have been painted when they were together in Rome. They had long left Italy before Patch's banishment and subsequent residence in Florence, where he made his name as a caricaturist.[14]

It is likely that neither Henry nor Reynolds thought it any disrespect to Raphael to borrow his subject and composition, which could be admirably adapted for Henry's purpose, a lampoon upon the pretensions of the connoisseurs. A pocket edition of Bellori's *Descrizione delle immagini dipinte de Raffaelle de Urbino, nel Palazzo Vaticano,* dated 1751, found among Reynolds' papers is evidence of the care and attention with which Henry gave his instructions to Reynolds. Bellori's interpretation, rather than Vasari's, of the group at the lower left of the picture, besides being the correct one, was better suited to the scheme: Pythagoras with pupils studying the principles of harmony, and not St Matthew with assistants copying the scriptures.[15]

Reynolds' list of those depicted, a list headed by Henry, follows perhaps the order in which the connoisseurs came for their sittings because it does not relate to the placing in the picture. Against a Gothic background, signifying northern vandalism, the connoisseurs take up their positions, while Henry, in the role of Raphael's Diogenes the Cynic, disassociates himself from the others and reclines, or rather lolls, on the steps apart.

Henry has turned his back to the protagonists, Plato and Aristotle and he holds in his hand a book entitled *LARRY GROG*. This appears to be an esoteric reference, the full meaning now lost, to the gentleman piper and ballad writer, Larry Grogan of Johnstown Castle, Co. Wexford. Grogan is best remembered for his ballad *Ally Croker*, composed in 1725, which told of a man who lived in Ballina Creasy, who wanted a wife to make him uneasy:

This artless young man just come from the schoolery
A novice in Love and all its Foolery,
Too dull for a wit, too grave for a Joker ...

and so on, the verses ending with the refrain 'Will you marry me, dear Ally, Ally Croker'. Perhaps for *Love* Henry substituted *Art*.[16]

Joseph Leeson is unmistakeably Plato and has for a disciple, Sir William Lowther beside him. Leeson points not to Heaven as in Raphael's picture, but raises instead his quizzing glass and the younger Leeson is clearly identified as one of his supporters. Lord Bruce, Alexander the Great, stands at the upper left and looks down from his height upon the assembly. In an allusion to the musical academy, we find Charlemont, Sir Thomas Kennedy[17] and Phelps in the Pythagorean group at the lower left.

The above placings are confirmed by a series of small caricatures painted by Reynolds and with names of the sitters given. Thereafter it is guess work.

Is it Murphy, now a great patron since his commission to Vierpyle for the busts of all the Emperors, who takes such a prominent place, seated at the table, a bottle of wine beneath, a pen in his hand, his glasses on his nose and intent upon his studies? For this ardent vulcanologist, it would be only fitting that he should be cast as Raphael's Heraclitus, who taught the world was created from fire.

Simon Vierpyle, on the grounds of a likeness to a later portrait, could be the seated young man in the right foreground with the dogs playing around him. Matthew Brettingham the younger, the architect and the protégé of Lord Leicester, may be the student arriving late, a portfolio under his arm; and perhaps it is Reynolds, who is said to have included himself, although he is not listed among the sitters, who stands facing him. Can it be Patch at the extreme right only his head seen, who takes the position of Giovanni Antonio Bazzi? Bazzi, nicknamed Il Sodoma by Vasari because of his disorderly and rakish life, was a role the wayward Patch, with his reverence for the earlier schools, might have been happy to play.

Somewhere among the twenty-six figures are Mr Dawson and Mr Maxwell (the Irishmen); Mr Stirling, Mr Barrett;* the jolly physician, Dr Irvine (attendant to the Old Pretender, but for his good sense and humour, popular with the Tourists); Mr Iremonger (the half-brother of Lady Fetherstonhaugh), and Abbé du Bois, the language teacher.

The smaller caricatures, based upon the grouping in the *Parody*, and therefore presumed to have been painted afterwards, confirm that neither Henry's concept of the connoisseurs as the Goths in possession of Rome nor Reynolds' depiction of individual physical idiosyncrasies, gave offence. John Ward, who is not in the *Parody*, appears twice, once with Lord Bruce, the younger Leeson and Joseph Henry, who on this occasion is absorbed in studying the plans of Cloaca Maxima, and again as an addition to Charlemont's group, still with their musical instruments. But now play is made upon the individual nationalities of these musicians; Charlemont disports a great bunch of shamrock in his hat, Ward a rose, Sir Thomas the emblem of St Andrew and Mr Phelps a well-grown leek!

After the diversions of the Carnival and then of the caricatures came the wagers, again as much a curiosity in their own way. Lest we begin to think the activities of Charlemont and his set were given up entirely to frivolity, there was the rain, which for more than three months continued unabated over Italy, and made pleasant excursions out of the question and even the daily pilgrimage to the ruins of Rome a duty to be eschewed. Moreover the news of Bouverie's death detracted sadly from the triumph of Dawkins and Wood in reaching Palmyra and this was followed by news from England of the death of the Prince of Wales, who only a short time previously had figured in their masque.

The first wager, or rather indenture, was made in Rome, 12 April 1751. It stated simply, 'I, Benjamin Lethieullier, promise to pay the

* Thomas Barrett of Belhus, Essex

sum of forty guineas to Lord Charlemont if I am married before him, as witness my hand, Benjamin Lethieullier and bore the signatures of Bruce, Thomas Kennedy, Pulteney and L.R. Iremonger'.[18]

This document constitutes the first hint of Charlemont's repugnance to matrimony, the reason for which, although he never refers either to his mother or her death, we can only suspect.

Incomprehensible to us today, but a pastime of men of fashion in the eighteenth century were those wagers upon the life expectancy of friends and acquaintances. These were set down in a most formal agreement to guard against long-term contingencies, or even short-term, since in one case the subject of the wager later turned out to be already dead when the bet was taken.

One such indenture was made between Lord Bruce and Charlemont on 26 September 1751 at Lucca. 'If Sir William Lowther of Holker in the County of Lancaster dies before John Martin jun. Esq of Overbury in the County of Worcester, Lord Charlemont is bound to pay the said Baron Bruce the sum of Fifty pounds, in case the said John Martin dies before the said Sir William Lowther, Baron Bruce is to pay the like sum of fifty pounds; and the parties aforesaid that in the case of General d'Olleune, Minister for his Polish Majesty dies before Lascelles Raymond Iremonger, late of Rome, Lord Charlemont is to pay Lord Bruce 10 pounds sterling and Lord Bruce is bound to pay the like sum in case of L.R. Iremonger dying before d'Olleune. Lord Bruce to pay if General Sallia, now of Florence, dies before the Duc de Nivernois, minister for the French King to the Pope and vice versa.'[19] A note protected any heirs of Charlemont or Bruce; at either of their deaths the agreement became void.

We know very little else of Charlemont's trip with Bruce to Siena and Lucca that summer. The theatre at Siena was, in July, completely destroyed by fire, but whether they were at Siena at the time is not revealed. Lord Bruce, re-visiting Siena only two years later wrote to Charlemont in Rome, 'the Sienese have rebuilt their theatre in a most elegant manner upon a plan of Bibiena's'.[20]

Not far from Siena there lived in opulent retirement the famous castrato Senesino, so well-known to the English for his historic appearances at the Haymarket in the 1720s. Confident of being well received as Englishmen, Bruce and Charlemont went to pay their respects. Their reception was as cordial as they could have wished. Senesino showed them around his villa and its grounds, fitted and laid out in the English taste. '*Ecco la Providenza Inglesi*' he crowed with understandable complacency and condescended to entertain them with a song.[21]

The vanity of the castrati, as much as the adulation which prompted it, made an impression on Charlemont, particularly that of Gizziello, who in a letter to the Marchesa Patrizzi, which she showed Charlemont, described his reception by the Royals of Portugal.* Madame Patrizzi was a principal patroness of the opera and the benefactress of Gizziello. Later Charlemont checked Gizziello's account and found it to be true that he was brought up the Tagus in the royal barge and escorted by a large body of horse guards to the palace. He was conducted into the presence of Jose I by the Lord Chamberlain, received by the king with the most cordial affection and led by him to the queen. Her Majesty accompanied him on the harpsicord while he sang an air. She was so moved that she took from her finger a diamond ring worth a thousand moideres and gave it to him. From her presence he was led to his apartments for repose. The apartments consisted of sixteen rooms, the last of these a dressing room, where he found upon a table a toilet set of massive plate and in one of its boxes a thousand moideres, a present from the king. The salary of four thousand moideres, which had lured him to Portugal, was effaced in these first few hours of royal munificence. It was hardly surprising that he ended his letter to his erstwhile patroness, 'I beg pardon, Madame, for the shortness of my epistle, but I am so interrupted and fatigued with the visits of the grandees that I have neither the time or the ability to write more'.[22]

Curious as this story of success was, and Charlemont obviously relished the anecdote, there were terrible consequences for others less fortunate. Seduced by the prospects of fame and fortune, thousands were emasculated who never attained any degree of excellence or fame. The Marchese Massimi told Charlemont of his family estates situated in a part of the Pope's dominions where 'this infamous ware was principally manufactured' and twice his father had been 'obliged to re-people their lands by sending colonies thither from the neighbouring countries, so effectively had the propagation of the human species been stopped and destroyed by this horrid trade.'[23]

On the way back from Lucca to Rome, Charlemont and Bruce are likely to have passed through Florence and perhaps heard from Mann, who had received the first news of Patch, while working on the views

* In Lisbon 1743 and again 1753.

commissioned by Charlemont, having run into trouble with the Bishop of Tivoli. Nobody seemed to know why and Patch had given no explanation. The Bishop's excuse for ordering him to leave his diocese on the grounds that a non-professing Catholic was prohibited from remaining more than eight days, was such a blatant quibble that Mann was at some pains to discover what was behind it, but Cardinal Albani could get no information. Patch, relying on his father's former connections with the Stuart court, applied to Cardinal Maresfeschi, who was Cardinal Stuart's auditor, and also to the Marquese Belloni, the banker who, apart from arranging payments to artists in Rome from their patrons in England, was in charge of expenses of the Pretender's household, but he could get no satisfaction.

By the time Charlemont was back in Rome, Horace Mann and Cardinal Albani had begun to think Patch's troubles were more serious than they had first supposed, and their suspicions were further aroused by the Bishop writing to Albani that had Patch kept within the limits of permission to make paintings of Tivoli, he would have been left to do so, as in fact had been the case the previous year. The Bishop's hint of some unmentionable crime so gross that his conscience forbade him to allow the perpetrator to remain in his diocese, discouraged further enquiry.

Patch did not confide in Simon Vierpyle, to whom among the artists he was closest, but it seems that he gave some sort of explanation to his patron and Charlemont was content to accept it. There the matter rested until it was dramatically revived three years later.[24]

At the time of Charlemont's return to Rome three events occurred, which in varying degrees affected him. The first was the death of the Prince of Orange. This would probably have done no more than recall to him, Ward, Sir Thomas Kennedy and Lord Middleton, serving officers in the Scots Brigade, their time together at The Hague. The second was the birth of the Duke of Burgundy, the heir to the throne of France. The third was the eruption of Vesuvius.

Murphy, that ardent vulcanist, immediately set off for Naples. He was unaccompanied by Charlemont; as he explained in a letter to Adderley, 'my Lord being obliged out of politeness to stay at Rome to see certain feasts made by the French Ambassador on the occasion of the birth of the young Dauphin'.[25]

Murphy, happily riding the chief of his hobby horses, in his letter to Dublin of 16 December touched briefly upon expressions of seasonal goodwill and discoursed over two closely written pages upon Vesuvius and the 'fiery eruption'. Fearing his letter might 'prove too long' it seemed that it was but an introduction to what he intended should follow. 'I shall here preface it by observing to you that this Mountain which has its center about 8 miles distant from Naples to the East, is a cone of 30 miles Circumference in the Base and about 3 eights of a mile perpendicular height, not to its vertex (for considered as a cone it has not a top of such a figure) but to its Summits; which are 2 in number in the shape of a shugger-loaf with about one third cutt off the Top, and another equally high, surrounding said sugger loaf at the distance of 3/4 mile so as to form a sort of Theatre round it the North and N. East side.'[26]

The above being no more than an introduction to Murphy's discourse, it is not surprising that Charlemont was found by Murphy to be sadly apathetic about his most favourite subject and, more especially, as it would appear that Murphy had made a collection of specimens of lava, which he wished to present to Lord Bruce or failing that, he wanted carried in their bulk to Ireland.

The French Ambassador to Rome, the Duc de Nivernois,[27] had been about to depart for France when news of the birth of the Dauphin arrived. Madame de Nivernois had already left and was not to be present at those celebrations, which both astonished and delighted the whole of Rome, and reached their climax in a masked ball at the Palazzo Farnese on 24 November 1751.

In the forecourt the fountains poured wine, red and white, and of no mean quality, for the populace. Within, armies of servants waited upon the guests with the finest of wines and carried to them, throughout the evening, plateaux of hot and cold viands.

The Princess Borghese, in the absence of Madame de Nivernois, did the honours. Seventeen cardinals and all the nobility of Rome, were present. Musicians, raised upon a platform apart, accompanied the dance; but amidst all this splendour nothing was so remarkable as the transformation of the Grand Saloon of the Palazzo Farnese for this occasion.

An army of artisans and artists, assisting Panini, had created architectural facades to cover the walls and the pilasters were painted to simulate lapis lazuli. At one end of the great room were hung the arms, the cyphers and the blazons of France and at the other symbolic figures of France, Peace, Abundance and Religion. Dolphins and putti disported, festoons of fresh flowers in abundance hung from the capitals of the pillars, and pier glasses reflected the lights of the crystal chandeliers and the massive, standing candelabra. Over all hung the allegorical sunburst.[28]

NOTES

1. See *A Dictionary of British and Irish Travellers in Italy 1701-1800* compiled from the Brinsley Ford Archive by John Ingamels.
2. PRO, London SP 98.56. Mann re Dawkins May 14th 1748 NS and Bouverie Aug. 1 1749. Lewis, *Connoisseurs and Secret Agents*, p. 25.
3. Harpton Court papers, National Library of Wales, MSS.
4. Ibid.
5. RIA, 12.R.6. p. 405.
6. Sir W. Lowther, Bt. of Holker, (1727-1756). F. Russell 'Thomas Patch, Sir William Lowther and the Holker Claude', *Apollo*, Aug. 1975, pp. 115-119.
7. St John Gore, 'A Grand Tour Collection', *Country Life* Dec. 2 1965, National Trust Guide booklet 1981 for Uppark.
8. William Bagot of Blithfield (1728-1798) 1st Baron Bagot of Bagot's Bromley, Staffs. 1754.
9. Thomas Dawson, created Baron Dartrey 1770, Viscount Cremorne 1785.
10. Wynne, 'The Milltowns as Patrons', p. 106.
11. F. Haskell & N. Penny, *Taste and the Antique,* Newhaven & London, 1981, p. 178.
12. D. Sutton, 'The Roman Caricatures of Reynolds' *Country Life Annual* 1956, p. 113.
13. Formerly Coll. Anthony M. Clarke.
14. C. O'Connor, 'The Parody of the School of Athens', *Bulletin of the Irish Georgian Society*, Vol. XXVI, 1983, p. 18.
15. E. Wind, 'A Source for Reynolds' Parody of the School of Athens, *Harvard Library Bulletin*, Vol. III, Spring 1947, No. 2.
16. Capt. F. O'Neill, *Irish Folk Music,* Chicago 1910, p. 170.
17. Sir Thomas Kennedy, 4th Bt. of Culzean, 9th Earl of Cassilis 1759.
18. RIA, 12.R.9, no. 4.
19. HMC, Rept. 12, App. pt. X, pp. 183-4.
20. Ibid, p. 186.
21. RIA, 12.R.5, n. to p. 56.
22. Ibid, p. 56.
23. Ibid, p. 55.
24. L. Lewis, p. 172.
25. RIA, 12.R.12, no. 8.
26. Ibid.
27. Hardy, pp. 89-90.
28. F. de Navenne, *Rome et le Palais Farnèse,* Vol. 2, 1923, pp. 60-4. B. Scott, 'Little Known Drawings from the French Provinces', *Apollo*, Feb. 1975, p. 142.

12

A HOUSE IN ROME 1752

It was not until 1755 that Charlemont returned to Ireland and during the winter of 1751-52* there were as yet no thoughts of his turning his face towards home. We find him in Rome, having taken a house for himself and his friends in that quarter where the English inevitably gathered, around the Piazza di Spagna. Hardy tells us Charlemont was one of the first amongst the English to set up household during their stay in the metropolis, and that Murphy was of great assistance to him in superintending the whole business of housekeeping. While we know that Joseph Leeson had already set the example and Charlemont was merely following him, Murphy's new role is confirmed by the parish registers of 1752; he is listed as *Odoardo Smorfi, Magr. Duomo Inglese* to *Milor Giacomo Sciaramon Inglese* at the second crossing following the Strada de la Croce towards the Corso.[1]

Also registered, apart from the Italian servants, a cook and a *perrucche*, are *Gio: Bacca Inglese* and *Barnardo Barni Came. Inglese*, names that appear again in the register of 1753. *Bacca* has not been identified, but *Barnardo Barni* is undoubtedly Barny, Charlemont's Irish servant. We do not know under what circumstances, how and when Barny had first come to Rome, and it is a matter of some curiosity that an Irish valet should be of the entourage. It is possible that Charlemont with his own comfort in mind arranged it as a sort of apprenticeship into the ways to which Charlemont was now accustomed, and was not prepared to forego at the hands of untrained Irish servants on his return to Ireland. Nevertheless it speaks for trust and loyalty between master and servant and we find Charlemont arranging for Barny's brother, a Dublin tailor, to go to Paris to better himself.[2] But when it came to his table, Charlemont fell back on the simple solution of borrowing, for his return to Ireland, a French cook from Lord Bruce, who did not need his services at that time.

As Charlemont settled in Rome, in the spring of 1752, the Leesons

* The year that began on 1 January and not, as formerly, on 25 March.

departed for Ireland and, by April, Richard Marlay was reporting from Dublin that 'the *Fair Penitent* is to be acted in town by some ladies and gentlemen, Leeson is to play Lothario, they say he will do it very ill, he is reckoned to have a good deal of the freeble in him, whether true or false I cannot say'. Marlay, of course, is referring to the younger Leeson, who whether a fribbler or not, was more suited to the part of the young seducer than was his father. Marlay's other news was that Burton was very well, 'as good-humoured as ever, he has got a daughter'.[3]

The gap left by their departures was soon filled with the arrival of Lord Tylney,[4] Thomas Scrope[5] and, from Ireland, Ralph Howard[6] of Shelton, Co. Wicklow who was accompanied by his tutor, Mr Benson.

There was also Charles Turner of Kirkleatham Hall, Yorkshire for whom the well-known portrait group of Grand Tourists in front of the Colosseum and the Arch of Constantine was painted. The artist remains unknown, but the figures now have been identified: left to right, Sir Thomas Kennedy, Charlemont, Charles Turner, Sir William Lowther, Thomas Steavens and Lord Bruce.[7]

It was at Kirkleatham Hall that the Earl of Ailesbury (Lord Bruce) in 1792 rediscovered Patch's caricature of himself and Charlemont. It was then in the hands of an upper servant of the late Sir Charles Turner, which suggests it was Turner who commissioned it from Patch, and gives further strength to the argument that it could only have been painted in Rome.[8]

One of several artists to whom the Grand Tourist group has been attributed, James Russel[9] assumes some importance for us in his being Howard's agent in Rome. His letters to Howard have survived and are a record of Howard's expansive patronage and those paintings and works of art which were destined for Shelton in Co. Wicklow. Moreover, the letters are in gossipy vein and describe many of the activities of Charlemont and his friends after Howard had left Rome.

It is Russel who reveals that Reynolds' caricature of a ludicrous incident from Ralph Howard's travels was commissioned by Howard, and that Reynolds was required to alter it before his patron was satisfied. Therefore, Marchi, Reynolds' assistant, was correct in his assertion that the caricatures were not painted by Reynolds for his own amusement and at the risk of giving offence to his prospective patrons, as had previously been assumed.

But however much information can be gleaned from Russel's letters to Howard, on one subject he was noticeably reticent. He never mentions Charlemont's newly founded Academy. Whether this was due to a certain jealousy of the appointment of another as its director, or to Howard's not being involved, we do not know.

A notice that appeared in the *Daily Advertiser* of 8 June in London, under the heading of May 12th Rome, outlined Charlemont's proposal. 'The English noblemen and gentlemen at this place on their travels, having taken into consideration the disadvantages young students of their nation in Painting and Sculpture lie under here for want of the foundation of an Academy, without pensions for encouragement for those whose circumstances will not permit their studies for a sufficient time at their own expense, have begun a generous subscription towards the foundation of an Academy and have appointed Mr John Parker, history painter to be receiver and director thereof. The generous promotors of this foundation are the Lords Bruce, Charlemont, Tylney and Kilmurray, Sir Thomas Kennedy Bt., Messrs Ward, Iremonger, Lethieullier, Bagot, Scrope, Cook, Lypeat, Murphy, and as all nations in Europe particularly the French have academies and great encouragements, it is hoped that all lovers of the Arts will promote this generous design.'[10]

The scheme was as zealously patriotic as Charlemont's design for the Carnival and was yet another of his tilts at French power and influence in Rome. The Academy survived for a mere three years. Quarrels between Patch and an obscure artist called Warner hastened its end.

On 6 June Russel wrote to Howard and, without any reference to the Academy, gave him news of its promoters. 'I have lately had the pleasure of attending a party of gentlemen, to Tivoli, Palestrina, Antium etc. which consisted of my Lord Bruce, Sir Thomas Kennedy, Messrs. Iremonger, Lethvullier and Mr Scroop; these Gentlemen at present are at Naples; and Rome now is very thin; there being only my Lord Charlemont and Mr Bagot. At Adrian's Villa we saw a place where the Marquis Gabrielli has been at the expense of digging, is put upon that spot where the famous Centaurs were found, where it is supposed Adrian's principal residence was. There was discovered several fine mosaic pavements, which the Marquis has cut into tables, and has transported to Rome; one of which he has made a present of to my Lord Charlemont.'[11]

Thus we find Charlemont in Rome with all his friends in Naples. Singled out by the Marquese Gabrielli, the attractions of Rome apparently outweighing those of Naples and the good company of

Lord Bruce and John Ward. In an attempt to inveigle Charlemont to join them, Ward, at the instigation of Bruce, wrote Charlemont an amusing account of their doings there, but Charlemont remained obstinately in Rome. Neither Russel nor Ward indicate any particular reason unless it was, as described by Russel, the recent archaeological finds and the erection of the statue of St Michael upon Hadrian's Mausoleum, the Castle of St Angelo.

In his letter to Howard, Russel wrote, 'In digging in a vineyard near the Catacombs of St Sebastian, were the other day discovered several bodies, together with them were found three very rare fine medals, two of Commodus and one of Marcus Aurelius. The Pope has purchas'd them, they are to be plac'd amongst his rare collection at the Vatican. A very fine cameo, an inch and a half over, representing Bacchus and Ariadne, has fell into the hands of Sgr. Borioni, of exquisite workmanship; it was lately found among some rubbish, in making the foundation of the Convent of S. Augustin in Campo Marzo. They are at present erecting upon the Castle of S. Angelo, a brazen statue of S. Michael sheathing his sword; it is about 23 feet high, and the action and air of the figure seems to be taken from the famous picture of Guido's at the Capuchines.'[12]

Charlemont's dealings with Borioni, the apothecary and collector, are not documented but we have evidence that Borioni was Charlemont's chief source of cameos and medals for the collections he made in Rome. Charlemont himself admitted to the collector's mania and it is possible that the discoveries were sufficiently interesting to keep him in Rome.

As with Marlay's letters from Dublin, we find in Ward's letter a reflection of Charlemont's mind, and indeed more so since Ward's letter was intended to draw Charlemont away from the attractions of Rome, with an account of what Ward knew would most amuse, interest and divert Charlemont were he to join his friends in Naples.

> 'My dear Lord
> My first reason for writing to you is that I am ordered by Lord Bruce, who thinks no man well employ'd unless in writing, the second is that I imagine you'll be glad to be inform'd a little what we are doing here and the third that I shall in some measure oblige you to a correspondence which I'm very ambitious of.
>
> If I thought any exaggerations would entice you to come to this place, I should not be so nice an addresser to Truth in the character I should give of the Opera. The Dance is very indifferent, the Sabbetina and

Nina de Sales are the chief Performers. Visconti, first woman, ugly, old and lame, but an admirable Actress, and in my humble opinion the best Woman singer I have heard on any stage. Caffariello either can't or won't sing well, however we are the sufferers let it be how it will. Ottani the Tenor has a very fine voice, accompanying his ignorance of musick with a matchless impudence. The second Soprano eletto Cornachini has very agreeable voice and sings well. The Fickle Countess Shenfield, unmindful of her Cafariello has already broken three fans in his Praise. Tho' it's not much the fashion to like the opera I must own that upon the whole it pleases me. The Carboniera, that you must have seen and heard at Mr Wiseman's* concert, does the last part in mens Cloaths, so much for the Opera. There are likewise two little Theaters, one of which is not bad.

We were very surprised a few days since by the return of Cook from Caprea, after he had sojourned there for 9 weeks, he has forgot his own language and French, so that finding it very disagreeable living among a People whom he could neither understand nor be understood by, he has by signs persuaded Sr. Thos. Kennedy to return to Caprea with him as Sr. Thos. loves the Sea and shooting I fear he'll stay there so long that he'll forget his english likewise, in that case the Abbé du Bois must look out for an other corrector of the Press for the English part of his works.

The Princess Francavilla desired me to bring her the Man who had made Love to the Regiana in so violent a manner. I suppose she flattered herself with the Idea of seeing a ravisher, but when poor Scroope came to her presence she could no more believe he was the man than K. Charles wou'd believe Butler the author of his beloved Hudebrass.

I'm ashamed to own it but I have not been to Herculaneum yet, all I know of it is it was debated if they should not divide a poor Janus found there, two heads being better than one.

It was wisper'd this morning that his Majesty had caught two very large fish yesterday, but the report is not confirm'd. What is certain is that his Majesty did not come to Naples Sunday fortnight, hearing there was a great flight of Quail on the other side of Portici.

I think you would amuse yourself here very well for a little Time. I'm not quite without hope of seeing you here. Ld. Bruce desires his compliments and says he has wrote to you, pray remember me to honest Murphy, and believe me, my dear Lord, your sincere friend and very humble srvt.

Naples June ye 10th *J. Ward*

If you should chance to be at Frascati give my respects to the Princess

* Charles Wiseman (*fl.*1738-*d.* 1778), composer and English music master in Rome.

[Borghese] and say a great many fine things for me. I believe I need not tell you that Lord Bruce is impatient to hear from you. Direct me at the Dutch Consul's.

Voila une lettre à la glace.[13]

A lively, witty letter from one fashionable young man to another, it is for us, in spite of some esoteric allusions, a revealing document. It throws light on a scene with which Charlemont was familiar from visits prior to and after the voyage. It tells of Charlemont's most intimate circle, the activities of his friends and also of his acquaintances and of interests in common. Characters begin to emerge who before then were little more than names; names that are associated with Charlemont in Reynolds' caricatures, in Charlemont's design for a masque for the Carnival, in the promotion of the Academy for British artists, and which were finally to come together again in their patronage of William Chambers.

First there is Ward himself, son of Lord Ward of Sedgely Park, Staffordshire (afterwards Viscount Dudley and Ward), whom Charlemont first met as a serving officer in Holland and who had pleased Murphy then for having his classics in his pocket and quoting his authors. He is confident of his ability to amuse Charlemont, whose interests and an acute sense of the absurd he shares, but he defers to Lord Bruce as the closer friend. He writes to Charlemont because he has been directed to do so by Lord Bruce, who may have complained as Marlay did, of Charlemont's not answering his letters.

Charlemont loves opera and so Ward obliges with a critique of the performances in Naples where women played their parts on the stage, and not as in Rome, sang only at concerts, and remembering Charlemont's visit to Senesino, recounts the present caprices of the spoilt *castrati*.

Sir Thomas Kennedy we know already to be a lover of music like Charlemont and Ward. A member of the Music Society, he appears with them and with Phelps in the caricature, but until now we have not seen him as a sportsman, who loved sailing, fishing, shooting and racing. This explains the wager of April of that year, 1752 on a match to be run on the Isle of Man on the first Tuesday in July 1755 between mare or gelding, bought for less than forty pounds, the stake a hundred pounds. Sir Thomas evidently had confidence in his own judgement of horseflesh, and Charlemont was game enough to challenge it.[14]

Mr Cook, of whom we know nothing except that he appears in

the caricature by Reynolds,* with Mr Charles Turner, Mr Woodyeare and Dr Drake, and appears in Reynolds' list of sitters as Mr Cooke of Bedford Square, London, and that he was among the promoters of Charlemont's Academy, now becomes a character in thrall to Capri and unable to communicate with his erstwhile comrades.

The shadowy Abbé du Bois, who appears in the *Parody*, is engaged upon some literary work, to which Sir Thomas has given his interest.

Thomas Scrope is revealed as a gentle, perhaps insignificant looking young man, who has got himself into a pickle over an actress or opera singer, and through this we learn that the tourists are well received by the Princess Francavilla, so famous for her lavish entertainment.

But what is most interesting, and somewhat surprising, is the first hint of the contempt in which this set held his Neopolitan Majesty, whose passion for sport is depicted by Goya in his famous portrait of him as Charles III of Spain, with his fowling-piece in his hand and his dog at his feet. The portrait shows how apt was the nick-name given him by Richard Phelps[15] – Ram's Head, although his features had presumably become more accentuated by the years. Ward, of course, is implying that the great flight of quail had come between the king and his customary presence in Naples on Sunday for mass; an omission of duty to his people as much as to his church, which might be whispered of but not talked of openly.

The king took the keenest interest in the excavations at Herculaneum, conducted under his auspices, but in the opinion of many, and not only the Grand Tourists, without proper method. In poking fun at the irregularities of the dig, Ward was echoing the general consensus and probably was assured of a sympathetic ear from Charlemont, who as we know received from his Majesty the early volumes of *L'Antichita di Ercolana* and showed no interest in acquiring the consecutive volumes to complete the set.[16]

Finally there is the implication that Charlemont was unlikely to be languishing with only Bagot for company in Rome, but was likely to attend the Princess Borghese's *villeggiatura* at Frascati. The Princess's entertainments were famous and even more lavish than those of the Francavilla.

Ward's letter epitomizes for us the euphoria of the fellowship of the British Grand Tourists in Italy. It happens that it was written at the peak of Charlemont's fortunes and sadly it presages their decline.

* Now in the Rhode Island School of Design

Charlemont did not join his friends in Naples although he was to go there once more before he left Italy, a visit that is referred to by Lord Bruce in a letter dated August 1753. This visit was possibly made with the object of inspecting the progress of the building of Caserta, of which the foundation stone had been ceremoniously laid in January 1752.[17]

By the end of the summer, Charlemont's set in Rome were nearly all dispersed: Lord Bruce with his bearleader Mr Lipyeatt was travelling around Italy; Lord Tylney had gone to Florence where he was eventually to settle for the remainder of his life; Iremonger and Lethieullier, after visiting Paestum, a new departure for the Grand Tourists, had returned to Rome and then left for home, and only Thomas Scrope was to remain with Charlemont until 1754.

With nearly all his English friends departed a new phase began in Charlemont's life in Rome. Fresh flocks of English tourists came and went, but Charlemont seems to have given no more time to them than politeness dictated, and his life began to revolve in a very much more serious orbit.

The new phase began dramatically with a violent attack of that illness which was to dog Charlemont at intervals for the remainder of his life. We hear of this first from Russel in a letter to Howard, dated 20 September 1752. 'As the present time is the hot season ... we have no English gentlemen here except my Lord Charlemont, who has been extremely ill of a rheumatism, & is not yet recovered. Mr Cook & Sir Thomas Kennedy left this place yesterday on their way to Florence and Lucca, where it is reported is a great flock of English.'[18]

Hardy tells us of that illness and the friendship that developed through it with the Duc de Nivernois, who until then Charlemont had considered 'merely as an elegant gentleman, and one who carried the fashion, and the *bel air* of Paris, to the utmost extremity. But a nearer connection soon developed in him considerable erudition, a refined taste, soundness of judgement, and, far better than all, an excellent heart. Towards the end of autumn, and the close of 1753, Lord Charlemont was confined at Rome, by a long and very severe indisposition, during which the Duke paid him several visits, and soothed many a weary hour by the amenity and agreeableness of his conversation.'[19]

Hardy is not correct about the date, which he has confused with the ensuing illness of the following year, after the Duc de Nivernois's embassy to Rome had ended, but there is no reason to doubt his account. We do not have to seek far to find the source of their compatibility, in spite of all Charlemont's prejudices against the French. Louis Mancini de Nivernois was regarded by Charlemont as a Mancini of illustrious Roman connection and he chose to ignore the French side rather as an accident. Moreover Nivernois' poetical imitations of Virgil, Horace, Ovid, Ariosto and, above all, of Milton were close to Charlemont's heart. We find in his own library, a collection of Miltoniana and his own translations and variations upon the same classical and Italian poets.[20]

It is from Hardy too we learn of Charlemont's being kindly noticed by Cardinal Passionei, whom Hardy refers to as the librarian of the Vatican, although that appointment did not come until three years later. As a bibliophile he was legendary. He kept no catalogue of the immense collection (said to be 300,000 volumes) in his house in the Quirinal and made it a point of honour to know the exact place of every volume, every manuscript in his library. He came of the illustrious family of Fossembrene in Urbino and had behind him a distinguished diplomatic career. The courtly manners of this remarkable old gentleman were such that he dispensed with formality: visitors were not required to rise or doff their hats at his entrance and he treated those that shared his interests on equal footing. Among other eccentricities was his avowed hatred of the Jesuits, a pretended sympathy with the Jansenist movement, and the tolerant countenancing of Voltaire's atheism.

According to Hardy, Charlemont visited Passionei sometimes at Frascati. Visitors were lodged in cells, one-roomed dwellings scattered about the gardens among the shrubberies, and over the door of each a saint's name, which for the length of the visit, bestowed upon the visitor canonization. Hardy pleads ignorance as to whether Charlemont was enrolled in their calendar. But we know that amiability rather than holiness was the qualification, that the Cardinal had visitors of both sexes, and that Voltaire's friend Madame du Bocage was among his saints, and that in this state of blessedness, formal attire was disregarded. Guests assembled for dinner in the main building wearing shifts and slippers.

If Charlemont's lost essay on the years in Italy were ever found, we should hope for a detailed account of the regime at the villa on the hillside above the ruins of Cicero's villa at Tusculum overlooking the Roman plains, and perhaps a description of the garden. Also, since Hardy counts among Charlemont's eminent friends in Rome yet another Cardinal, the famous Allessandro Albani, it would be interesting to know more about a friendship which is not evident from such documentation as we possess, and through Albani a connection with Winckelmann.

Hardy's claim that 'that amiable, and, perhaps, that best of all Pontiffs, Benedict the 14th' paid Charlemont not only civility and attention, but regarded him 'with a kindness and benevolence that was almost parental' is likewise unsubstantiated. Nevertheless, we should remind ourselves that Hardy, who had access to papers no longer extant and had known Charlemont in person, was, apart from some minor dating errors, and an understandable partiality to his subject, very reliable.

It is likely when Charlemont had first arrived in Rome that he had been seized upon by Abbé Peter Grant and led off for an audience with the Pope. As we know Charlemont had dealings with Abbé Grant, as had the majority of English visitors to Rome. A representative of the Scots Mission and well-known to have Jacobite sympathies, he was nevertheless very popular with the Tourists. Over four decades he supplemented his income by acting as cicerone, running errands and generally making himself useful, to the detriment of his official duties and often in defiance of his bishop. Lady Mary Wortley Montagu described him in the 1730s as an honest North Briton, and as late as 1778 Henry Swinburne was taken by him to an audience with the Pope when the Abbé talked so much the Pope could barely get a word in.[21]

One may suppose that once the ceremony of kissing Benedict XIV's toe was over, Charlemont was encouraged by the Pope, with his great interest in antiquity, to speak of his travels and, Charlemont revealing himself to be a very agreeable as well as a very learned young man, made an impression to the extent that from time to time there was a kindly word or an enquiry after his health. But there may have been more. The Pope was the friend of Montesquieu, whom Charlemont went out of his way to visit at La Brède after he left Rome.

In Charlemont's papers we find one reference to the Pontiff and that not in the context of any personal relationship, but as a note to his observations on the *castrati* and self-mortification. The story is not for the squeamish. The incident occurred during Charlemont's time in Rome. An abbate in a frenzy of piety castrated himself and 'sent the spoils of his virility, in a gold box, to the Pope. Benedict received this strange present, surrounded by cardinals and prelates. Looking round on the attendant eminences and monsignori, he dealt with his and their embarrassment as wittily and good-humouredly as his reputation could have justified. '*Coglioni a me sciocco*' he exclaimed. '*Eh, non mancano cogliono.*'[22]

NOTES

1. Archivo del vicariato di Roma, State delle Anime S. Lorenza in Lucina 1752, 1753. Information kindly communicated by Sir B. Ford.
2. RIA, 12.R.12, no. 8, a note on the reverse in Adderley's hand reads 'Paid Barny's brother Taylor on account of Milord 5 gns'.
3. HMC, Rept. 12, App. pt. X, p. 184.
4. 2nd Earl Tylney (1712-84) of Wanstead, Surrey. From 1752 lived in Florence and Naples. See Ford & Ingamells *Dictionary of Travellers in Italy* pps. 959-90.
5. Chambers designed the Temple of Romulus and Remus for Scrope at Coleby Hall, Lincolnshire in 1762. See *Dictionary of Travellers in Italy* p. 844.
6. Baron Clonmore 1776, Viscount Wicklow 1785. *See Dictionary of Travellers in Italy* pps. 528-530.
7. Sergio Benedetti, The Milltown Exhibition, National Gallery of Ireland, 1997, pp. 48-9.
8. RIA, 12.R.20, no. 58.
9. His *Letters from a Young Painter Abroad* was published anon. 1748.
10. D. Sutton, 'The Roman Caricatures of Reynolds', *Country Life Annual*, 1956, p. 115.
11. Wicklow papers, National Library of Ireland, MSS Pc 227. Copies of Russel's letter to Howard are with the Paul Mellon Centre for Studies in British Art, London.
12. Ibid.
13. HMC Rept. 12, App. pt. X, p. 185 as 'apparently from Edward, Lord Howard'. The MS letter is clearly signed J. Ward, HMC, 12.R.12, no. 13.
14. RIA, 12.R.12, no. 9.
15. Ibid, 12.R.11, no. 4, Ailesbury (Bruce) to Charlemont, Aug. 28, 1779, 'Ram's head was the Name poor Phelps gave his Neopolitan Majesty'.
16. HMC, Rept.13, App. pt. VIII, p. 365. Charlemont to Ailesbury in an undated letter, 'I have first four volumes of the Herculaneum Antiquities, which were given me by his Neopolitan Majesty, whose munificense being exhausted stopped there'.
17. The State Archives Naples, C.R.A. fasc. 1257, 14 June 1753, entry of Charlemont with Murphy and Potter. Information kindly communicated by N. Figgis.
18. Wicklow Papers.
19. Hardy, pp. 29-30.
20. RIA 12.R. 1-4. Translations and a history of Italian poetry. *Select Sonnets of Petrarch* was published Dublin 1822.
21. B. Skinner, *Scots in Italy in the 18th Century*, Edinburgh 1966, p. 18.
22. RIA, 12.R.5, n. to p. 55.

13

GATHERING CLOUDS

Based in Rome throughout 1753, with all his English friends except Scrope departed, Charlemont would seem to have made very little contact with the fresh flocks of Tourists who crowded the city in January, among them the Lords North and Dartmouth and two Irish gentlemen, Mr Rochfort and Lord Lanesborough's son, Mr Brinsley Butler. Lord Bruce was still in Italy and wrote with faithful regularity from Florence, from Lucca and Siena, but showed no disposition, nor was he encouraged, to rejoin Charlemont in Rome. When Bruce left Italy in August for Germany, it was the beginning of the travels which would take him to Vienna, to Russia, Poland and Denmark, and then back across Europe to Spain and Portugal. He and Charlemont would not meet again until they returned to England.

It was Charlemont's last year in Rome, a year that is poorly documented, but as yet there was no talk of departure and Charlemont seems to have moved rather more than hitherto in Roman society. He was more active as a patron than formerly, if we are to judge from the many commissions to be attended to by Parker after Charlemont's eventual departure.

Hardy tell us, without specifying any date, 'Lord Charlemont was a kind benefactor to several young artists then at Rome. Sir William Chambers, whose fortune, at that time, was very limited and his friends, or acquaintance not many, he particularly distinguished, and was of signal service to him ...'[1]

This is particularly interesting because, although it is generally assumed that Charlemont first met his future architect in Italy some time between 1750 and 1754, no direct documentation of that meeting has been found. The links are many but the evidence circumstantial.

Research continues into Chambers' movements during his years abroad, but we do know that on 24 March 1753, while Charlemont was still a resident there, Chambers was married by a Church of England presbyter in Rome to Catherine Moore and that the witnesses were George Potter, James Murray, Abbé Grant and Colonel

J.H. Oughton.[2] Some curiosity is attached to two of the witnesses being Jacobites; James Murray was the personal physician of the Old Pretender and Abbé Peter Grant made no secret of his political sympathies. But it is the first witness, the obscure George Potter, who attracts our particular attention. A protégé of Charlemont, he was a familiar of the house in the Strada de la Croce, if not actually living there, and eventually he was to accompany Charlemont back to England.

Another close link between Chambers and Charlemont was Thomas Scrope, the last remaining member (apart from the later addition of Lord Pembroke), of Charlemont's original set in Rome. Scrope had pretensions to some talent as an amateur architect and was to recall to Chambers years afterwards, 'We are brother Genius's in the Architectural way; we viewed old Rome together and I remember your doing me the honour to ask my opinion on different subjects'.[3]

The young Earl of Pembroke did not arrive in Rome until the end of 1753, but he came as a neighbour and friend of Lord Bruce in Wiltshire. Probably he had already met Chambers. He had been at Siena with Bruce, Tylney and Mann in August and at the beginning of September, Chambers with Joseph Wilton and Simon Vierpyle were with Mann in Florence. Bruce, writing to Charlemont, recorded that Mann, Pembroke and Tylney had been with him at Siena and returned to Florence on the morning of 8 September.

By December, Chambers with Vierpyle was back in Rome and Lord Pembroke had arrived in the city to find in Charlemont a ready friend. Russel, writing to Howard, told him that Vierpyle had completed his commissions, two tables, six statues of gesso, a faun and an Apollo, and was now employed upon the *Fighting* and the *Dying Gladiator*, the former for Lord Charlemont and the latter for Lord Pembroke.[4]

In 1753, or maybe earlier, Charlemont acquired a bas-relief Venus by Guglielmo della Porta, and at the same time had a copy made of the relief *Antinous* in Cardinal Albani's collection. Both, as we know from Parker, were embedded into sculptured frames by Vierpyle. One of the few works heard of again from Charlemont's collection of sculpture, mostly dispersed and without trace, the Venus was, at the beginning of this century, recorded as being in the collections of the descendants of Francis Johnston, the Irish architect. Then it was described as a Venus by della Porta, dated 1512, set into an octagonal plinth decorated with panels of trophies, and a very poor photograph showed a pedestal in situ at Kilmore, Richill, Co. Armagh. With the sale of the 'Johnston Heirlooms', the Venus again disappeared and so we are unable to confirm what was then purported, that the plinth was designed by Sir William Chambers. If this was in fact so, it would be the strongest possible evidence for Charlemont's having met Chambers in Rome, and would have the added interest of being the first known work by Chambers for Charlemont.[5]

When, in 1759, Chambers' *Treatise on Civil Architecture* first appeared, the plans and elevations for the Casino took prominent place; but there were also designs inscribed to members of Charlemont's set in Rome, Lord Bruce, Lord Tylney, Lord Pembroke, Sir Thomas Kennedy and Mr Ward. Chambers could have met these gentlemen in England after his and their return, but it is much more likely that in inscribing the designs, he was paying tribute to the gentlemen who had noticed him in Rome or, in the case of Lord Tylney, through Mann in Florence.

Robert Adam, writing from Rome, 18 April 1754, was envious of Chambers' success, '... all the English, who have travelled for these five years are much prepossessed in his favour and imagine him a prodigy for genius, for sense and good taste ... he is in such great esteem, so intimate and in such friendship with most of the English that have been in Rome that they are determined to support him to the utmost of their power, amongst whom are Tylney, Huntingdon and others of great consequence and even reckoned of great taste'.[6]

It was shortly before Charlemont's departure from Rome, although Piranesi says earlier, that Piranesi approached Parker with the proposal of dedicating his forthcoming work, *Monumenti Sepulcralia,* to Charlemont. Charlemont, for all his interest in Roman antiquity and his reputation as a lover and patron of the Arts, was the one man in Rome who had seen the Greek monuments and was likely, if it came to the crunch, to be predisposed in their favour. Nevertheless, Piranesi had at his back the vast success of his *Opera Varie*, his reputation and standing in Rome, and was well under way to be able to flatter himself that he, not the patron, was conferring the favour. When all did not go smoothly and Charlemont was less accessible than his vanity would accept as his due, Piranesi's sense of grievance began slowly to fester, unobserved by Charlemont until the eruption came three years later.

The details of the notorious row have been many times discussed and published, starting with Piranesi's own account. Hardy, who might be supposed to have heard something of it from Charlemont himself, is ambiguous. 'Piranesi he [Charlemont] endeavoured to encourage, but that eminent artist was self-willed and often violent in his temper. He took something amiss of Lord Charlemont (what I know not, nor is it now of any consequence;) but, after he had dedicated three or four of his prints to his Lordship, he struck the name out, and inserted that of the two Adams's. Not content with that he published an abusive letter to Lord Charlemont; some copies were sold, and dispersed, before any one had heard of the quarrel; but several persons in authority at Rome were extremely angry with Piranesi, when they read his pamphlet, and he would have been treated with some severity, had not Lord Charlemont's usual good nature interfered. Piranesi made an apology, the pamphlet was suppressed at Rome, and the belligerent parties were again on amicable terms.'[7]

When we come, in due course, to investigate the ramifications of the above, we shall find that Charlemont himself took no action in the quarrel, apparently, as became a nobleman who finds himself unwittingly at the centre of a broil, aloof from the vulgarity of a common dispute. It has always been taken that Piranesi's accusations, directed at Parker, were an indirect indictment of Charlemont and that Piranesi, if in this instance alone, was politic, and careful to absolve Charlemont from all responsibility for the actions of his agents. As Craig succinctly puts it in *The Volunteer Earl*: 'His tone is similar to that of a political pamphleteer, who protests loyalty to a king while regretting that he is hoodwinked by his ministers.'[8]

So many of Piranesi's statements, as we shall find, are unreliable that even his partisans then, as today, are hard put to disentangle the threads of truth and reason from the skein of his fury. But what if Piranesi meant what he said, that Charlemont's agents kept the matter from him until it was beyond their control and, as Hardy says, Piranesi's abusive letter was published before anyone (Charlemont?) had heard of the matter? Then, if there was a villian of the piece, it would be honest Murphy, whose well intentioned efforts to spare Charlemont at a time of illness and crisis, were misdirected.

The exigences of Charlemont's situation at the beginning of the dealings with Piranesi have not been taken into account because so few facts are known about those months preceding his departure from Rome. Charlemont was again seriously ill in September but by

December Lord Bruce could write of his relief at hearing of his full recovery.

This would appear to be the second attack of that recurrent illness, from which Charlemont would suffer intermittently for the remainder of his life. It gave rise to a scandalous story, that his departure from Rome was 'hastened by a disorder contracted as is supposed from poison administered by the jealousy of a woman with whom he had an amorous intercourse'.[9]

On the surface at least, apart from this attack of rheumatism, all was well. If Charlemont was inaccessible to Piranesi, when he called repeatedly at the house in the Strada de la Croce with the designs for the dedication plates for his approval, Charlemont may have been indisposed or out on some other business.

It was about this time that he sat to Batoni for his two portraits (one of which only is known) and attended to the unfinished business with Vernet, that Charlemont had left to the eve of Vernet's departure for France. Vernet's book of *commandes* show that in 1751, at the height of his patronage by Leeson, Sir Matthew Fetherstonhaugh, Joseph Henry, Ralph Howard and Thomas Dawson, Charlemont had approached him for six paintings, but without specifications. The entries for 1753 record, with Charlemont's name immediately above Lord Pembroke, for whom Vernet was to paint '*un petit tableau*' that there was required for '*milord Charlemont quatre tableaux toile d'Empereur qui doivent representer les quatre parties du jour, en sujet de marines, le prix est de cents cinquante livres sterlins les quatres qui doivent m'être payés par Messrs. Sollicose et Crowe Banquiers à Marseille, à qui je dois remettre lesdits tableaux.*' There is no evidence of the delivery of this order, which seems to have been a revision or amplication upon the earlier vague commission of 1751.[10]

Charlemont continued to add to his collection of medals and visited Borioni, ostensibly to inspect new additions to the apothecary's collection, but also in the hope that Borioni would part with some treasure, which on occasion he was known to do.

Murphy, in one of his quaint letters to Charlemont, refers to Borioni. Written after Charlemont's return to Ireland, when Charlemont was in despair at his disagreeable situation, Murphy reveals himself as no stranger to these moods of black depression and exhorts Charlemont to bestir himself. 'Shake off that abominable Listlessness … Don't you remember how many anxious Minutes Borioni and Medals have saved you? Do: be a good Boy and busy yourself and I'll give my heads* off my shoulders if you be not soon a much more joyous youth.'[11]

Although Murphy continued to treat Charlemont as an orphaned child when he was a young man of twenty-six, he could scarcely have lived in close proximity with him for nine years without being aware of Charlemont's gallantry, and if not the number of his many dalliances at least something of his more serious amours or affairs. Charlemont need not have made a confidant of Murphy, but Murphy must have known that their abrupt departure from Rome was due to a crisis in one of Charlemont's love affairs.

We do not know what that crisis was. There is no evidence of a jealous woman administering poison, or as some said, a lovephilter. The only woman mentioned in the documents is the unidentified Magdalen (perhaps his nurse tender through his illness) for whom Charlemont arranged a pension to be paid by Parker. But we do know that Charlemont had a liaison with a Roman noblewoman,** and she is almost certainly the Roman marchesa, whose letters Charlemont, on his death bed, requested to be burnt with those of the Italian contessa he had loved and then left at Turin.

On the little evidence available, and Charlemont's denigration of cicisbeism as 'a dangerous practice', we are left to conclude that he had flouted the conventions and for the sake of the lady's reputation and his own peace of mind decided to quit Rome.

Earlier in 1753 a scandal involving Lord Tylney's brother, Joshua Child, had aroused wide-spread interest in England and in Italy. The matter was much discussed and there was a striking divergence of opinion between the two countries, and as a warning to Charlemont, and as an illustration for us of the conflicting points of view, the story is not entirely irrelevant here.

In February news came to Lord Tylney from England of 'the terrible accident that had happened'[12] to his brother. The family had long dreaded Mr Child's ruin through his association with Mrs Wymendfal, and began to believe him to be on the point of heeding the warnings, when the husband brought an action against Joshua Child for his criminal conversation with his wife, Henrietta, a daughter of Lord Luxborough, laying the charge for damages at twenty thousand pounds sterling.

* A reference to Vierpyle's copies of 78 busts of the Roman Emperors.

** Although there is no concrete evidence, it is tempting to assume that this was the Marchesa Gabrielli.

British circles in Italy were alarmed by the amount of Charles Wymendfal's claim, which even the vast incomes from the Wanstead estates could not easily bear, and hoped for Lord Tylney's sake he had secured the money.

Italian society was astonished. They could not understand a criminal case before the Court of the King's Bench at Westminster. They looked on the woman only to be at fault, and a more practical solution, the customary one of their own nation, was to confine an erring wife to a villa; or if the fault merited more than banishment to a country estate, to put her in a convent.

The outcome of the affair was, as it happened, less painful to Lord Tylney's resources than at first had been feared. Mr Child's criminal conversation cost two thousand five hundred pounds. The lady was divorced. Mr Child married her and, to spare the family any further embarrassment, took her abroad.

Charlemont was well received in Roman society or, as Hardy puts it, 'To mention the various persons of rank and estimation at Rome, to whom Lord Charlemont was well known, would be to give the names of the most respectable of the Roman or Neopolitan nobility'. In effect, that meant he moved in the circles of 'superior splendour' of the Princess Borghese, her daughter, Contessa Viani, of the Gabrielli, the Patrizzi, the Bolognetti and the Corsini.

Roman ladies were bored by young English gentlemen, even young noblemen, who did not speak their language fluently, but Charlemont, as Hardy wrote, was 'on that account, as well as the variety of his accomplishments, truly acceptable to all persons of rank and fashion ...'[13] A commoner, like Robert Adam for instance, seeking advice about an entrée, was told by Robert Wood, 'I do really think it will be rather a loss to you as an advantage, as you don't know the language and as it will surely consume your time in some degree as it will draw you into gaming which you don't know and must lose at'. And though an introduction to the Princess Borghese could be arranged and the answer would be that anybody Robert Wood brought would be extremely welcome, there would still be his own countrymen who would be the readiest to put him out 'as they did to a gentleman of above £5000 a year because his father, who was dead, was a brewer in London'.[14] In this context the Leesons can be seen at a disadvantage.

Whatever the cause of Charlemont's hastened departure, his wavering course, as he moved restlessly between Turin and Florence during the early months of 1754, reflected his state of indecision. His

Irish correspondents, Marlay and Adderley, were in some perplexity as to where to direct their letters, but only Marlay seems to have thought he might return to Rome.

His Roman correspondents were better informed. Charlemont's propensity for helping lame dogs over stiles brought him in touch with many whimsical characters and, judging from a letter written to him at Turin from George Potter in Rome, Potter must have been one of the oddest and fondest of his creatures.

The letter is not quite so odd if one is familiar with the idiom; Lady Mary Wortley Montagu wrote to a recalled ambassador in similar vein. 'Your Excellency is dead, but as I do not doubt it is only a removal to a better life, I ought rather to congratulate than condole.'[15] The implications of Potter's letter are more difficult to interpret. Are we to understand that Charlemont's retreat from Rome with Murphy, his servant Barny and Badine, his favourite whippet bitch, constituted no defeat or rout but a noble action?

Potter wrote, 'My dear Lord, Be it known to you that you are dead and that I ought to be in Mourning for you, but I will not indulge you so far, as I am not sorry you are departed *this life*. This *here world* deserv'd you no longer. I regret no soul that I leave behind me, but I envy one that had the happiness to quit this vale of misery before me. Now at Death's Door; let the words of a dying man have some weight with you, and believe me that it is no Affectation in me to declare this kind of Death has, for me, no terrours, and that I would not give a sixpence to live here longer. What gives me boldness in these my last moments is that I have Hopes to be again joined in blessed Immortality to those I loved in *this here world*.

'However I have not been in this lower World so incurious a spectator as not to observe some kind of difference of Merit among the People that Fate has thrown in my way. Let us then judge of men by the most critical point in Nature (that of their Death). Some men went off like the snuff of a tallow candle: but I, who have a good nose, smelt you out, and you died *en odeur de Saintité*. I have therefore already made you a Saint *in petto* and when I find two others of equal merit I will publicly declare you one; but I know you intend to disappoint me, and throw men to the Distance they ought to keep.'

'... My dear Lord, I love Murphy for his own intrinsic worth, but I love Mr Barny, because he belongs to you and I love Badine because I always called her my own.

'I could write you an account of an affair that would make you laugh but I have tears in my eyes always when I think of you. I have prevented a duel that was never intended to be fought between Lloyd and Mitchell. The Event was that one behaved like a linnen Draper and the other like a Woolen Draper. Make my good friend Murphy write to me.

Yours sincerely, George Potter'[16]

Whereas Potter directed his letter to Charlemont at Turin, Abbé Grant's of 30 April was addressed to Florence, for Mr Mann to hold for my Lord Charlemont. Charlemont was again on his way south. It is evident that he had already been in correspondence with Peter Grant about Potter, referred to by Grant as 'our friend George'. George Potter was still in Rome. 'The only impediment to his leaving this place was the emptyness of his purse', Grant reported. He had given George to understand that, although far from being a wealthy man, he, Grant, had friends and credit, for which George returned him 'infinite Thanks' and 'many fine speeches' and had agreed to go that very day with Mr Scrope to Frascati for three or four days before he went off, leaving his servant in the meantime to get in all the accounts he owed. This the fellow had done. The debts amounted to about two hundred and twenty crowns in all but 'I am hopeful to chop off at least 10 crowns and satisfy his creditors with 210, which added to the 30 sequins your Lordship is so good as to allow him over and above, make in all the sum of 270 crowns, which I have this very afternoon received from Mr Parker having judged it better for the sake of secrecy to make use of him, rather than of Belloni or Abbé Wilkins directly.'[17]

'George' had given Grant his word that he would get out of Rome on Tuesday or Wednesday next, along with Mr Scrope, and take the route of Tuscany. Scrope intended to proceed from Siena to Genoa, but George's servant, interrogated by the Abbé, had acquainted him that his master intended leaving Scrope at Siena and proceeding to Florence. From 'this piece of intelligence', Grant forecast George would soon 'be beating up at your Lordship's quarters'. But this was not all of Potter's troubles. He might yet be answerable for 50 pounds to Belloni on two bills of 25 pounds each; the first, drawn towards the end of January, on being presented in England, had been rejected. Until Abbé Wilkins, Belloni's clerk, heard further from London, he refused to hand out any more money for bills. It was upon this first refusal that Grant had begun to discover that melancholy in George, mentioned in a letter to Charlemont, two posts earlier.

The story of George Potter, as far as we know it, ends happily.

Robert Wood, writing from Rome to Charlemont in London, in January 1755, sent his respects and compliments to Murphy and Potter.[18]

Somewhere along the route of Charlemont's retreat he had met Wood, who was bearleading the young Duke of Bridgewater, and Wood had become Charlemont's confidant. Wood had advised his not returning to Rome, and had undertaken to explain the reasons when he had reached Rome, and delivered Charlemont's letter and messages to the lady. Wood's letter of January 1755 is sufficiently discreet as to give no hint of her identity except that she moved in the most elite circles and that he believed her worthy as well as beautiful and her character unjustly maligned.

Meanwhile every inducement was being made to persuade Charlemont to return home. Adderley was kept posted by Murphy, who may have intimated the need for some greater incentive. At any rate on 5 June 1754 Adderley wrote to Charlemont of 'having built a house at Donneycarny in the opinion of all who have seen it not inferior to any near Dublin either with respect to situation, taste or convenience' and his hope that 'your Lordship will in a most particular manner honour & oblige me by yr acceptance of it'.

On the face of it the offer was extraordinarily generous. 'I must once more request & entreat your Lordship will be pleased to make me very happy in complying with the favour I ask: it will add greatly to the many unmerited obligations your Lordship has already conferred on me'. Adderley wished he could say the land was free, but there was a reserved rent of a hundred pounds a year, which to a common farmer it was worth, and it could be expected to mow 350 load of hay off the 17 acres, sufficient for Charlemont's horses.[19]

Charlemont, without having seen the house, would have known the situation, which commanded a splendid prospect over the city and Dublin Bay to the Wicklow mountains beyond, a site which inspired thoughts of building and additions to the tiny estate. A further inducement in Adderley's eyes was a gallery in the house, 72 feet by 20, large enough for 'yr whole collection of curiosities'. About this Charlemont almost certainly, even at this early stage, had very different ideas. His acceptance of the offer was taken by Adderley as an indication that at last he was about to turn his face towards home. On 11 October Adderley wrote acknowledging 'the honour your Lordship has been so good to confer on me'. On Murphy's advice he directed the letter '*Alla locanda de Signor Carlo Hattfield in funduccio di Santa spirito*', with a covering note to Hatfield that in Charlemont's absence he should forward the letter to Paris.

The decision having been made, Charlemont began again to act with purpose. His new course took him to Vicenza, where early in September he and Murphy were seen by Matthew Brettingham jun. measuring up the Rotonda. This could be dismissed as a purely academic exercise, had not Charlemont written to Parker about this time instructing him to apply to Luigi Vanvitelli for designs for a building described by Vanvitelli as a *palazetto abitabile*.

As it happened the letter Parker wrote to Vanvitelli on 10 October 1754 was not received by him until at least six months later, and Vanvitelli did not reply until 4 July. He directed his letter to Monsieur Jean Parker, *fameux peintre,* Cafe Inglese in Piazza di Spagna, Rome and gave explicit directions as to how he, himself, should be correctly addressed, '*a Luigi Vanvitelli Arch*^{to}, *Ingeg*^{re} *di Corte e Dirett*^{re}, *Generale delle fabriche di Caserta, Capua per Caserta*'. Yes, it would be possible for him very soon to do the drawings, plans, elevation and section for the *palazetto abitabile* desired by the Irish cavaliere. He would apply all his skill and diligence and once the plans were done, he would communicate with Parker so that payment of 100 zecchini could be lodged with some secure merchant or banker at Naples, to whom on receipt of that sum, he would consign the drawings.[20]

By the time Charlemont had heard from Parker of Vanvitelli's 'exorbitant demand', he had seen the little estate of Donneycarny and was contemplating other ideas.

How seriously Charlemont considered the Rotonda we are not told, nor if this journey took him to Venice, but notes and an appendix to his *Essays on Italian Literature* tell us of his visit to Marchese Scipione Maffei at Verona (erroneously recalled by him as possibly in 1756).

Maffei was already very old (he died at the age of 80 on 11 February 1755) but still 'healthy and vigorous'. He lived in retirement in a very pretty palace, where, according to Lady Mary Wortley Montagu, he delighted in receiving young people for discussion and classical instruction. He would set them upon a hunt through his cabinets of medals and antiquities to find those items most appropriate to the date and illustration of the subject under discourse. There was a hall for debate, a main gallery and a library, but also a room for dancing and for cards, although gambling was forbidden.

On Charlemont's arrival at Verona, he was immediately 'with the most condescending Politeness, invited to his house'. Among the many favours Maffei conferred on him, he had 'the unmerited Honour of assisting at an Academy, which met there weekly under his auspices – The Assembly consisted of the principal Literati of the City and its nai'bourhood, many of whom brought with them Essays upon various Subjects, written during the previous Week, which were read to the Society, and not only learnedly, but impartially criticized, a Trial which the Authors seemed to expect'.

At his departure, Charlemont was presented by Maffei with 'a quarto Edition of his *Merope,* together with Translations of the same into French and into English, a Token of his Goodness towards me which I preserve as an invaluable treasure, especially as it is in many places corrected by his own Hand'.[21]

NOTES

1. Hardy, p. 27.
2. J. Harris, *Sir William Chambers*, London 1970, p. 6, n. 15.
3. R.I.B.A. CHA. Box 2, Journal, p. 5.
4. Wicklow papers.
5. R.M. Young, *Belfast and the Province of Ulster*, Pike Century Series 1909, pp. 224-5.
6. Fleming, p. 160.
7. Hardy, p. 28.
8. Craig, p. 86.
9. *Public Characters of 1798*, Dublin, p. 180.
10. L. Lagrange, *Les Vernets, Joseph Vernet et la Peinture au XVIIIe siècle,* 1864, see *Commandes* and *Recus*, p. 335 & 339, entry nos. 155 & 156.
11. HMC Rept. 12, App. pt. X, p. 221, 'Don't you remember how many anxious Minutes Borioni and Medals have served you?' For *Served* read *Saved* as in the MS letter RIA 12.R.12, no. 22.
12. Walpole Correspondence, Vol. 20 pp. 355-6.
13. Hardy, p. 26.
14. Fleming, pp. 148-9.
15. R. Halsband ed. *Select Letters of Lady Mary Wortley Montagu*, London, 1970 p. 298 when in 1761 James Stuart Mackenzie, Lord Bute's brother, was recalled from Turin.
16. RIA, 12.R.12, no. 14.
17. Ibid, 12.R.9, no. 15.
18. RIA 12.R.9, no. 75, postscript to letter pub. HMC Rept. 12, App. pt. X, pp. 199-200.
19. HMC Rept. 12, App. pt. X, pp. 196-7.
20. RIA 12.R.9, no. 35.
21. RIA 12.R.3, n. to p. 375 & 12.R.4., p. 353.

14

THE JOURNEY HOME

It seems that Charlemont's first intention was to go by way of Lyons straight to Paris, but there was a change of plan. Letters awaiting him at Lyons were sent on to Paris by a M. Claude Tolozan (perhaps his host there in 1749 when Charlemont was on his way to Turin), who assured him any more that came would be promptly despatched to Paris to await his Lordship's arrival there. He and Madame Tolozan, who sent a thousand compliments, often talked of Milord. She was impatient for news of Charlemont's whippet, and a happy outcome to the impending accouchement.[1]

Instead it seems he sailed for Spain, maybe taking with him Murphy if not Potter, Barny and the pregnant whippet (Badine?). At Genoa he stood for the last time on Italian soil. The only reference to Genoa among all his papers is to the foolish and dangerous practice of ciscisbeism, 'which however it may be sometimes perverted, and from natural propensity must always be dangerous, is undoubtedly founded upon the chastest and most innocent ideas'. He continues 'While I was at Genova, a Lady of the highest Rank and of immense Fortune, was married to the representative of the Balbi Family, one of the most noble and ancient of the Republick and was allowed by her Marriage Settlement, among sundry other stipulated Advantages, two coaches for her Cicisbees; That is to say, a public and expensive conveyance for eight Gentlemen under this Denomination, who were to attend in her train wheresoever she went. Wou'd such a contract on the part of her Husband, or indeed of the Wife, have been possible if anything of we call gallantry had been understood by Cicisbeism?'[2]

Apparently an impersonal note on Italian manners and probably written many years later, the conclusion must always have been the same: it was a dangerous custom. But Charlemont, even while his own experiences were painfully fresh in his mind, could not fail to have been amused by Lord Bruce's account, written in July of the same year from Lisbon, of how matters were so differently conducted there, 'No Portugese women are allowed to speak to any Men except their Husbands, and very nearest Relations, all Cousins are excluded; for the jealous fool who finds his wife talking with another Man looks upon it as the same thing as if he had found them in bed together. The Moors [?] here have much more liberty than married women.'[3]

Lord Bruce had followed the route Charlemont had taken along the south coast of France as far as Barcelona, and made use of the many hints Charlemont had given him for that itinerary, but from Barcelona Bruce had continued on through Spain to Portugal. Charlemont, having 'an ardent desire of seeing and knowing' the great philosopher, Charles de Secondat, Baron Montesquieu, procured his passport for France and turned his face towards Bordeaux.

Charlemont having seen the Roman ruins at Nimes, Bruce evidently thought it unnecessary to comment upon the amphitheatre, Maison Carrée and the Pont du Gard, but the inconvenience of travelling in Spain (a country not as yet frequented by the Tourists) was all he had been led to expect, he wrote Charlemont, and the collection of virtu at the Escorial exceeded all he had imagined. Later from Lisbon, he wrote, 'Mafra, a Convent built by the late King for Franciscan Friars (about thirty miles from thence) ... is well worth seeing: the Church, particularly the Dome part of it, is one of the most elegant pieces of architecture that I ever saw.'[4]

Somewhere along the way, Charlemont met 'the excellent Mr Elliott', the source of all the ridiculous stories about Philip Stanhope, having in his childhood shared the tutelage of Mr Harte. Charlemont in his account of their visit to the ageing Montesquieu, testified to the more serious side of Eliot's character. 'A gentleman of Cornwall, whose excellent understanding, cultivated and improved by the best education, and animated by a mind of the most pleasing cast, rendered him the most agreeable of companions.'

On arrival at Bordeaux they were greatly disappointed to hear Montesquieu was not there and had gone to reside at a country seat four or five hours distant. There was long deliberation as to what they had best do, and, finally determining upon a 'bold stroke', and putting aside 'timidity, perhaps propriety', they sat down and composed a joint letter, giving their reasons for coming to Bordeaux, telling of their sad disappointment and their eager wishes for the honour of his acquaintance. They begged to wait upon him at his villa.

They had not long to wait and when the answer came it was favourable. 'The first appointment with a favourite mistress' could not have rendered their night more restless; they were up before dawn and out so early that they arrived at La Brede before Montesquieu had risen. A servant showed them into the library.

A book lay open upon a table, turned down beside an extinguished lamp, 'Eager to know the nocturnal studies of this great philosoper, we immediately flew to the book; it was a volume of Ovid's works, containing his elegies, and open at one of the most gallant poems of that master of love.' Before they could overcome their surprise, the President entered and 'instead of a grave, austere philosopher, whose presence might strike with awe such boys as we were' the person who now addressed them was 'a gay, polite, sprightly Frenchman', who, after a thousand genteel compliments and thanks for the honour they had done him, desired to know if they would not breakfast. Having eaten at an inn not far from the house, they declined his offer, whereupon, as the day was fine he suggested they walk, and he would show them his villa, which he had endeavoured to lay out in the English taste.

Following him into the farm, they soon arrived at the outskirts of a beautiful wood, 'cut into walks and paled round, the entrance to which was barricadoed with a moveable bar, about three foot high, fastened with a padlock'. Montesquieu, searching in his pocket and not finding the key, thought it not worthwhile to wait, they could leap as well as he could and 'this bar shall not stop me' he said, and running at the bar fairly jumped over it. They followed him 'with amazement, though not without delight,' to see the philosopher likely to become their playfellow, and indeed this had the effect Montesquieu probably intended. Charlemont and Eliot lost their 'awkward humility' and the conversation became as free and easy as if they had been his equal in years.

The discourse turned on matters of learning and taste, and the Baron asked about the extent of their travels. When he heard of Charlemont's voyage, he fixed his attention particularly upon him and questioning him, lamented his own fate which had prevented him from seeing these curious regions. '"However", said he, "I, too, have been a traveller and have seen the country in the world which is most worthy our curiosity – I mean England."'

He told them of all the civilities he had received there. No country produced 'so many great and shining characters as England' nor as many 'singular ones'. The very eccentric Duke of Montagu, under the pretext of it being the custom to thus introduce ambassadors, had him ducked over head and ears in a tub of cold water and, though at the time Montesquieu had thought it odd, he had felt it incumbent upon him to take the world as he found it and submitted gracefully.

Having seen the farm and the gardens imitated from the English style, they returned to the house. They were received most politely by Madame la Baronne and her daughter in the drawingroom. Madame was elderly and apparently never handsome. The daughter was 'a sprightly, affable, good-humoured girl, rather plain, but, at the same time, pleasing'. The president's secretary joined them as they sat down to a 'plain and plentiful' dinner. He spoke nothing but French, but, as they afterwards discovered, he was an Irishman and Charlemont and Eliot thought how 'disagreeably trapped' they could have been in their private conversations had they said anything except in praise of the President, which, of course, they were not inclined to do. It was only on their way back to Bordeaux, when the secretary was escorting them, that he declared himself Charlemont's countryman.

At Montesquieu's insistence, Charlemont and Eliot stayed for three days. Throughout their visit his conversation continued 'as sprightly, as instructive, and as entertaining as possible'. Although he was still styled President, he had lately resigned his judicial office in opposition to a plan, whereby the streets of Bordeaux were to be 'laid out in the most sumptuous manner, of great breadth, and in lines directly strait', but without any consideration for the owners of houses, gardens and vineyards that stood in the way, and with no fixed indemnification, so that hundreds were to be ruined to make Bordeaux the most magnificent city in France.

In some discussion on Irish politics, the President advocated a union between Ireland and England, which he believed would be to Ireland's advantage. It was a move that Charlemont came in later years to detest, and to resist as vehemently as Montesquieu had the new advantages to Bordeaux.

After staying at Bordeaux 'a competent time' Charlemont and Eliot parted, and Charlemont set out on a course for Paris, where he found Montesquieu had arrived ahead of him. Montesquieu came several times to see him and they met frequently in company. The President was as lively, as polite, as sprightly as ever, but Charlemont did notice he seemed a little absent-minded at dinner with the British Ambassador, Lord Albemarle. Being engaged in a warm dispute, though never carried beyond the bounds of good-breeding, he was so intent upon the controversy, he gave back seven clean plates to the servant behind, apparently unaware he had not used them.

As Charlemont came to leave Paris, Montesquieu fell sick and, although Charlemont left him with infinite regret, it did not occur to him that the illness would be fatal. Soon after Charlemont's arrival in England, word came from Paris of the President's death. There were stories of his having been tormented by priests and asking for a few minutes to himself; he had lived long enough to know how to die. Charlemont was certain he was not a 'papist'; and Madame de Montesquieu, he knew, was of the reformed religion.

It is not easy to assess the accuracy of Charlemont's account of the philosopher in that last year of his life. Others told of Montesquieu being nearly blind and not nearly as lively as Charlemont related (or rather, as quoted by Hardy from the missing manuscript, although we have no reason to doubt Hardy's transcription).[5]

During Charlemont's stay in Paris he renewed his friendship with the Duc de Nivernois, who presented him to his father, the Duc de Nevers, and also to a number of distinguished academicians, among them the Marquis de Mirabeau, the political economist, father of the great Mirabeau; and the hedonistic philosopher and man of letters, Claude Arien Helvetius. Entertained by the Comte d'Argenson, to whom Diderot and d'Alembert dedicated their *Encyclopédia*; and the Duc de Biron, Charlemont was introduced to polite society and saw, for the first time at the Duke of Albemarle's, Count Poniatowski, whose manners fascinated him, *les manières nobles* of the future King of Poland.

But, at times, Parisian society shocked him. That ladies of fashion should talk before gentlemen of the natural functions of the body surprised him, and he found distasteful 'the painted and powder'd Dolls' who filled the front rows of the boxes at the Opera.[6]

He had some doubts, too, about business methods in Paris. Adderley had trouble over one of Charlemont's bills and suspected Selwyn the banker of not having acted scrupulously! There had also been the business of a Vernis Martin snuff box Charlemont had ordered a year before from Rome, and although M. Tiron the Paris goldsmith seemed to be blameless, it was thought there had been carelessness, if not dishonesty, on the part of Mr Woolf and Selwyn in their handling of the transaction.[7]

With no further desire to linger, Charlemont was in London when Adderley, from Paris, received a letter from Lord Tylney's brother Joshua Child. It was in reply to a letter written by Adderley under Charlemont's instructions, perhaps because Charlemont felt it would be indelicate for him to deal directly in a money matter with Child himself. Charlemont had almost certainly met Child in Paris, where he now resided, married to the lady who was the cause of 'the accident'. Child was much in vogue for having introduced to the Parisians what Horace Walpole called the '*fureur des cabriolets*', the English one-horse chairs that the French drove everywhere about Paris. They even had cabriolets embroidered on their stockings and painted upon their waistcoats. Child's letter was date-lined Paris 25 February 1755.

'Sir, Till the receipt of yours last post I never heard that Lord Charlemont had any inclination to my saddle Horses, and was quite unacquainted with my groom having accompany'd his Lordship the first post from Paris, it is from that on my buying 4 Coach Horses of Ld Euston I told my Groom that I would dispose of my saddle Horses not having sufficient stabling for them all, but I am much surprised he should have offer'd them for 70 Louis deliver'd in London, as it was a liberty I never gave him, besides which he knows I refused a greater sum for them here sometime ago; however the difficulty I am put to for stable room has determined me to part with my Grey Horse for 40 Louis and my Bay for Thirty, if I sell them separately, or if I dispose of them the two together Sixty Five Louis, so that if it is agreeable to Lord Charlemont to have them at that price I will deliver them sound here at Paris, into the hands of any person his Lordship shall direct immediately on receipt of his answer. I have only to add Mrs Child's and my compliments to Lord Charlemont and yourself, J. Child.'[8]

Charlemont was on the look out for saddle horses, the scarcity in Dublin being so great Adderley had informed him that 'very indifferent cattle bear an exorbitant price',[9] however one concludes that following so stiff a letter, no deal was made and all we know is that Charlemont and Lord Tylney's friendship continued as before.

There were coach horses, which if Charlemont would accept, Adderley would deem it an honour; there was family plate and sufficient linen. But appearances had to be kept up and some formality had to be attached to Charlemont's homecoming, although, with so little pleasure did he look forward to his return, that he lingered for five months before bringing himself to cross the Irish sea and this without any idea of what disagreeable times were there in store for him.

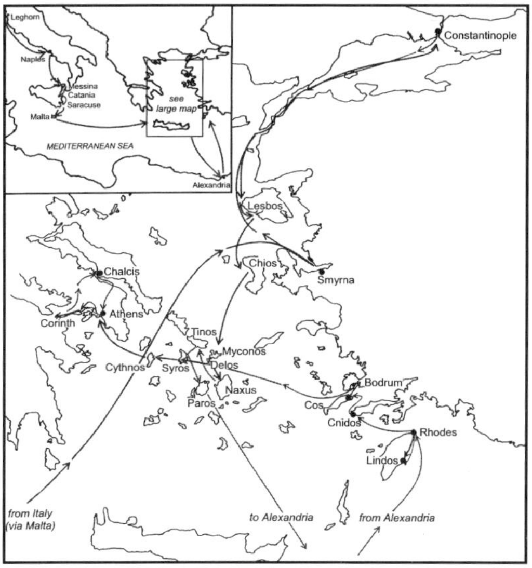

The Voyage of L'Aimable Vainqueur
Department of Geography, University College, Dublin

The friezes from the Mausoleum in the castle of the Knights at Bodrum
Travels in Asia Minor, Society of Dilettanti, 1775

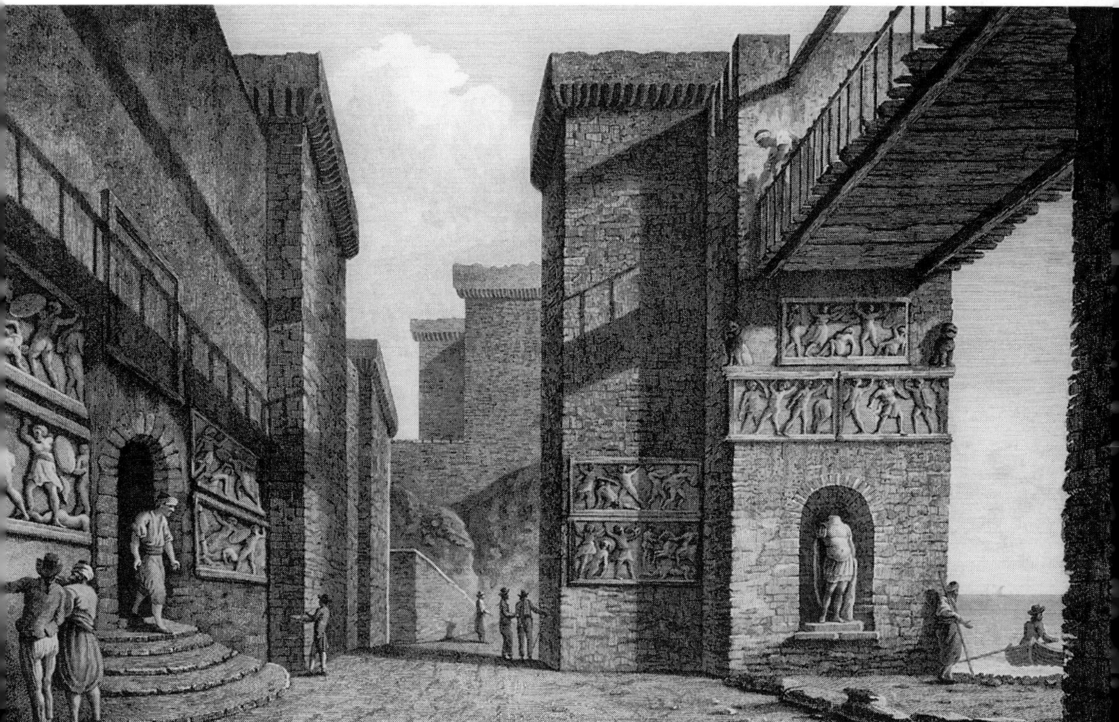

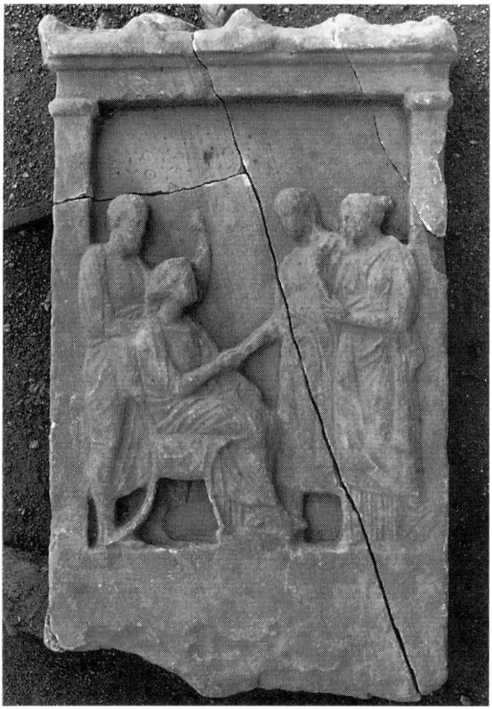

Attic Stele, mid 4th c. B.C. as found in the grounds at Marino before restoration
Photograph John O'Connell

Johann Heinrich Müntz's 'Plan of the Egyptian Room at Marino'.
The Lewis Walpole Library, Farmington, Conn.

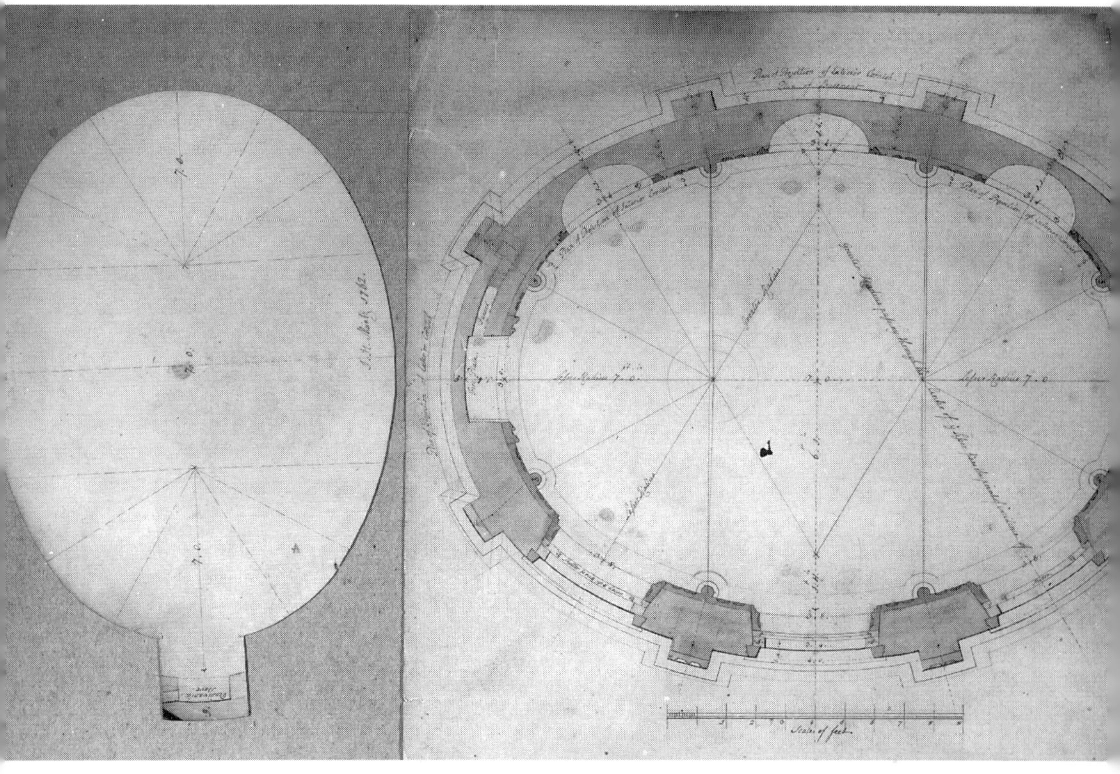

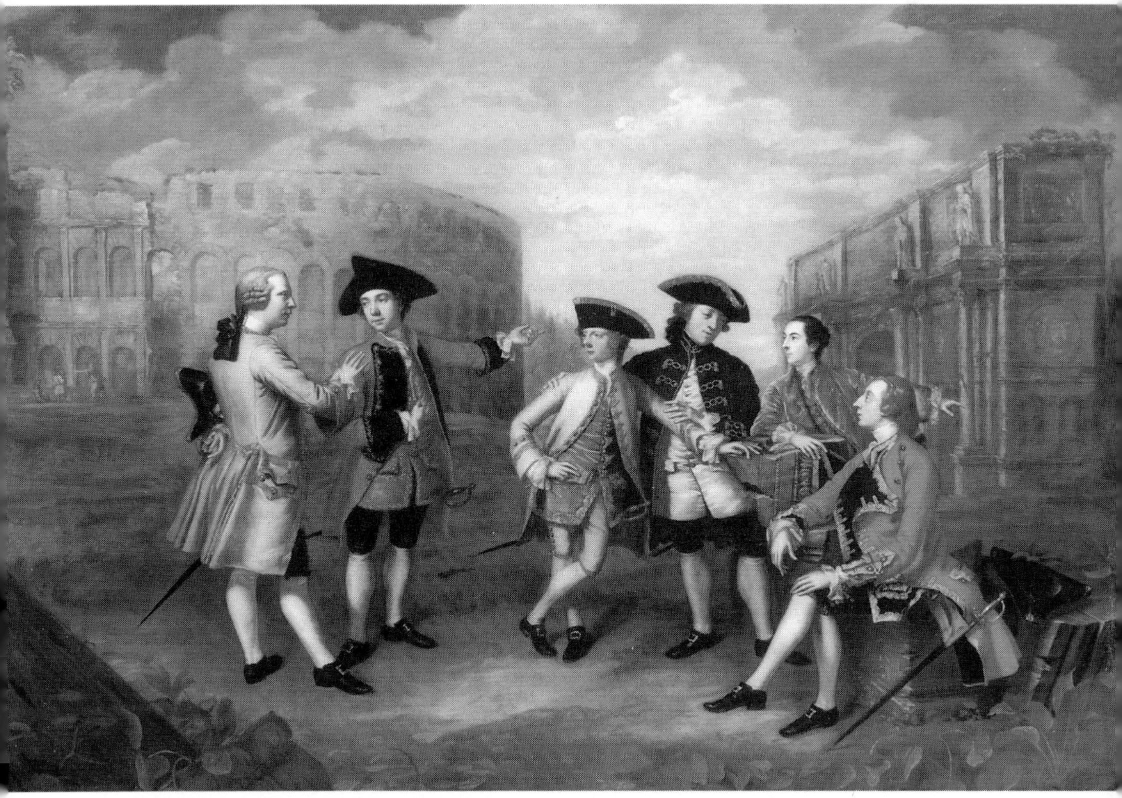

British School of Connoisseurs in Rome *c.* 1750 (Figures identified by Sergio Benedetti)
l. to r. Sir Thomas Kennedy, Lord Charlemont, Sir Charles Turner, Sir William Lowther, Thomas Steavens and Lord Bruce
Yale Center for British Art, Paul Mellon Collection

J.H. Müntz's Section of an Egyptian Room designed for Lord Charlemont
Courtesy of the Lewis Walpole Library, Farmington, Conn.

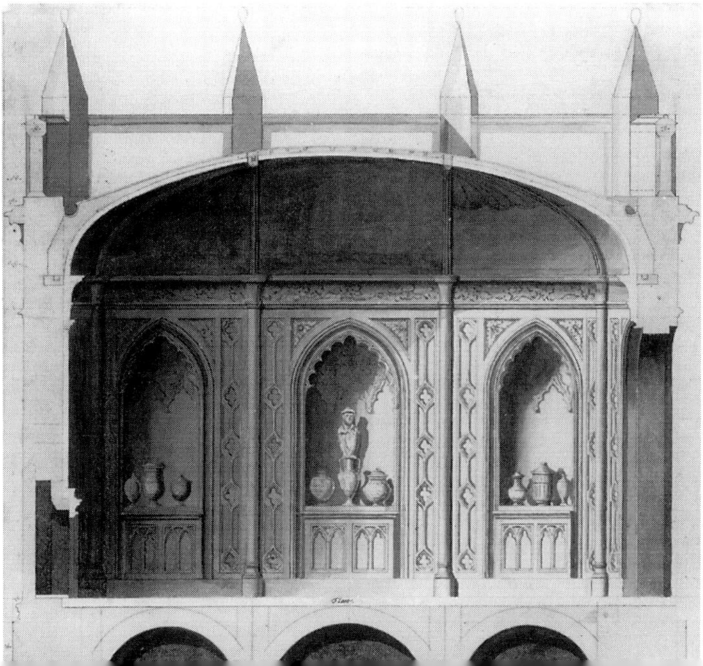

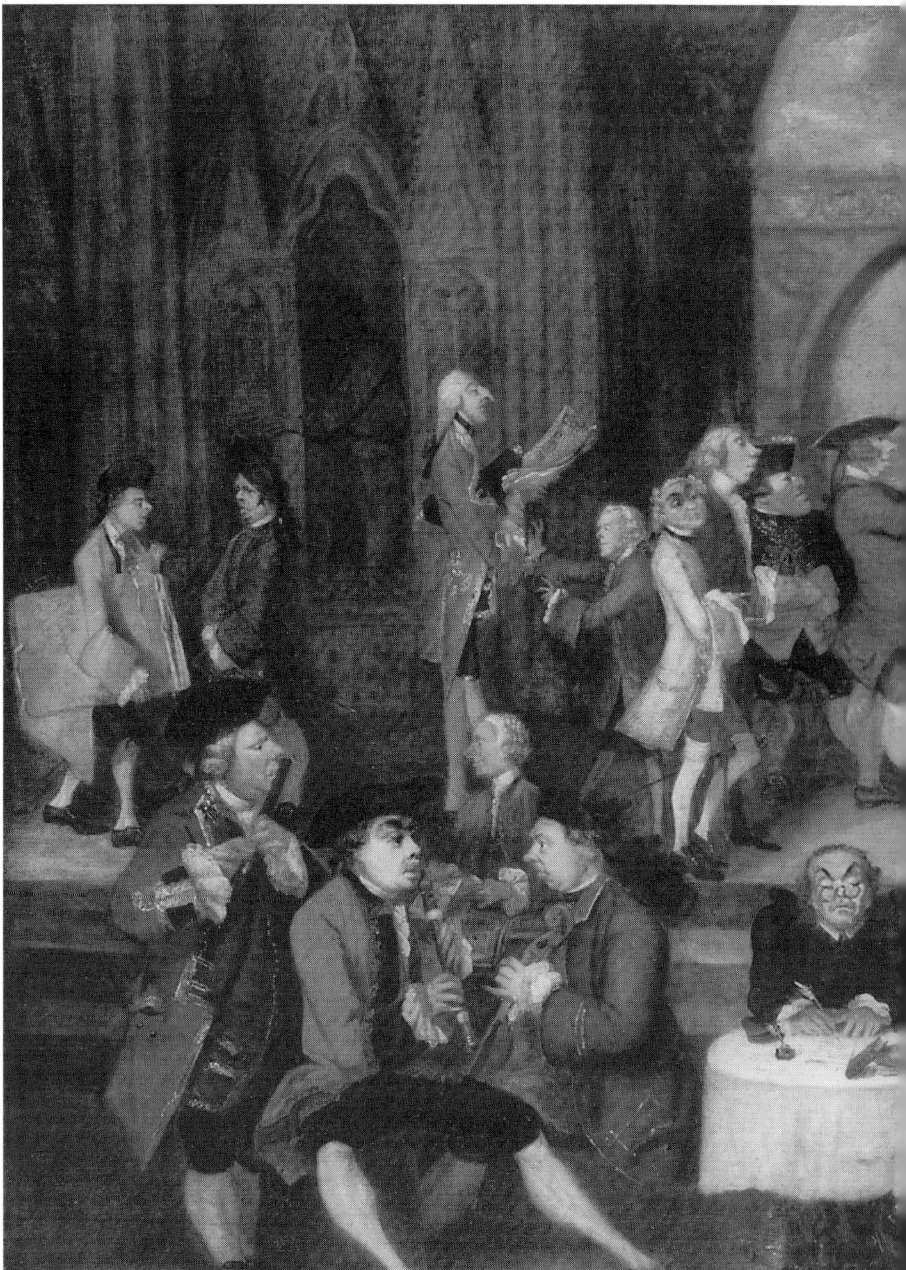

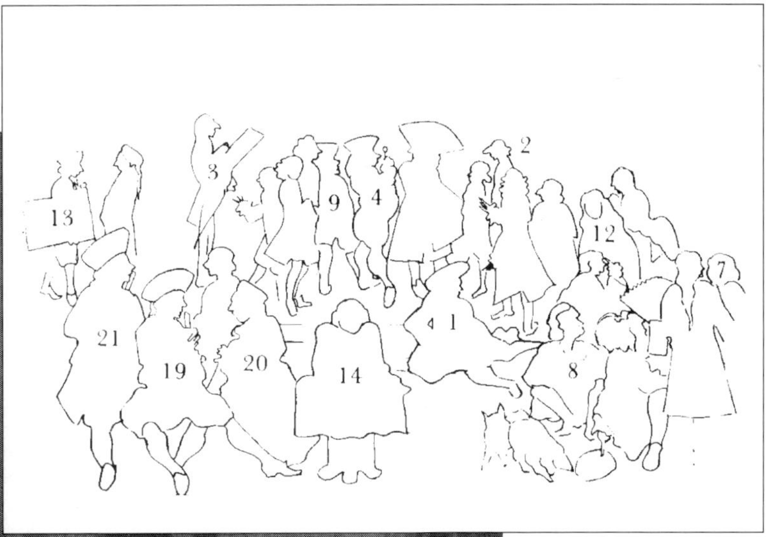

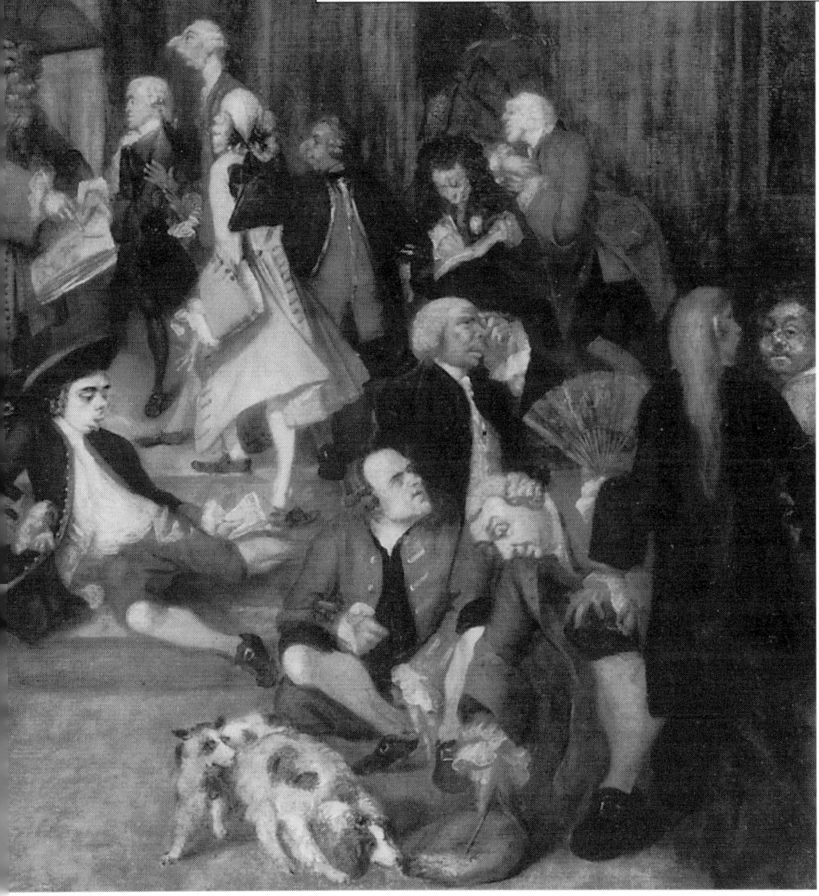

Reynolds' *The Parody of the School of Athens*
Courtesy of The National Gallery of Ireland

Key to diagram (above): Numbers are in order of Reynolds' list of sitters. 1. Henry as Diogenes. 2. Leeson junior, a follower of Aristotle. 3. Bruce as Alexander the Great. 4. Leeson senior as Plato. 9. Lowther, a follower of Plato. 19. Charlemont as Pythagoras with 20. Phelps and 21. Kennedy. Possibly Patch is 7, Vierpyl 8, du Bois 12, Brettingham 13 and Murphy 14

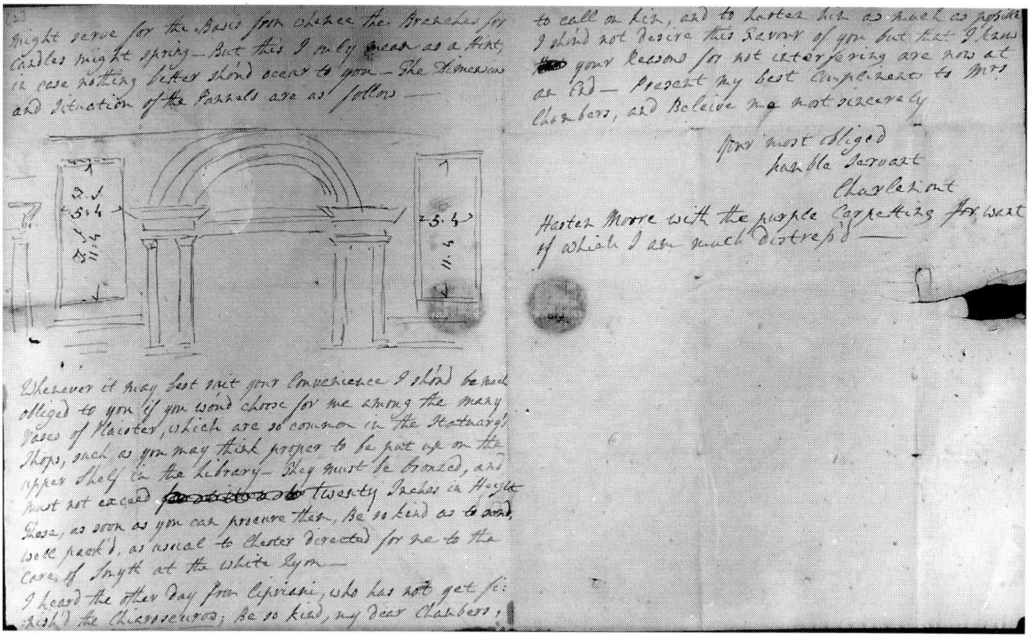

might serve for the Basis from whence the Branches for Candles might spring — But this I only mean as a Hint, in case nothing better shou'd occur to you — The Dimensions and Situation of the Pannels are as follow —

Whenever it may best suit your Convenience I shou'd be much obliged to you if you wou'd choose for me among the many Vases of Plaister, which are so common in the Statuary's Shops, such as you may think proper to be put up on the upper Shelf in the Library — They must be Bronzed, and must not exceed ~~[illegible]~~ twenty Inches in Height. These, as soon as you can procure them, Be so kind as to send, well pack'd, as usual to Chester directed for me to the Care of Smyth at the White Lyon —
I heard the other day from Cipriani, who has not yet finish'd the Chiaroscuros; Be so kind, my dear Chambers, to call on him, and to hasten him as much as possible I shou'd not desire this Favour of you but that I know ~~[illegible]~~ your Reasons for not interfering are now at an End — Present my best Compliments to Mrs Chambers, and Believe me most sincerely

Your most obliged
humble Servant
Charlemont

Hasten Moore with the purple Carpetting for want of which I am much distress'd —

Detail of an undated letter from Charlemont to Chambers re Charlemont House
Courtesy of Royal Irish Academy, Dublin

Elevation of Medal Cabinet with instructions from Chambers
Courtesy of Christie's

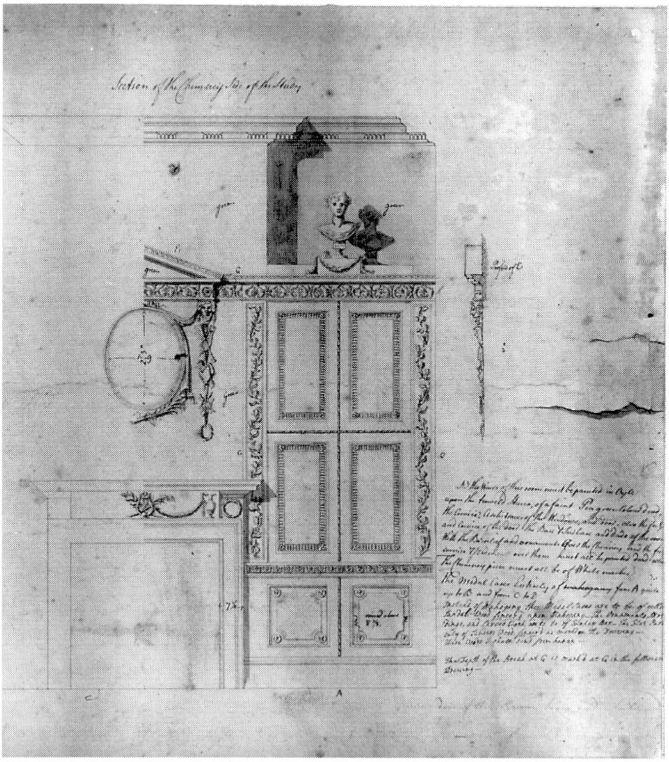

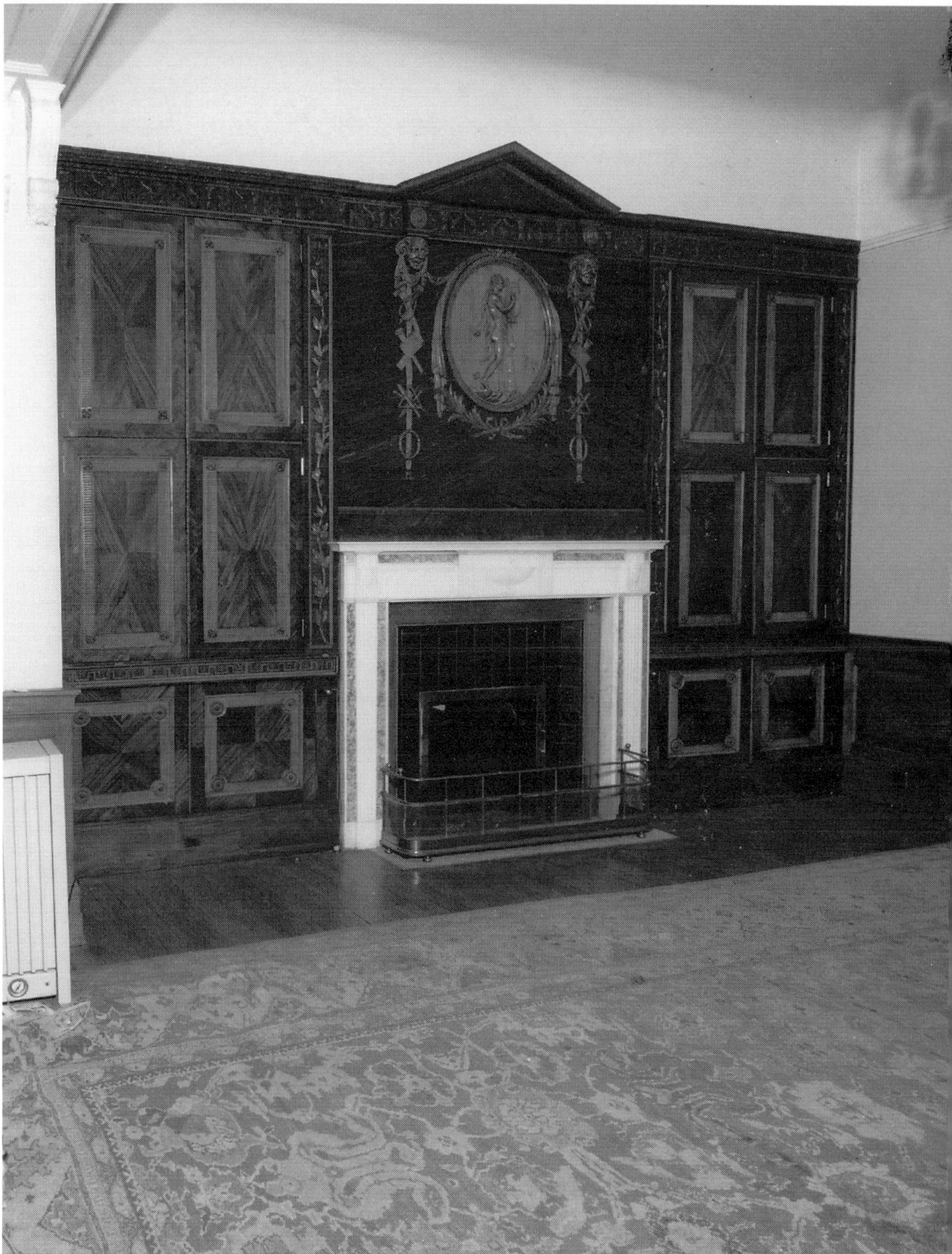

The Charlemont House Medal Cabinet – Elvedon Sale
Courtesy of Christie's

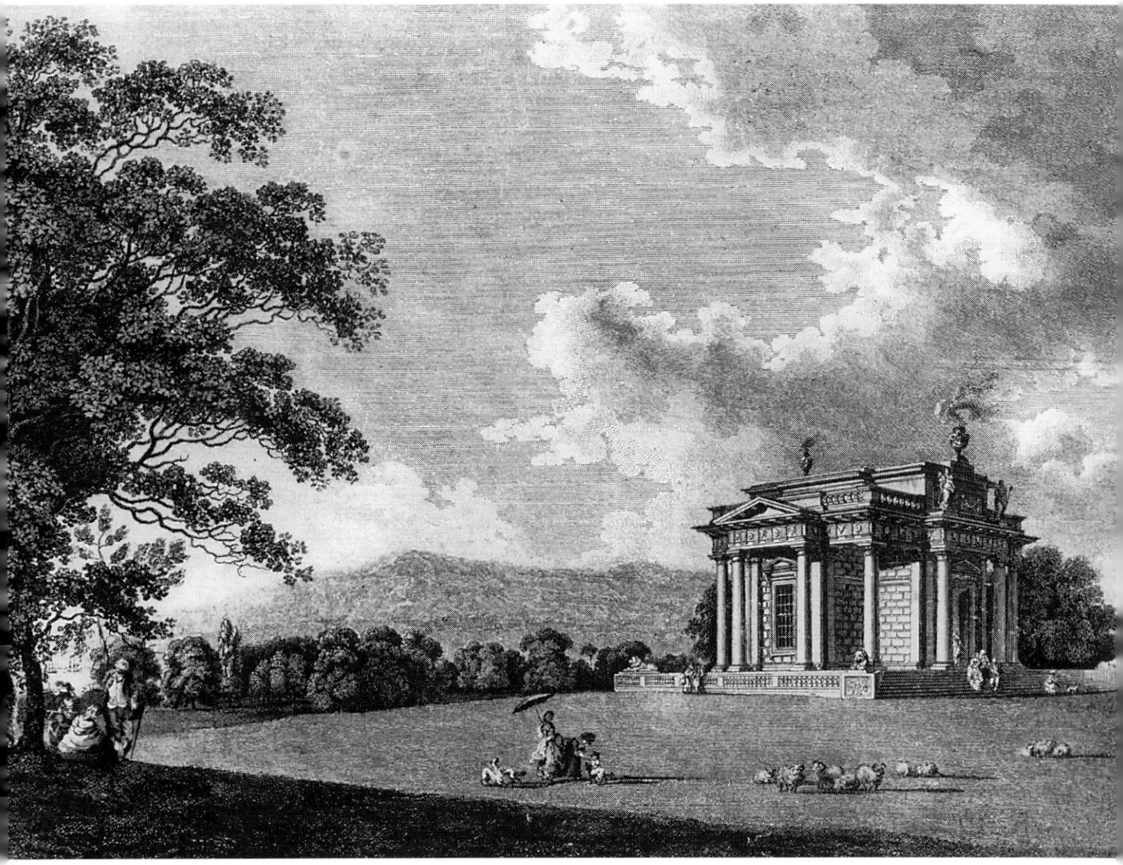

Francis Wheatley
Thomas Milton *View of Seats*

Corner of the Saloon at the Casino
Photograph by John Redmill

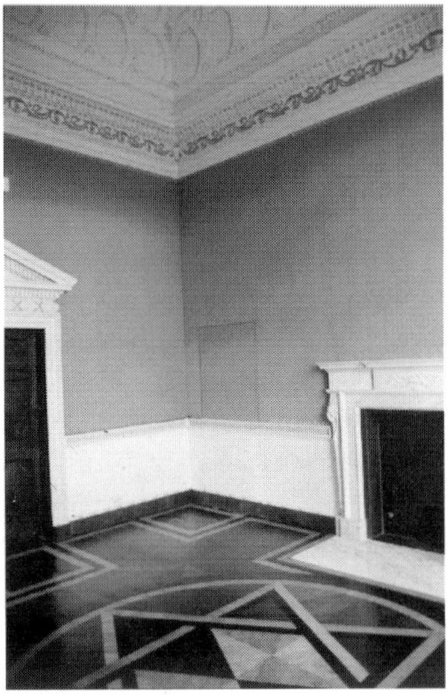

The Vestibule of the Casino
Photograph by John Redmill

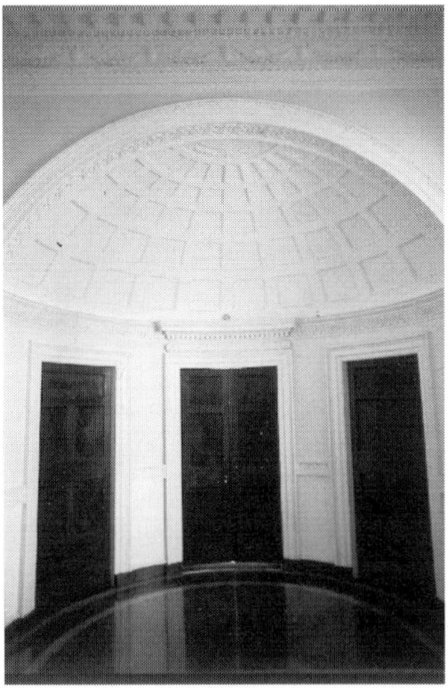

Perhaps he slipped almost unobtrusively back to his native land. Certainly he would never have displayed any of the airs and ostentation of that erstwhile traveller and former companion, St Leger, who on his return from his Grand Tour was seen wearing 'a white surtout, a crimson cape, a French waistcoat, his hair *en papillote*, a feather in his hat, a *couteau de chasse* by his side, with a small cane hanging to his button, and attended by two Italian greyhounds.'[10] When Jack St Leger fought a duel over some imagined insult, and nearly killed his opponent, Charlemont must have felt he had a good excuse to drop his acquaintance, as thereafter we only hear of St Leger as a former companion of his youth.

NOTES

1. RIA, 12.R.9, no. 21.
2. Ibid, 12.RE.2, p. 471.
3. Ibid, 12.R.9, no. 48.
4. Ibid.
5. Hardy, pp. 32-38. Edward Eliot 1727-1804, Baron Eliot of St Germans 1784.
6. RIA 12.R.5, p. 7.
7. Ibid, 12.R.9, no. 16.
8. Ibid, 12.R.12, no. 20.
9. Ibid, 12.R.9, no. 29.
10. Bellamy, Vol. 2, p. 82.

15

BOOTY

Prior to Adderley's offer of the house at Donneycarny with a room sufficiently large for the whole collection of Charlemont's curiosities, a shipment of Charlemont's 'Boxes etc.' had arrived in Dublin from Leghorn and, in accordance with Murphy's written orders, they were lodged in the Customs House stores. Adderley wrote on 19 April 1754, 'The place in which they lie being very moist & likely much frequented by vermin viz Custom-house officers & Rats & many goods belonging to several people scatter'd amongst them, which when they are removed, the Boxes necessarily must be disturbed' had led him to apply to one of the officers for permission to lock them up and secure them separately until Charlemont himself came to have them viewed. This request had been refused to Adderley's 'mortification' by a person, he had lately 'laboured to serve'.

However he was hopeful that when other commissioners came to town, he would obtain his suit and the boxes would be laid in the large parlour at Jervis Street, where they might be frequently aired by fires, 'for I much fear by the Nails in some of the Boxes being almost eaten thro' with Rust, they have laid long in some damp place'.[1]

It would seem that these cases contained the fruits of the voyage about which Charlemont was so reserved in his *Traveller's Essays*. Adderley mentions that the captain had not been happy about taking delivery of a damaged box, but on being informed it contained a mummy and that no injury had been offered it, he was prevailed upon to take it, but apart from this souvenir of Charlemont's visit to Egypt and two bales of coffee, there is no precise evidence of the number of cases or what they contained.

Nevertheless, it is most probable that the Greek stele was included in the first shipment and, though we hear nothing of any other antiquities until they were presented to the Royal Irish Academy by Charlemont's grandson in 1868, also 'an Egyptian basalt with hieroglyphics'; an 'Egyptian basalt with relief of emblems' and the case of an Egyptian animal idol, 'which almost certainly identifies with the mummy.'[2]

A second shipment from Leghorn (referred to by Adderley in his letter of 5 June 1754 offering the little estate at Donnycarney), was explicitly of 'ten cases of Statues and Busts'; and on 11 October Adderley reported having attended the landing of Charlemont's Venus and a box of books on the Customs House Quay.[3] Adderley continued to do all in his power to have the cases removed from the stores and lodged at Charlemont House in Jervis Street. The Venus could only have been Joseph Wilton's copy of the Venus de' Medici; the little Venus by della Porta had not yet been embedded in its frame by Vierpyle, and is accounted for in a letter from Parker.

On 9 January 1755 Adderley wrote to Charlemont who was still in London. 'I have this instant rec^d an acct of the arrival of your Cloths etc. from Leghorn' and that he would attend the landing the next day.[4]

During all this time, things were going badly in Rome. Parker, acting as Charlemont's agent, was engulfed in misfortune, difficulties and delays. On a visit to Ischia for the baths, he had contracted an ulcerous leg and been laid up at Naples for ten months, the expense of which had nearly ruined him. He had been unable to finish his Lordship's commission 'of Milton etc.' and that troubled him most. Murphy was able to inform him that Charlemont had not only accepted his excuses, but that he had generously ordered Murphy to tell Parker that, in consideration of his present unhappy circumstances, he might take up a hundred sequins for his assistance.

This was generous because, due partly to Parker's absence from Rome, and partly to Patch's quarrels with another artist called Warner, Charlemont's Academy had not prospered and had more or less disbanded itself.

Two months later Parker was again in fear and danger of losing Charlemont's protection. He had run into trouble with Murphy for not furnishing proper accounts of payments through the banker Belloni, of items packed and despatched, and of items wanting. On 26 July, he wrote to Charlemont giving the details of monies paid to himself, Patch and Vierpyle, which amounted to more than one thousand and eighty eight sequins, and also a list of the contents of the cases already sent. He had heard of his Lordship 'having been frightened about the Case of Medals' which Charlemont thought had been missing, but had been found, Parker hoped, in good condition.

There had been two large boxes, one full of books only, the other, besides books, 'contained in a case at bottom yr. marble mosaick table, the case of medals & walnutree case with Draws for the Medals'. Also sent had been the Farnese globe and, under it, the bas relief of Minerva teaching the use of olives, bedded in a frame, Etruscan vases, boxes of lava (Murphy's), the marble busts of Swift, Homer, Brutus the elder, ditto the younger, the antique Faun, modern Faun, girl's head from Alexandria, and Agrippina, each in separate cases.[5]

As for the list of things wanting: all bronzetti, Gladiator, two Centaurs, Silenus, Antinous, bas-relief of Venus by Guglielmo della Porta; these he had not sent, some not being in order. The Venus, which Vierpyle was to bed in a frame, was not yet done, no more than the busts of Brutus, Pompey and Caesar in bronze that Vierpyle was to do, and the busts in red marble. 'I have often recommended them to him – if not yet done no fault of mine. I suppose he will do them when the Gladiator is finished, which he says is very forward. I have not seen it as I am still unfortunately kept in bed with my wounds.'[6]

Some unspecified pictures bought by Parker for Charlemont had not been sent. Parker had intended to send them with Patch's and Pompeo's 'to have one Expense only in the license for them & Bronzos', but Pompeo had not yet finished, 'nor can I get the portraits out of his hands, he is p'd the half of the great one'. Patch had never let him know he had finished, nor would he have known the pictures were sent but for Belloni's account, 'nor do I know the reason for sending them away unknown to me.'

Parker's misfortune and illness made him, understandably, pettish, but his attempts to justify the delays by shifting the blame were clumsy. Charlemont would have known that Vierpyle was honest, conscientious and hardworking, that Pompeo had a reputation for tardiness and that Patch was wisely keeping out of Parker's way.

By the end of the year the Gladiator, busts of Caesar, Pompey, Brutus and Diogenes, the bas-relief Antinous and della Porta's Venus in their frames and the bronze Centaurs, the Faun with Bacchus, Gladiator and Antinous together with two models for window curtains had all been sent.[7] Besides there were all Murphy's heads of the Emperors and statues.

Murphy was in London when the heads of the Emperors were to be landed in Dublin. He wrote to Charlemont, 'I am in mortal fear about those cases being opened by any Hands but my own. I should break my heart did any unlucky accident happen to one of those Heads.'[8]

As it happens the heads have for the most part survived and are today in the collections of the Royal Irish Academy. The same cannot be said for Charlemont's statues and busts, which were dispersed in the nineteenth century and are so far untraced. This is not so surprising since copies after the antique were a commonplace of any extensive Grand Tour collection, but there was also 'the marble mosaick table' which can almost certainly be identified with the table made from the paving from Hadrian's Villa, which according to James Russel, the Marchese Gabrielli had given to Charlemont. There was the little Venus by della Porta, which, as already mentioned, was last heard of at the beginning of the century, when it was described as framed in an octagonal plinth with trophies, designed by Sir William Chambers.

Further, there was a bust of Swift, which might be that mentioned by Mann in a letter to Horace Walpole, 9 November 1753 as a fine work by Joseph Wilton. That bust has never been traced and does not appear in catalogues of Wilton's works.

The mystery of the dispersed heirlooms, for that is how Charlemont designated the statues and busts in his will, has never been fully solved. At this stage, we are only concerned with those works of art, listed by Parker, that we may have some idea of what they consisted, and how they were to be fitted into Charlemont's future schemes for Marino and Charlemont House in Dublin.

Considered in terms of bulk only, apart from a quantity of marble and bronze busts, two granite and one mosaic tables, Charlemont had on his hands Wilton's full-scale copy of the Venus de' Medici, the landing of which had been overseen by Adderley; Vierpyle's Fighting Gladiator, which as we know from Parker was held at Leghorn to await a suitable vessel rather than risk it being carried on the deck of a small ship. There was also the Mercury, about which Parker had been disappointed when Cardinal Albani failed in his promise to get permission to mould the statue in the gardens of the Villa Medici, but which nevertheless appears in a photograph taken in 1865 of the great corridor of Charlemont House as the bronze Mercury by Giovanni di Bologna.[9]

The pictures Parker purchased on Charlemont's behalf were likewise large. On 28 February he wrote he had bought more than two of those he had described, 'I got them I think very cheap, viz. the two figures singing and one playing on a guitar by Michael Angelo Carravagio; two, a man singing and woman playing on the lute by Tintoretto; and two half length figures, companions, hieroglifical, both by Gerard Huntorst called Gerardo delle Notte.

The above four pictures are all figures as large as life.'[10]

Before word reached Parker that no more pictures were to be bought, he had acquired two fruit pieces: one by Michael Angelo di Campidoglio and another, smaller, by Gobbo Carracci. There were also copies of unspecified pictures in the Farnese Gallery and later, a miniature painting by Rosalba. Parker was particularly pleased with this 'little jewel', a self-portrait of the artist with her master, Abbate Ramelli, in masking dress.[11]

We know that Charlemont acquired many of his pictures on his return from Rome, in London, including his Zuccarellis, but there may have been other paintings, which, like Patch's views, were not handled by Parker and it is possible that a pair by Orizonte, a small Gaspar Poussin and three Italian views by Richard Wilson, all at Charlemont House or Marino in the nineteenth century, were purchased or, in the case of the Wilsons, commissioned by Charlemont in Rome.

Books sent by Parker were not catalogued by him. Engravings, views, etc., were not listed and were sent as portfolios of prints. The medals, about which Charlemont had been anxious, were contained in cases and, though Parker may not have known of what they consisted, they were precious to Charlemont. He was to commission for them one of the most magnificent medal cabinets of the eighteenth century.

The evidence for the medals having been acquired mainly from Borioni is inconclusive, but when Borioni died, Parker was instructed by Charlemont to treat with Borioni's heir, Niccolo Conti and reported 'The table was sold to the Margrave of Bareith.'[12] Is this another example of Parker's procrastination or the difficulty of interpreting instructions from Charlemont relayed by the cautious Murphy?

NOTES

1. HMC, Rept. 12, App. pt. X, pp. 191-2.
2. RIA.12.R.13 preface.
3. HMC, Rept. 12, App. pt. X, p. 197.
4. RIA, 12.R.9, no. 24.
5. HMC, Rept. 12, App. pt. X, p. 218.
6. Ibid.
7. Ibid, p. 222.
8. RIA, 12.R.9, no. 44.
9. HMC, Rept. 12, App. pt. x, p. 222.
10. HMC, Rept. 12, App. pt. x, p. 350.
11. Ibid.
12. Ibid, p. 227.

16

THE TRIBULATIONS OF PARKER AND PIRANESI

Parker may have had a feeling that Charlemont was not entirely satisfied that the collapse of the Academy was brought about by Patch alone. At all events, we find Parker patently triumphant when in the letter of 24 December he comes to tell of Patch being in serious trouble.

'I must inform your Lordship that this day we lost Patche, who was obliged to leave Rome in twenty-four hours … by an order from the holy office directed to the cardinal secretary of State, who signed it, and sent it to the governor of Rome with orders to put it into execution. He sent for Patche, who was ready to s—. He went to Abbé Grant (supposing it to be about some academy affair) first and got him to go with him there. The order was absolute and the matter must be so bad as he could not get a respite of a day or two to settle his things, though Mr Stevens did all he could with his friend Monsignor Piccolomini and he with Cardinals Corsini and Valenti for this respite. I heard of this order from the office, and went to Patche to see if true. He took no notice to me at all of it, and left Rome without so much as letting me know either by word of mouth or line; nor has he left his things in Virepoyle's care, but to almost a stranger. It is judged by us the reason to be, from the confession of something his girl of Tivoli or his boy, who died lately at the hospital of St John Lateran must have confessed that had passed between them, and when dieing they would not give the boy absolution till he discovered the actions etc. to the holy office; and Patche said to Virepoyle he could not imagine what it was, if not a thing he did which only he and his boy knew, nor should anyone else ever know. His behaviour of late has been so extraordinary that the most favourable construction is to say he is mad. Crazy he always was. Sir William [Stanhope] bought two landscapes by him to assist him in his journey. Mr Stevens, I am told, offered him money, but he had lately received £100 from Sir William Lowther. He is gone to

Florence. He confessed to several he was afraid to be shot or poisoned every day. I shall endeavour to learn the true reason of this affair if possible I can and let your Lordship know.'[1]

On 28 February, 1756, Parker wrote again, 'Mr Patche's disgrazia hindered me from his further friendship; he is now in Florence. Various are the storys told of the reason of his banishment. Some say B—y, others giving a potion to a nun to make her miscarry, must be something confessed by his boy (who died a few days before the order for his banishment in the Hospital of St John Lateran). He has told strange storys to Mr Stevens and Sir Horace Mann that they have tried several times to poison him, that his dog eat of a minestra set before him by some particular people and died immediately, this happened at Terni and his boy who ate of it never recovered; both false, his dog died in Rome several months after he returned to Rome, and his boy of the pox, other story that he had several guns fired at him by order of the Monsignor who now keeps his Tivoli girl.'[2]

Parker evidently got no encouragement from Charlemont; on 22 May he wrote agreeing that his Lordship was probably right. 'I am of your Lordship's opinion that his oddities and loose way of talking in all companies was the cause of his exile.' But, he added slyly, that if Charlemont wanted to hear more, Vierpyle who was by then on his way to Ireland, could tell him.[3]

Charlemont had in the meantime heard from Patch himself, who had also written in similar terms to Sir William Lowther, who was now back at Holker and well satisfied with Patch, who had acted on his behalf in the acquisition of a fine painting by Claude Lorraine.[4]

Patch's letter to Charlemont was dated Florence, 2 January 1756. 'I must beg your Lordship's pardon for the liberty I take after so long neglecting my Duty towards your Lordship, but it proceeded from knowing that you had a continual correspondence in Rome wch. gave me frequent Pleasure of hearing that your Lordship enjoyed perfect Health and perhaps I should not have been so Bold now had it not been for an Accident that had Lately Befall'n me wch. perhaps may Appear in Bad Light when you are told I am sent out of the Pope's State.

'For this reason I think myself under an Absolute Obligation of Vindicating myself to you more Particularly than any one liveing as your Lordship was pleased to Honour me wth. your Patronage whilst in Rome.'

'On the twenty second of October I was sited to appear before a

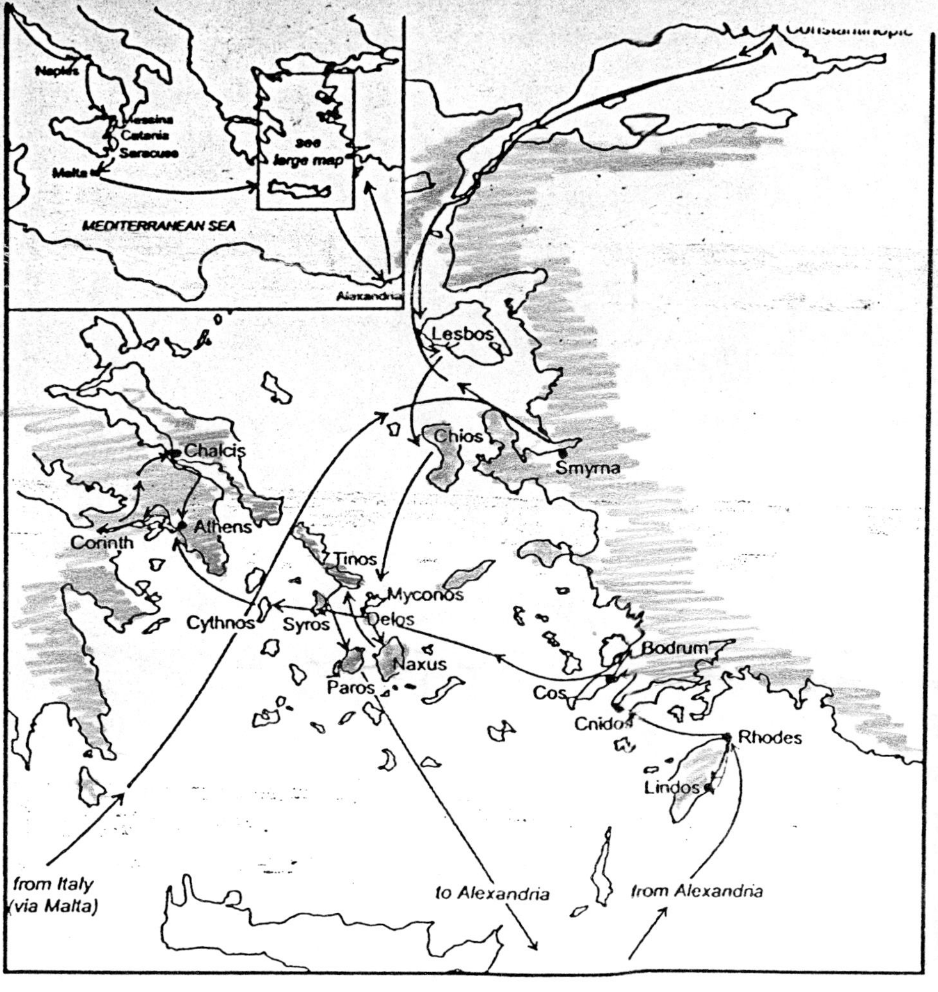

The Voyage of L'Aimable Vainqueur
Department of Geography, University College, Dublin

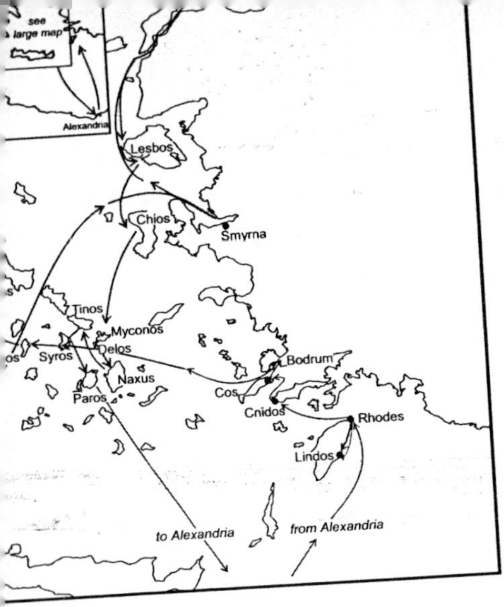

of L'Aimable Vainqueur
Geography, University College, Dublin

from the Mausoleum in the castle of the Knights at Bodrum
Minor, Society of Dilettanti, 1775

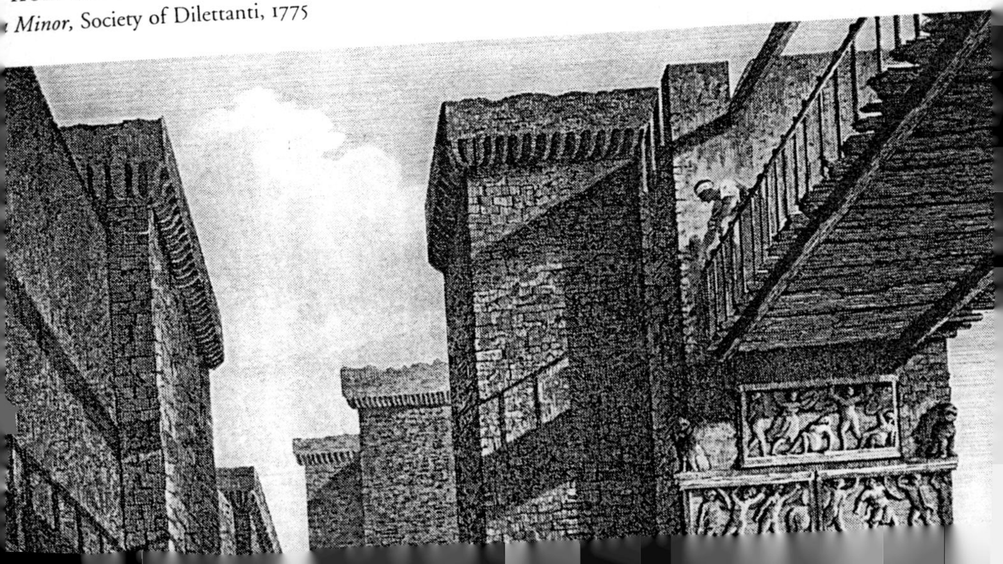

Notary Belonging to the Governor of Rome I beg^{d} of Abbe Grant to Accompany me wch. he did and was soon Informed by a Petition made from the Santo Offizzio to the Cardinal Secretary of State, for to Exile me out of the Pope's dominion, but without mentioning any Reason wch. surprised me much as I cannot recollect any one thing possible for them to take Hold on unless the old affair of Tivoli, whitch has been before acquainted wth and for more than a Twelvemonth the past I have not Been in any Italian Company and as little as Possible my own Countrymen, never had any Dispute of any kind, whatsoever nor talk about Religion. I had but four and twenty hours to stay in ye State wch. gave me more Trouble than that of Leaving the Country, wch. I hope I shall have no reason to Regret as Mr Stevens had taken Particular Notice of me on account of my haveing been before Honour'd wth your Lordship's Protection. So on this Affaire, wch. I acquainted him wth immediately, assisted and did all that Lay in his Power for me by strongly recommending me to Monsignior Piccolomini who has Given me a Letter wth the Strongest Recommendation to the Count Rochford here in Florence as has Mr Stevens to Mr Mann … by home I have been received wth extreme Politeness and promises of his Protection. So that I am in hope of Soon finding Florence more Agreeable and Profitable to me than Rome and shall be entirely Happy when I can be assured of Lordship's being Persuaded of my innocence in this Affair."[5]

Here we leave Patch, soon by Parker's account 'abridge-painting' for Lord Huntingdon, and soon to be successful and happy under the protection of Mann at Florence.

Amidst the scandal, and some gossip about cameos from the Prince Borghese's collection being stolen by a favourite footman and offered to the Prince before the theft had even been discovered, came the first rumblings of the dispute with Piranesi.

On 22 May 1756, nearly a month after publication, Parker wrote to Charlemont, 'Pyronese has at last published 4 vols. of Antiquities, the whole dedicated to my Lord Charlemont and is a very fine work, he has ordered to be bound two setts to send your Lordship. I could not persuade him to send them loose, he would bind them *con magnificenza per mostrare & ca*, he sells the 4 vols. unbound 15 sequins & tells me they will cost him 8 crowns per tom, the binding, he offered to return me the 100 sequins I gave him & for which I have his note of hand, this I refused till I had yr. Lordship's further orders, as soon as delivered I will forward them.'[6]

Parker in specifying the whole of the work being dedicated to Charlemont brings us to the crux of the argument. When Piranesi had first approached Charlemont, correctly enough through Parker as his agent, it would appear that he was looking for backing for a less ambitious work, seemingly an extended edition of *Camera sepulcrali degli Antichi Romani*, a short series of engravings, which he had published circa 1750.[7]

But in 1752 the Comte de Caylus had produced his magnificent *Recueil d'Antiquitiés* and, by tentatively suggesting Greek superiority, had opened the controversy. The following year Wood's *Palmyra* had appeared and in 1755 Allan Ramsay's *Dialogue of Taste* and Abbé Winckelmann's *Gedanken über die Nachahnung der griechischen Werke*. The latter work, particularly, being of deeper content than its predecessors, had incited Piranesi to defend his position, and drawing upon ten years of work and study on the subject, he set about establishing Roman superiority in the production of *Antichità Romane* in four volumes.

Thus was Charlemont brought involuntarily into the controversy on the side of its greatest Roman champion when his own inclinations were more probably for neutrality and a middle-of-the-road path.

Two years had elapsed since Piranesi's first proposal to Charlemont. One of the closest observers of Piranesi's behaviour was Robert Adam, who shortly after Charlemont's departure, had found good reason to regard Piranesi as erratic. Greatly flattered at first, by Piranesi's proposal to dedicate to him, a young and unknown architect, a plan of ancient Rome and the plate of the Campus Martius, Adam had then been teased by Piranesi's apparent cooling off. 'That Piranesi is a most changeable, interested madman, whom there is no depending on' he wrote. But from the first Adam had known the dedications would cost him money and also that, in his professional capacity, he could get the first copies off the press in London and on sale at a profit before Piranesi was selling them in Rome.[8]

The instructions that Parker awaited with regard to the two sets and their extravagant binding came probably not from Charlemont but from Murphy, and amounted to telling Piranesi that if he did not agree to the binding being cancelled, his Lordship would have no need for his dedication.

Piranesi was furious. He wrote directly to Charlemont himself what he described as a humble remonstrance. It was, of course, nothing of the kind, and if Charlemont ever received it he did not reply. A second letter was despatched by Piranesi and met the same fate. One letter only, the second, is extant among Charlemont's papers. It runs to five thousand, five hundred words, which were later to be more or less summarised in Piranesi's formal statement or recantation in Rome.

Piranesi pleaded for a hearing from Milord. He had been reproached for writing him directly, but had not Horace written letters to Augustus, Catullus to Caesar, the architect Apollodorus to the Emperors Trajan and Hadrian and received replies? With such illustrious examples might not he take the liberty of addressing Milord and expecting an answer? Might he not become despicable in his Lordship's eyes if he continued to show himself insensitive to the insults publicly heaped upon him by his lordship's unworthy agents; although Parker had told him everything he said was as from Milord? He swore he was ignorant of any convention which required him to submit fully to an agent, especially when that agent was less renowned than he, who could claim the celebrity of his works all over Europe and was heard of even in England.

This much established, Piranesi went on to retrace the entire range of the events of the past two years. He recalled having been advised of Milord's fame as a protector of the Arts, and the establishments he wished to set up in Rome for their encouragement and, with this in mind, he had spoken to Mr Parker, who had the honour of being known to Milord. He had waited a year and then at a single meeting with Mr Parker, he had been assured of Milord's goodwill and protection. A date was fixed for him to show Milord the epigraph. He took particular care to come to Milord's house at the appointed hour, but was denied entry. He called again and again, but it was evident that Mr Parker had seen to it that the door was closed to him.

However Milord had called once at his lodgings, but in the company of others and he had not been so indiscreet as to complain before them, especially as Milord, he thought, could not have been the author of his being refused admittance or he would not have considered him worthy of a visit.

He was grieved that Milord had departed from Rome without saying more, leaving him improperly instructed as to his intentions, and without any definite order although he had been induced to hand over the drawings for the dedicatory plates to Mr Parker to show

Milord, or under the pretext of their being shown to him. A different version of this appeared in his public recantation: a servant of Charlemont had brought back the first draft as unsuitable, with instructions that it would have to be shorter and more modestly phrased.

Time went by and, according to Piranesi, he heard nothing and went at last to Parker for confirmation of approval, or further instructions with regard to what we know to have been the second draft. Mr Parker, after keeping the drawings for four months, disdained to comment, but handed back the drawings to him with an inscription, purported to have been written by Milord himself; and this Mr Parker had ordered him to follow as if he was ordering his lackey to bring him a glass of water.

Mr Parker had also informed him that he was empowered to give him two hundred scudi from Milord, but would not entrust him with the full sum and wanted a receipt made out to himself because Mr Parker feared that in accordance with Italian habits, he, Piranesi, would not keep his promise. How then was he treated? Was he taken for one of the mob of rogues? Was he a suspicious character? This insult he had been forced to accept from Mr Parker, who claimed to be worthy of his regard as the conveyor of Milord's sentiments, but was a man so base that he saw only merit in protecting Milord's monetary interests, and could not see that his behaviour was an affront to Milord's generosity and high principles.[9]

Parker was, as we know, acting under Murphy's instructions and Murphy was wary of Italian business methods and strongly protective of Charlemont's interests. It is doubtful if at that stage Charlemont had any knowledge of the details of a transaction which he had left entirely in Murphy's hands.

According to Piranesi, he was then advised by a friend to try to find out whether the aforegoing was due to Milord's indifference, or to Mr Parker's disregard of Milord's instructions and accordingly he had returned to Mr Parker and asked him for the two hundred scudi. This he swore he had no use for nor indeed could have used, as could be proved by his having taken the credit notes, countersigned by Mr Parker to Milord's banker, which Belloni had refused to accept.

As soon as the first proofs had come from the press, he had taken two copies of his work to Mr Parker and asked him how he should act with regard to Milord. How many copies should he send? He had also told Mr Parker that he had given two copies to be bound in

Moroccan leather and he was having the Charlemont arms engraved to imprint them on the covers. By asking Mr Parker's advice, he was entrusting himself to his judgement but Mr Parker had said he did not wish to give advice because he ought to hand over some copies for Milord in exchange for the two hundred scudi lent or advanced on Milord's account. He told Mr Parker that he would rather return the money than hand over six copies with twenty scudi to balance the account.

It was then that Mr Parker had told him that Milord had no need of his dedication. Was it true that Milord despised his dedication? Why then had he been allowed to go to great expense and take such pains on the supposition that his work would give pleasure to Milord? A great gentleman had desired it and such an offer might have been tempting had he not been a slave to Milord's word. Finally why make him write the epigraph Patron of the Arts when Mr Parker now said Milord was not really given to the Arts and when forty copies had now been distributed under Milord's name?

Yet again he had returned to Mr Parker in another attempt to discover Milord's true feelings. In answer to his enquiry what Mr Parker himself thought of the work, Mr Parker was so discourteous to say that he had not opened it. How was this possible? Mr Parker piqued himself on being an antiquarian and had not opened his work when milord Stanhope [Sir William], perhaps as high-ranking a gentleman as Mr Parker, had taken the trouble to come to his house to see it, when critics in Rome had acclaimed it and two hundred copies were already ordered from Paris.

It was then that he had first written to Milord and when his letter was on the way to England, there had come to his house by chance Mr André (Anderson), a friend and confidant of Mr Parker's. He had thought it fitting to discuss his letter with a man who flattered himself he knew the intentions of Milord. Whereupon Mr André had reproached him for addressing Milord, rather than his agent, and he had replied that knowing the public outcry in Rome against Mr Parker's treatment of others, he doubted he would be better done by.

Mr Parker had refused to pay for the white marble busts commissioned from the sculptor, Maini, (who had died before finishing the work); likewise he had refused to pay the pension of two paoli a day granted by Milord's generosity to the master of languages (Abbé du Bois) although this man had complained strongly of such treatment and was in dire need. It was left to Mr Oudry (Robert Wood) to help him. Unbeknownst to Milord, while he was still in Rome, Mr Parker had kept artists from his door. After Milord's departure, some artists with commissioned work on their hands and payment agreed before the undertaking, were partly cut on receipt of their works, as had happened to the carver, who had made a model of the Falconieri gates and had one and a half scudi deducted from the agreed six sequins. All the Englishmen who had benefited from the Academy accused Mr Parker of being the author of the disturbances. There were some people who believed the story that it was Milord himself who did not want to pay the language master and the lady's (Magdalen's) promised pensions; he, Piranesi, had defended Milord and told them Milord would be shocked if he knew of such things.

All things he said against Mr Parker he could prove with witnesses, as he did not doubt he had been depicted to Milord as an odd man and one to whom Milord need pay no attention. Why else had Milord sent to another, and one of the most ignorant architects in Rome, a commission for a design for gates?

Until he had an answer from Milord, he would not send the two hundred copies ordered from Paris, because if Milord was no longer pleased with the work, he was prepared to cancel the epigraph. He would do more. He would show to the public that it was Milord who had refused the work so that it would not be shocked at seeing it appear under another name. He would, for greater effect, have printed before the preface this letter to Milord so that the public might be informed as to the strange reason why some copies were dedicated to Milord and others to a great prince and people would not think that selfish interests had induced him to dedicate the work to someone else offering more money. The world was so malevolent that it would not hesitate to think that he had received a considerable gift from Milord, but had the meanness to prefer a richer and more powerful patron.

He did not doubt that Milord would allow him this justice, but if he refused, he would appeal to his contemporaries and posterity. He said posterity because he ventured to believe that he had finished a work that would pass to posterity and be placed in every public library. He would send copies to every sovereign in Europe, to the academies of the fine arts in Paris, Berlin and St Petersburg, etc., and with the copy destined for the Vatican library, he would place the original manuscript beside the printed letter, the better to authenticate his justification.

Was it the delay in publication that had displeased Milord? But had Milord wished to have his name at the head of a work, mediocre, because it was hurried? Posterity would not seek to find out if Mr Parker was dissatisfied with the delay, but would notice only whether the work was good or bad and if it was worthy of its patron. When Milord was in Rome the work was only to be one folio volume, now it was compiled into four and increased fourfold. The great plate alone, showing the aquaducts, had taken him six months to prepare. Such painstaking labour on that and the other plates, with the particular research involved, should have drawn on him praise, not reproach.

As for the sacrifices and expenses incurred on behalf of Milord, he mentioned them not to show off his zeal nor to attempt to excite Milord's generosity. He was well enough off from his work to be raised above the level of an attachment to money, so that his inclination was to spend three times as much again in order to protect himself from the malevolent treatment he had received up to the present.

The paper alone for the four frontispieces, sixteen thousand sheets, as he customarily printed four thousand copies of his works, amounted to six hundred and forty Roman scudi. He could not have etched one of those frontispieces for three hundred scudi, but a moderate estimate for the four was twelve hundred which with six hundred and forty, brought the total expenditure to one thousand eight hundred and forty Roman scudi. The Pope had released him from the import taxes on two hundred bales of paper to encourage him in the continuation of the work, but Mr Parker had not entrusted him with an eighteenth part of the whole, nor even a sixth part of the costs of Milord's dedication plates. Who had acted more nobly? He, who had spent one thousand eight hundred and forty scudi to put Milord's name in good standing, or Mr Parker, who had attributed to Milord the caution of a banker in dealing with one who could find ten thousand scudi in Rome without difficulty if he need.[10]

One letter only, as outlined above, is extant and today preserved among the Charlemont papers. Probably an earlier and milder version had been intercepted by Murphy and concealed from Charlemont. But these renewed complaints, with Piranesi's threats of imminent and damaging publication, could not be so lightly dismissed, nor Charlemont kept any longer in ignorance. But what was to be done? The matter had gone beyond a conciliatory reply and Charlemont could not be expected, in the face of Piranesi's insults, to stoop to a personal letter. Parker had lost all use as an emissary.

Besides it must have occurred to Charlemont that, despite misrepresentation, at least some of Piranesi's accusations were not without foundation. Murphy had been perhaps over zealous in his efforts to save Charlemont money, but with the best intentions, as we shall find, following the failure of Charlemont's Irish bankers and Charlemont's ill health and depression at the time.

With the introduction of Abbé Peter Grant, probably at Charlemont's suggestion, the situation, already explosive, erupted dramatically. Had Peter Grant used half the diplomacy with which he had previously on Charlemont's behalf extracted George Potter from his creditors in Rome, the matter might still have been resolved. Instead he went into battle with counter threats and, at a meeting with Piranesi, as he reported to Charlemont, told him, 'with all the smoothness and coolness' possible, that if he did not desist from publishing, he could expect 'the vigourous and severe penalties of galleys'. Piranesi, who had taken the precaution of concealing a witness, perhaps told the truth when he swore that the Abbé went further and threatened that if he published his letter to Charlemont, Milord would have him 'assassinated'.[11]

Piranesi's next move was to write another letter, recounting the scandalous harangue, and address it to Grant, threatening to publish it also as a preface to *Antichità Romane*.

On 13 June, 1757, Grant succeeded in getting a formal precept entered in the books of the office of government, which restrained Piranesi from publishing anything in writing or in print which might reflect on Lord Charlemont or Abbé Peter Grant. But to Parker's chagrin, Mr Grant and Monsignor Cenci neglected to take care for his character also. Parker's name was not inserted in the order.

Ten months passed before Grant sent a copy of the mandate to Charlemont with a footnote, '... after this none but a madman could have done what Piranesi has since done: and the truth is that he really and truely is out of his senses'. It was not until April of the following year that a full report from Rome reached Charlemont. The report, for fear of tiring his Lordship, was divided into two letters, one from Parker to Murphy, the other from Abbé Grant to Charlemont himself.

Undeterred by the mandate, Piranesi continued to sell the four volumes of *Antichità Romane* with his letters to Charlemont annexed as a justification for his having erased Charlemont's name from the dedication; but without the substituted dedication to a great prince, whose identity was still a mystery. Parker, who had been complimented originally with a sepulchre in the Via Appia beside the tombs of Robert Adam and Allan Ramsay, discovered that his encomium had been defaced.

It was Parker's turn to take the initiative and, acting on information received, he went to the Governor's Lieutenant, Signore Cherubini, to draw his attention to Piranesi continuing to publish his letters to Charlemont and preparing to print the letter to Abbé Grant, which was very scandalous against Mr Grant and Mr Murphy. There were, besides, some satirical engravings, which were already off the press. To Parker's request that Piranesi's house be searched for the copies and the plates, Cherubini could do nothing unless Parker could produce a witness, who could swear he saw them there; and the gentleman who had seen them refused to appear as a spy. A few days later Piranesi published.[12]

Piranesi's *Lettere di Giustificazione* was produced as a pamphlet running to twenty-eight pages. Those who received a complimentary copy perceived their names inscribed upon the frontispiece in a space provided and surrounded by emblems of eternity, elegantly engraved. The title page read *Lettere di Giustificazione scritte a Milord Charlemont e a di lui Agenti di Roma dal Signor Piranesi, Socio della Real Societa degli Antiquari di Londra intorno la Dedica della sua Opera delle Antichita Rom: fatte allo stesso ed ultimament soppressa.* A notice to the public followed under an engraved head-piece of Time discovering Truth, showing Parker, 'a fat fellow with a swelled leg, his hat fallen off'; Murphy in 'a despairing action' and Peter Grant in clerical garb.

Piranesi's letter to Grant revealed that the concealed witness was Baron d'Hanau, who had overheard Grant's threats of the galleys or assassination and an admission that it was not worth while Piranesi writing to Milord, as Parker and Murphy were in agreement and stopped his letters. Moreover Murphy kept Charlemont's seal and forged his hand and the letter shown Piranesi at the meeting between him and Grant, was one such forgery, purporting to be Charlemont's instructions to Grant.

Although misrepresented, this was probably not an entire fabrication: Charlemont was at the time so crippled with rheumatism that he was unable to lift a pen.

Following the letters, was a plate of the Campus Esquilinus, the burial place of slaves, with figures carrying bodies under the latinised names, Parker, Murphy and Grant with three pairs of *coglioni*. The original dedication plate was printed and again with Charlemont's name and coat of arms erased, as appeared in the second impression of the four volumes.

The final plate was Piranesi's new dedication, not to a great prince, but to the public and posterity, with Charlemont's name erased* from a column in the Circus Maximus and replaced with Marti Ullori, one pair of *coglioni* above and two below.

In February 1758, the scurrilous pamphlet was sent, 'industriously' to all the cardinals, monsignors, and other persons of quality, and to the Pope himself, besides English noblemen and gentlemen, including the Lords Mandeville, Brudenell and Garlies, Sir Brook Bridges and Mr Compton and to others as they arrived in Rome and also to English, French, German and Italian painters.

Then began for Parker and Grant 'two months in continual agitation and perpetually running about'.[13] Together they called on Cardinal Cenci to see what might be done. His advice was to have a lawyer draw up a full account of the affair for formal presentation to the Governor, Monsignor Caprara. This document they had prepared by 'a clever lawyer' and brought it back to Cardinal Cenci. He presented it to the Secretary of State and an immediate order was put out for Piranesi's arrest.

Piranesi, however, had forestalled this move by procuring through 'some interest' the protection of the Cardinals Corsini, Orsino and Albani. Piranesi had given copies of his works to them and their dependants and nobody dare move against him under their patents of protection. Cherubini, the Governor's Lieutenant, admitted to having received such a present, but was, according to Grant, on the side of Charlemont with Cardinal Cenci. Parker, on the other hand, suspected his duplicity throughout; he had only moved against Piranesi when it was already too late, and seemed to be looking for a reward, which Grant thought he deserved. Parker became more suspicious when Cherubini told him it was he who had once done Milord a favour by giving up his room at an inn in Perugia to him.

Cardinal Cenci was 'most active' but all he was able to do was to have the plates of the letters seized and Piranesi's bookseller ordered to deliver to the Governor all loose copies in his hands and to tear from the bound volumes the remainder. The governor thought this

* The 4 volumes with the original dedication reached Charlemont and appeared in the sale of the 3rd Earl's library in Dublin, 1892.

barely enough, that Piranesi deserved corporal punishment, but was soon 'given to understand, that therein, he was not to be gratifyd.' The reason for this, Grant thought, was that with a change of Padrone Supremo imminent, everybody was on the make, with the cardinals not knowing their next master. The Abbé, complacent and confident as ever (he had survived, for more than twenty years, the disapproval of his bishop) and without fear of treading on the toes of any cardinal, wrote Charlemont that, believing in the justice of their cause, he thought it unnecessary to offer a farthing to anybody.

A compromise was at last thought to have been found. The fellow, as Grant called Piranesi, was to be obliged to publish something in the way of a recantation, which would be acceptable to those injured or abused. But Piranesi was not easily induced and some fifty or so different drafts were written and submitted to the Governor, who returned them as not sufficiently contrite. Finally Piranesi sent a message that if Monsignor Caprara was not satisfied with the last draft, he could expect nothing further. The Governor, 'finding himself overpowered' accepted it, but insisted Piranesi should put his name to it and have it printed. The fellow 'struggled hard', disappeared for five days and then threatened to throw himself in the river rather than sign and 'make honourable mention of those he had abused'.

The Governor however was adamant. Piranesi signed and the recantation, printed in Italian and French, appeared dated Rome, 15 March (a significant day in Rome's history!), addressed to the Governor, but it read more as a summary of his letter to Charlemont than a recantation and it was thus, as Parker wrote Charlemont, that most people saw it. In defending himself, Piranesi wrote he had also taken on the defence of Milord, but if in his writing, full of praise for Milord, there escaped some phrase or word that might be interpreted otherwise, he reiterated before all the world his veneration for Milord and his esteem for Abbé Grant, for Mr Parker and for Mr Murphy, who apart from their own personal qualities, had the recommendation that they were esteemed and loved by Milord, a very enlightened nobleman, who had recognized their merits.

The recantation was fairly meaningless: it admitted no exorbitant demands and withdrew none of his accusations against Charlemont's representatives. The offensive satirical plates were not withdrawn and the engravings continued to be circulated in Rome. Piranesi had not concealed his anger at finding himself in the hard necessity of justification, a situation, for all the gold in the world, he could not have wished. The document ended, '*Voìla tout, Monsieur; ne m'en demandez pas d'avantage, & soyez persuadé que je vous aime du meilleur de mon coeur, Piranese" and in the Italian version, "Eccovi informato di tutto, senza che voi stiate a cercar d'altro, e resto con vero affetto tutto vostro &c. Gio. Batista Piranesi.*' It was as much to say that this was all, and not to ask any more of him.[14]

The matter might have ended there had not it made such a noise in Rome that it came to the ears of the community of Irish friars, who took up the cause of their Protestant compatriot and prepared a long address to Cardinal Corsini, 'the chief and most zealous stickler for Piranesi'. Seven of the friars signed, attesting that Milord Charlemont was one of the first peers of Ireland and universally beloved and adored in that kingdom and in England.

According to Parker, now greatly concerned for his own reputation, the Irish friars found Cardinal Corsini almost ignorant of the affront to his Lordship and, so misled by Parker's rivals, James Russel and Thomas Jenkins, into confusing him with another Parker, who had been banished from Rome, that the Cardinal wondered at the friars appearing in favour of such a villain. Corsini ran on about the other Parker deserving several times the galleys and the friars had difficulty in persuading him they were pleading for a different Parker, whose only fault was being the agent of Milord.

When at last Cardinal Corsini was persuaded of the injury he had done to his Lordship and Parker by his unquestioning protection of Piranesi, who had falsely informed him in the matter, he gave his considered judgement, which was to send the published recantation to Milord and tell him that if he was not satisfied, he had only to let Cardinal Corsini know and he would have Piranesi punished, he promised, as his Lordship thought fit.

Charlemont evidently took no action. Cardinal Corsini and a Father Nolan sent messages of goodwill and devotion to him. The Governor's Lieutenant, Cherubini, received for his trouble fifty Roman crowns, a sum agreed between the Cardinal and Peter Grant. As the Abbé pointed out, Cherubini had taken possession of the satirical plates, which he would hand over on something handsome being given him and who was to know, with all the changes in Rome, that on the Lieutenant being replaced, the matter would not come up again. Peter Grant survived unscathed, in spite of Sir William Stanhope reminding him he was not completely cleared of connivance in keeping letters from Lord Charlemont. The same might have applied to Murphy, but he was safe in Charlemont's affections and too far away from Rome. All the harm and hatred of Piranesi's revenge fell on Parker.

Parker's later letters to Charlemont became cries of anguish. Bereft of his reputation and his living, Piranesi saw to it, Parker believed, with the aid of Russel, Jenkins and the young architect Robert Mylne, that patronage from Lord Brudenell and others did not come his way. He was almost destitute. Surely, he begged piteously, Charlemont owed him this, that he write to Sir William and clear his name. All the English painters except himself were employed and Lord Brudenell, who had formerly asked him to dine on several occasions, had now closed his door against him and shunned him as an ill man. He had not enough money, including what his father sent him, to leave Rome and go to Venice. 'I must wait here till it shall please the Almighty to open to me some way to gain by work wherewithal to get forward.' In the past, as we know, Charlemont had provided and perhaps he did again now because in the following year Parker was writing more happily to Charlemont from Rome.

But Parker, though it was poor consolation, had in his way the last word. He wrote to Charlemont, 'I am now able to inform yr. L. that the prince that Pyronese says in his libel well-known to yr. L. & that was to have been a witness for him against Abbé Grant & who was the person taken stealing of the Termini in the Villa Negroni, is now run away afoot from Rome, having robbed and taken in people for considerable sums ... he has left the woman called his wife with child and talk of Rome is that he was *valet de chambre* to the Prince of Lichtenstein and this woman the laundress ... he was remarkable for the linen he wore and lately kept a coach and two servants ... and was the constant companion of the English these two years and always dined with Lord Brudenell. He called himself Baron d'Hanau.'[15]

The point about the fine linen and the laundress would not have been lost on Charlemont, but as with those other cases, Dalton, Patch, and now Parker and Piranesi, when patronage was shown to be fraught with trouble and pitfalls, Charlemont kept his own counsel. He was from time to time to run into similar difficulties, but none of his protégés were to prove as adamantly awkward as that turbulent genius, Piranesi.

NOTES

1. HMC Rept. 12, App. pt. X, p. 222. See also Watson, *Walpole Society*, vol. XXVIII (1939-40), pp. 16-50.
2. Ibid.
3. Ibid, p. 228.
4. 'Landscape with Apollo guarding the Herds of Admetus and with Muses', National Gallery of Scotland, Edinburgh. F. Russell 'Thomas Patch, Sir William Lowther and the Holker Claude', *Apollo*, Aug. 1975, pp. 115-9.
5. RIA 12.R.9, no. 52.
6. HMC Rept. 12, App. pt. X, p. 227.
7. *Exploring Rome, Piranesi and his Contemporaries*, Catalogue by C. Denison, M.N. Rosenfeld, S. Wiles, Pierpont Morgan Library and Canadian Centre for Architecture, 1993 pp. 99-104.
8. Fleming, p. 230.
9. HMC, Rept. 12, App. pt. X, pp. 231-240.
10. Ibid.
11. Ibid, p. 241.
12. Ibid, pp. 245-6.
13. Ibid, p. 241.
14. Ibid, p. 243.
15. Ibid, p. 254.

PART THREE

Ireland

17

HOME-COMING

With the Roman scandals as yet in the future and no hint of trouble with Piranesi, Patch or John Parker, Charlemont arrived back in England. It had occurred to Lord Bruce that the charms of London would detain Charlemont longer than he anticipated, but even Lord Bruce, still in Lisbon, was surprised to hear of Charlemont still in England in early June. This gave Bruce some hope of seeing him there in September, or earlier should there be a declaration of war between France and England, in which case he planned to come direct from Portugal on the Falmouth packet.

Rumours of war continued and there were reports of hostile incidents in the English channel and elsewhere, but Lord Bruce saw no need for haste. When he eventually reached England, Charlemont had gone.

During the five months he was in England, Charlemont had a house in Suffolk Street and the household arrangements were much as they had been in Rome. Murphy was in charge, Barny in attendance, George Potter still about and a new addition, Lord Bruce's French cook, Longchamp, on loan to Charlemont until such time as his master should again require him.

Charlemont, by all appearances, was very content to be the fashionable young man, seen at Lady Hervey's receptions; the friend of the Marquis of Rockingham (as Lord Malton now was); of the Marquis of Hartington and of his brother, Lord John Cavendish (whom he had met on the Grand Tour); of the Earl of Tylney (at Wanstead for the last time before leaving England for ever to settle in Florence); and known to be the friend of the young Earl of Pembroke and of Lord Bruce, neither of whom had yet returned from their travels. But Charlemont, in taking up such grand connections, did not forget Richard Phelps, who was in low spirits, bored and depressed with his post of tutor to the Duke of Bedford's son and restless to get back to Italy. He went out of his way to meet Phelps again.

The time was yet to come when he would keep a house in

Hertford Street, be a leading member of the Society of Dilettanti, and join the circle of Dr Johnson's Club and count among his friends Topham Beauclerk and Edmund Burke.

For the present he would have been very content had he not been beset by a stream of letters from Adderley, a constant reminder that he must soon leave the delights of London and face the petty irritants, the boredom of unaccustomed responsibilities at home. Adderley saw clearly it would take some spirit to endure the anxieties and vexations of a change from a country as happy as England to one 'so lamentably wretched as this now is' but made little attempt to soften the prospect.[1]

Charlemont heard for the first time of the problems of management on the northern estates; a large tract of bogland was not bringing in a single farthing; two limestone quarries had been discovered at Moy and it had to be considered how these could be brought to advantage; an anonymous letter had been received casting doubt on the honesty of the hitherto entirely trusted land agents, and letters from them, protesting their innocence, followed.

In February Adderley had first mentioned the failure of Dillon's Bank and a run upon the other banks. On 4 March he wrote, 'One ruin draws another. On Saturday last Wilcocks & Dawson stop'd payment. Yesterday Lenox & French did same. Never did this city appear in such dejection – the most moving yet to come, the poor wretched peasants whose all consisted in a five, ten, or twenty pound note of these Banks, have not yet heard the fate of them.'[2] Added to this was a note that credit arranged for Charlemont in London might now be rendered useless.

A fortnight later Adderley wrote again, 'The cashier (Brewer), is now in confinement upon a writ marked for £60,000 at the suit of Wilcocks & Dawson; his papers are in the sheriff's hands ... The Public from the discoveries made of the knavery of Brewer, acquit his employers of any design to impose on the world, but are loud in exclaiming against their very great imprudence in allowing their servant to make such a command over the cash' and it appeared that Brewer had built and furnished a house for himself before attracting any suspicion.[3]

Adderley, having left Charlemont to understand that his losses might be considerable, now assured him that he would not suffer a single farthing and that he would settle the account with Wilcocks & Dawson as soon as he had the London banker's account of the money drawn by Charlemont on Dublin. Lodgements would in the meantime be paid to the bank of Alderman Dawson and his son, unless Adderley received instructions from Charlemont to the contrary. Adderley believed the bank to be as fully secure as any in Dublin. Charlemont let the matter stand: he knew Thomas Dawson, the Alderman's son (Dawson had been in Rome and appeared in the *Parody*) and Adderley confirmed in April that Alderman Dawson's credit with Knox & Craghead in London was in Charlemont's favour.

It is not clear whether Adderley made good the losses out of his own pocket, as the correspondence seems to suggest, or whether there was some adjustment of the revenue from the northern estates to provide for Charlemont's immediate needs and to settle the deficit in London. The incident, which probably disturbed Charlemont very little if at all, foreshadows the financial difficulties Charlemont was to run into in the future, palpably caused by his entirely fatalistic or careless attitude to money, which as yet had not become apparent and in this particular case, was through no fault of his own. Murphy's constant harping on costs from this period on reflects his recognition of the dangers of Charlemont's improvidence rather than the unhealthy state of his exchequer.

Before Charlemont left for Dublin he made out an order in Murphy's favour for 'the sum of one hundred pounds a year until such time as by preferment or otherwise, he shall be in possession of five hundred pounds a year'. On a slip of paper, dated 17 May 1755, Murphy acknowledged 'this high compliment and great mark of tender friendship and goodness from my dearest friend Lord Charlemont' and on another scrap of paper, Charlemont made a note to settle this affair in a proper manner as soon as he could inform himself about the proper legal procedure. It is notable that at the same time Murphy was owed the arrears of his salary over nine years and that a sum of thirteen hundred and ninety-five pounds, seven shillings and eight pence, was not paid until November 1757. The accounting then showed that Murphy had received in Rome in 1753 eight hundred and fifty-six pounds, seven shillings and six and a half pence, the greater part of which probably went to Vierpyle in payment for the Emperor's heads.[4]

Meanwhile Francis, Charlemont's younger brother, who had been discouraged from coming to Paris to meet him, was begging to come to London; Adderley hinted this might not be wise. In 1753 Adderley had, in Charlemont's absence, campaigned unsuccessfully for Francis as opposition candidate in the Armagh election. Now Francis, without aim or occupation, was feared to be easy prey for the hawks.[5] It still rankled with Charlemont that the election had cost him over one thousand pounds.

Charlemont, who did not necessarily lack family feeling, must have been dismayed by Adderley's constant references to domestic arrangements by which it appeared that his brother and his sister, Alice, were no longer Adderley's responsibility. This was not said specifically by Adderley, but implied in the information that the town house of Charlemont's uncle needed about three hundred pounds spent on repairs, conveniences and carpets, which would be better bought in England. The furniture was indifferent, and some of it belonged to Adderley, but he begged leave to present it. The plate all belonged to Charlemont and an inventory was being prepared. It all added up to Adderley's abdication as guardian of his step-children and their affairs.

We have no details of Charlemont's actual home-coming. Adderley had anticipated that thousands would await him and the chiefs of both parties would rejoice to kiss his hands in a country that was wasted by political unrest and strife, and Charlemont looked for as a peacemaker between the two camps.

Murphy, left behind in England to attend to outstanding business, the purchase and despatch of presents to Rome, carpets to Dublin, and innumerable other tasks, wrote on 26 June, 'How does the Air of Ireland agree with your Lordship. How work the Political Volcanos? Produce they smooth or firy Lava or are they extinguished? But I cannot expect from you answers to Lavatick questions. Fond as I am of such information, nor Aetna nor Vesuvius nor the Lavaqueous Globe can furnish me with any half so desired – as your Health & Happiness.'[6]

Charlemont had not yet confided his despair to Murphy, who wrote happily that he had heard with joy and pride that his Lordship was '*fort gouté en Irlandé*'. But the truth was that after his long absence, Charlemont had found few friends among a people whom he had thought of as his own, a people he had little in common with and whose manners and customs he could not view with the curiosity and dispassionateness of a passing traveller, since it was among them that he was expected to live.

That he confided some of the misery to Lord Bruce we know from comments in Lord Bruce's reply. 'You paint so lively that I have a strong idea of your present disagreeable situation and heartily Condole with you on it. Your picture of the Irishman is not less striking and I suppose meant to be of the Flemish school. You pay your Friends in England a great compliment by you saying seeing them again will be a relief to you ...'[7]

Some hint of the Breughelesque scenes which so offended Charlemont is given in his *Essay* on Turkey. Referring to the habits of the hard-riding fox-hunting Irish squires he writes 'After dinner the doors shall be locked, the keys laid on the table,' and the guests drenched with wine until they can hold no more; which out of 'pure Hospitality and Friendship is poured down their Throats' and they are 'left to wallow in Filth and Beastliness'.[8]

Turning to Murphy, Charlemont received a long, meandering letter with some sensible advice, however curiously expressed. 'Shake off that abominable Listlessness, or fly from it to the Coalmines of the North or the Cateract of the Shannon, or to both. Or take a plough and plough up all Ireland and build granaries. Or come hither and arraign this Senate of high Treason against the King and constitution for encouraging the French not the Irish Trade of Cloath in the Levant.' In short Murphy's advice was that he occupy himself, 'Do: be a good Boy and busy yourself.'[9]

Without further consultation, Charlemont took his advice and turned his attention to the improvements at Marino, which were ultimately to prove so expensive to him and, consequently, as he was to apologise in the Political Memoirs addressed to his sons, so expensive to his heirs. Murphy on hearing rumours of this, wrote that it did not sit easily on his mind and he thought the money could be put to better use elsewhere. Charlemont's own account of all this was summarised thus. 'As I had left Ireland when almost a child, I had few or no Acquaintances there ... all my connections and Friendships had been formed among Englishmen, the attractive force of which circumstances I quickly perceived and being thoroughly sensible that it was my indispensible Duty to live in Ireland, determined by some means or other to attach myself to my native country and principally with this in View I began those improvements at Marino.'[10]

But scarcely had Charlemont begun his plans when serious ill-health intervened. He was attacked by 'a violent rheumatism' which by his own account made him 'an absolute cripple' and for the space of two and a half years 'totally disabled' him from any sort of business.[11] During this illness Murphy took on all dealings with Parker and, as we have seen, ill-advisedly although with the best intentions, concealed the beginnings of the dispute with Piranesi. In October 1756 Charlemont was on his way to Aix-la-Chapelle in search of a cure and in such pain it was feared he would not be able to continue the journey. We hear of the many remedies suggested by well-wishers, quacks and clairvoyants and of his trying Gum Guiacum and the Balsam of Mecca,[12] which he had brought back from Egypt. We hear also of the concern of his friends in Rome; of Allan Ramsay reporting to them that he had seen Charlemont at Harwich, and that the sea-bathing had done some good and Dr Irwin, desiring his respects and advising 'nothing but the air of Italy'[13] could recover his Lordship perfectly. Once Mrs Delany* saw him in the Spring Gardens in 'a very weak way'.[14]

Many physicians were consulted and at last, although the condition was not completely eradicated, some relief was obtained through the tender care and skill of the doctor, politician, and author, Charles Lucas. He became, according to Hardy, the recipient of a pension of two hundred pounds a year – a token of Charlemont's gratitude to God and a wise physician – but the pension would seem to have been more in the nature of a retainer. Dr Lucas was to be often in attendance and mention continues through the years of the old enemy rheumatism, of nervous disorders, and eye-trouble. Dr Lucas prescribed sea-water bathing, and that was an added incentive to continue the improvements at Marino. It was close by here that Charlemont, daily, throughout the year, winter and summer, took the most popularly prescribed of eighteenth century medications, a dip in the chilly ocean.[15] The little estate of Donnycarny was aptly renamed Marino.

* Mary Granville Delany (1700-1788), accomplished 2nd wife of Swift's friend, Dr Patrick Delany, knew all the eminent people of her day. Celebrated for her 'paper mosaicks', meticulous copies of botanical specimens ingeniously cut out from coloured paper and pasted on a black ground, which are now in the British Museum.

NOTES

1. HMC, Rept. 12, App. pt. X, p. 208.
2. Ibid.
3. Ibid, p. 209.
4. RIA, 12.R.12, no. 23.
5. Ibid, 12.R.9, no. 26.
6. Ibid, no. 44.
7. Ibid, no. 49.
8. Ibid, 12.R.5, p. 8.
9. HMC, Rept. 12, App. pt. X, p. 221.
10. Ibid, p. 14.
11. Ibid, pp. 8-9.
12. RIA, 12.R.11, no. 10 and 12.R.9, nos. 62, 63. One Thomas Bulger, a quack faith healer, offered advice.
13. HMC, Rept. 12, App. pt. x, pp. 250-1.
14. Lady Llanover ed. Autobiography and Correspondence of Mrs Delany, London 1861, Vol. 3, p. 455.
15. *Memoirs of Nine Illustrious Living Characters*, Dublin 1799 pp. 937-8.

18

ANOTHER LORD BURLINGTON

The improvements at Marino were to become a life's work and culminated in the building of the Neo-Classical miniature masterpiece known as the Casino. The landscaping of the small demesne was designed as its setting. One of the great garden pavilions of the western world, it bears comparison with the Petit Trianon and Lord Burlington's villa at Chiswick. In the context of Chiswick, substituting Neo-Classicism for Palladianism, it is tempting to characterise Charlemont as the Lord Burlington of Ireland.

Such a characterisation might seem an over-simplification of the role Charlemont played in a movement which changed the face of Ireland in the late eighteenth century, had not an anonymous contemporary anticipated that this was the very part he was destined to play.

The unknown author of the Epistle addressed to Charlemont on his return from his travels may have been Richard Marlay. The Epistle was printed in Dublin and seems unlikely to have been written by one of Charlemont's English friends. It extolled Charlemont's virtues, his love of Science and his early fame. It is not until we come to the final couplet that we can recognize it as an adaption of Alexander Pope's Epistle to the Earl of Burlington.

Pope had written:

> You too proceed! make falling arts your care,
> Erect new wonders, and the old repair;
> Jones and Palladio to themselves restore,
> And be whate'er Vitruvius was before: …

Marlay, or another, wrote,

> 'Tis, Yours, sir, to enjoy such pleasing Hours,
> To make what Greece, what Rome can boast of, Ours
> To give to Arts success unknown before
> And fix the Graces on thy native shore.:[1]

Much can be claimed for these modest lines; that they marked the beginning of the Age of Neo-Classicism in Ireland and a renaissance such as the country with her troubled history, had not known since the flowering of Christian Art in the Dark Ages. The unknown versifier had given Charlemont his cue: to champion the cause of Virtu and to preside, like the Minerva of his design for the Carnival in Rome, over the arts and sciences of his own country.

If Charlemont, and he was not without vanity, had any such grandiose ideas about his own capabilities and the future, his first response was weak and showed little resolve about accepting the challenge. The ill-fated approach to Vanvitelli, the survey of the Rotonda at Vicenza, were indications of an ambitious vision that had been rudely dispelled by his first confrontation with the realities. If he were to stay with his purpose, the overriding question had now become how?

The potential of Marino, its beautiful situation overlooking Dublin bay and its close proximity to the city, was an incentive to build there. Shortly after his return, Murphy had wondered if Charlemont would remain at home and 'really finish up your Gallery', which probably meant Charlemont was contemplating alterations to the long room of Marino House, in order to accommodate, however temporarily, his collections. Only a month later rumours reached Murphy of money being laid out at Marino, which, as already mentioned, did not sit easily on his mind. At the same time, under Charlemont's instructions, Murphy, as we shall see, was making overtures to James 'Athenian' Stuart.

Money was spent on acquiring more land. At the cost of £3400, the little estate was increased to about 100 acres. The land transactions of Marino are unusually complicated, and the acreage fluctuated according to the leasing and re-letting of outlying farms. None was freehold and all of it under a head rent to the City of Dublin; but a parcel of 30 acres to the north east of Marino House was held on a lease of lives renewable for ever. It was upon this 30 acres that Charlemont was to concentrate his plans.

Marino House stood outside the selected site; it had no architectural pretensions and, apart from the convenience of having a dwelling close at hand, did not enter into Charlemont's schemes. The overall concept was a *villa* or even a *vigna* in the original Italian sense of the words, a sort of suburban garden or small farm with a little house, a *casino*, to provide a retreat during the summer months; to this plan Charlemont more or less adhered.

In spite of the location and a prospect that to travellers recalled the Bay of Naples and to Charlemont, perhaps, those Greek edifices raised above the sea and distant mountainous islands, open to the sky, the light and the winds, the site would have been regarded as impractical in Ireland, where gentlemen built in hollows rather than on heights, in consideration of warmth and shelter. Marino may have first have been thought of as a summer retreat, but Charlemont's sea bathing regime would alter that.

The additional acres ensured access to the strand and the sea and were not, as might be supposed, for the greater seclusion of the demesne. There were to be no estate walls because Charlemont intended to recall the *Lex Hortorum* of Renaissance Rome, and would open the gates of his 'terrestial paradise' to the citizens of Dublin to walk wherever they chose. This was an unprecedented privilege in Ireland and a testimony to the liberality of his ideas. Obviously open to abuse, it was to be some time before other landowners adopted the practice.

Work began with the kitchen garden at the north end of the thirty acres close to the stables and convenient for the cartage of manure. It was laid out as a five-sided polygon of nine acres enclosed by 12 feet high brick walls. The walls were angled for the best advantage from the sun, and provided with a built-in system of flues to protect the fruit trees from frost. The flues, graduating from the widest at the base to the narrowest at the top, were lined with stucco throughout.

Within the walls, paths radiated from an off-centre hub recalling the lay-out of Renaissance gardens Charlemont had seen in Italy. Hydraulics played their part in an elaborate pattern of stone-vaulted conduits which supplied the kitchen garden with water, before gushing out over a grotto to feed the lake constructed below to the south west. A great stove or hot house, 170 feet long, was built within the walls for the cultivation of exotic fruits and plants, and the housing during the winter months of tender flowering shrubs.

Charlemont's consultant gardener was Matthew Peters (father of the painter the Rev. Matthew Peters) who advertised himself in *Faulkner's Journal* as a gardener and seedsman who 'Designs, draws and executes improvements for gentlemen in the most natural and rural taste in which business he was bred up by his uncle, who was chief gardener to Lord Cobham at Stowe'.[2] Having engaged him, Charlemont sent him to England to study the most up-to-date methods. By late 1756, work was in progress under Peters' direction, with the planting of trained fruit trees against the walls of the kitchen garden begun and the construction of the stove well advanced.

With the following summer came the first signs of disruption. Charlemont, in poor health, was in London when Adderley wrote on 11 June, 'Edgar the gardener has gone from Marino and by Peters' acc. has left all things in great disorder'.[3] Adderley was distrustful of Peters and when again in the following year Peters wrote his complaints, Adderley forwarded the letter to Charlemont with the warning that Peters might be looking for more money. But Peters in his recital of ills wrote, more in sorrow than greed, of the work which had been 'formed from my own Judgement and variety of enquiries when in England (for his Ldsip's Acct. two season's past) to form Walls agreeable to his Lordship's sentiments made known to me, and the manner most proper for the Training & advantage of the Wall Trees, not known here, and but by very few in England, must be Distressful to me to think such Trees should be abandoned to Distruction & such Walls after the great expense his Ldship has been at, furnished with ignorant management ... and the best stove ever constructed should also be put into the hands of ignorance.'[4]

Charlemont at Harwich decided to leave the supervision to Peters, who working without pay, restored order, and planting once more progressed at Marino. Gifts of seeds and plants came from friends and acquaintances, near and far, from then on: the seeds of the 'East India red-flower tree' procured by Adderley from Col. Bagshawe[5]; in 1762 Lord Arran presented 'fourty shining leav'd Laurustinuses' and offered Balm of Gilead, liquid ambers and cockspur hawthorn.[6] Shrubberies outside the kitchen garden walls began to take shape and forest trees were planted to clothe the lake. In August 1758 Charlemont sent the first pineapples from the great stove to Mrs Delany; 'as fine ones as ever I tasted' was her verdict.[7]

It is surprising to us today that progress at Marino attracted so little local attention. But however splendid the stove, the walls and the trained fruit trees, to say nothing of the unusual layout of the nine acres of kitchen garden, Charlemont was not alone in his horticultural aspirations. Pineries and orangeries were not rare in Ireland. There were the gardens at Moira, Co. Down, and Lord Kingston's collection of rare and exotic plants at Mitchelstown. Lord Trimleston personally supervised the raising of pineapples and bananas at Trimleston Castle, Co. Meath and Dr Patrick Delany, without benefit of a green-house or stove, grew orange trees at Delville, Co. Dublin.[8]

Mrs Delany was more interested in matchmaking and Charlemont's health than his activities at Marino. In September 1759 he, and his brother Francis, his sister and half-sister, dined at Delville. She wrote, 'He is perfectly recovered and a very agreeable (ugly) man, sensible, lively and polite. I wish he would fall in love with Miss Mary Hamilton, as she would make him a very proper wife.'[9] Perhaps Mrs Delany had been listening to gossip from England. In May, Lady Caroline Fox had written to her sister, the Countess of Kildare, 'I hear Lord Charlemont is violently in love with pretty Mrs Dunbar and that she don't discourage it, which I am sorry to hear, for she was a sweet, pretty modest-behaved woman as ever I saw; but everybody says he is so agreeable that very possibly she may like him, if that's the case she is to be pitied very much.'[10]

But by then, although they may not have known it, Charlemont had made his decision to spend less time in England and dedicate himself to the improvements at Marino. The three year period of vacillation since he had brought Simon Vierpyle from Rome to Dublin in 1756 was over.

In Rome Vierpyle had been employed by Charlemont in moulding wax ornaments for an exact model (in wood) of the Falconieri gates (the subject of one of Piranesi's calumnies). Parker, in forwarding other designs on the eve of Vierpyle's departure, had written, 'Vierpoyle will be about to assist your builders as to the execution without other models in wood'.[11] Vierpyle had arrived. A house had been made over to him in Henry Street and, apart from some outside commissions for statuary work, for which he had taken the precaution of shipping 12 blocks of marble from Carrara, he had been kicking his heels ever since. No decision had been made about gates for Marino and there were no builders for him to assist.

After the breakdown of negotiations with Vanvitelli, Parker had suggested two former pupils of Niccolo Salvi's and, at the same time, submitted a design of his own – 'in plain Dorick'.[12] Charlemont's further instructions, on hearing that Fernando Fuga had gone to Naples, and without considering Parker's own submission, were that if Vanvitelli came down in his demands, the drawings of the Santa Scala should be sent to him. The reference to the Santa Scala is not easily explained and we hear no more of Vanvitelli.

Charlemont's next thought was the Lanthern of Demosthenes (the Choragic Monument) for which plans (according to the *Irish Builder* of 1894) were prepared by William Chambers, and that

Murphy on seeing 'the engravings' had written, 'Have a care, my dear Lord, how you undertake this building. If the Lanthern costs you more than £200, or £250 at most, it will be an extravagant article ... in the original, the architrave and freize are all of one stone.'[13]

Murphy's letter is no longer extant, but on stylistic grounds alone, even without the sentiments, we can hardly doubt that the *Irish Builder* had access to a genuine document. The construction that was placed upon it however is questionable. Apart from Chamber's well-known antipathy to the *gusto greco*, and the unlikelihood of Charlemont consulting him on such a project, the word 'engraving' is the clue. The first volume of the *Antiquities of Athens* did not appear until 1762, but since 1755 Stuart had been back in London working on the plates. Weight is given to this supposition in Murphy's letter of October 1755 from Bath when he wrote Charlemont he had not yet heard from 'Mr Stewart'.[14]

NOTES

1. RIA, Pamphlet 254, no. 5.
2. Strickland, Vol. 2, p. 229.
3. HMC Rept. 12, App. pt. X.
4. RIA, 12.R.9, no. 67.
5. C. O'Connor, 'Gardening at Marino' *Moorea*, Vol. 2, pp. 29-37. For 'Wordsworth' read Colonel Wadsworth of Connecticut.
6. RIA, 12.R.12, no. 33.
7. Lady Llandover ed. *Autobiography and Correspondence of Mary Grenville, Mrs Delany*, London 1861, Vol. 3, p. 511.
8. E.C. Nelson, 'Some Records (c. 1690-1830) of Greenhouses in Irish Gardens', *Moorea*, Vol. 2, pp. 21-5.
9. Llandover ed. p. 566.
10. B. Fitzgerald ed. *Correspondence of Emily, Duchess of Leinster*, Dublin 1950, Vol. 1, p. 222.
11. HMC, Rept. 12, App. pt. X, p. 226.
12. Ibid, pp. 221-2.
13. *Irish Builder*, Vol. 36, Mar. 1st 1894, p. 50.
14. HMC, Rept. 12, App. pt. X, p. 221.

19

THE APPOINTMENT OF WILLIAM CHAMBERS

It is not known precisely when or in what circumstances began that association between Charlemont and Chambers which is so often held up as the ideal of understanding between patron and architect. The lack of documentation with regard to Chambers' appointment is undoubtedly due to Charlemont's constant presence in London. Discussions would have taken place at the house in Hertford Street or at Chambers' offices. The correspondence between the two men, as it survives, starts in 1763, by which time the foundations of the Casino had been laid and building had started on the town house in Rutland Square, Dublin.

Assuming Charlemont had already met and favoured Chambers in Rome, the renewal of that earlier connection was inevitable and the first indication of this appears in 1757. In that year Chambers published his *Designs of Chinese Buildings*, which he dedicated to George, Prince of Wales and Princess Augusta. Among the list of subscribers we find all the chief members of Charlemont's set in Rome: the Marquis of Rockingham, the Earls Tylney and Pembroke, Lord Bruce, Sir Thomas Kennedy, Sir Matthew Fetherstonhaugh, John Ward, Thomas Scrope, Charles Turner, Robert Wood and Philip Stanhope, besides Mr J. Reinolds (*sic*) painter and Joseph Wilton sculptor.

All of these, except for Lord Bruce, had subscribed for one set each. His and Charlemont's names stand out from the other subscribers for four sets apiece, and the list includes the names of Thomas Adderley and Richard Marlay, who, having had no previous connection with Chambers, would only have subscribed on Charlemont's recommendation.

Allowing for the interim between the proposal and publication would take us back to 1756 at the latest, and if in that year Charlemont had not already approached Chambers, we can at least assume that he was then giving him consideration. In September, while Charlemont was at Aix-en-Chapelle and still in poor health,

Lord Bruce was, to the consternation of the Adam brothers, travelling with Chambers in Scotland.

In Janury 1757 Charlemont and Bruce were in London and had their first sittings for their portraits by Reynolds. In April, while Charlemont was still in London, Chambers issued the Proposal for the *Treatise on Civil Architecture* and, taking into account the prominence given in the publication to the Casino, it may be assumed that, at the time of the Proposal, Chambers had already grounds for believing the commission his, even if there was not yet a formal understanding.

At all events, it would seem that Charlemont had come to a decision in the summer of 1757, when he took the momentous step of mortgaging various castles, manors, lands and tenancies in the counties of Armagh, Tyrone and Monaghan to commence building. A memorial of a deed dated 7 September 1757 records an agreement with William Harvey of Chigwell in Essex and James Colebrook of Gatten in Surrey for the consideration of twenty thousand pounds.[1]

By the standards of his English peers Charlemont was not a rich man and the income from his estates was probably not above eight thousand a year. Consequently the raising of the stake by another ten thousand in mortgages by 1760 placed him in a position from which there was no turning back without an enormous loss of face to himself as well as Chambers. The designs for the Casino had already been published in 1759, and described by Chambers as 'a magnificent Casino', designed by him for the Lord Viscount Charlemont's seat at Marino.

A drawing, which was originally among Chambers' papers, is thought to be a preliminary sketch for the Casino. It is not in Chambers' hand. The drawing is for a cruciform temple dedicated to the Arts, Sculpture, Architecture and Painting; jottings on the verso show a dome, two indistinct plans and the legend 'Recapitulation of the Event of the Year 1757. Prince Edward under Commodore How'. The inscription, apparently a reference to one of Howe's sorties in the Channel against the French, may have no particular significance, but the year agrees with Charlemont's raising of the first mortgage.[2]

The sketch cannot be convincingly claimed as Charlemont's, but we know from the later correspondence that it was not unknown for him to illustrate his own ideas for the designs he ordered with a sketch, however weak. Charlemont was always in command of the over all plan for Marino, which Chambers never saw, and although the Casino was to be the jewel in the crown, it had to be fitting to the whole.

The question arises whether Charlemont took a more active part in the design than is generally assumed. Hardy wrote 'The late Dr Quin*, who was himself an excellent judge of the fine arts, used to say, that he had just reason to believe, that Lord Charlemont himself planned the temple at Marino, and resigned the credit of it to Sir William Chambers.'[3]

In 1777, Thomas Campbell published his *Philosophical Survey of Ireland* in which he went further than Dr Quin and asserted that both Charlemont House and the Casino were designed by Charlemont. 'His Lordship is not only a patron of the arts, but also a great proficient in them; his house is of his own planning. And I have seen, at his beautiful gardens at Marino, near town, a temple of his design; of which a print was lately struck off in London.'[4]

Against all of this was Chambers' claim, or admission, that the design was 'originally one of the end pavillions of a considerable composition, made soon after my return from Italy, for Edwin Lascelles Esq'. Chambers had smarted under the humiliation of the rejection by Lascelles, and it is to be supposed that only the self-assurance that came with success enabled him to refer to it thus in the 3rd edition of his *Treatise*. And possibly, at the same time, to quell rumours about Charlemont's authorship.

Charlemont's overall scheme for Marino provided, as with other estates in England at the time, an approved route for visitors. Guests would pass, by meandering paths, from dark enclosed groves to open undulating lawns. They were led, at every turn, to yet another unexpected vista of the mountains in the distance, Dublin Bay, the city or the temple, the Casino itself, from another angle.

It can be seen, in the painting of Marino with the Casino by Thomas Roberts (formerly attributed to William Ashford), that Charlemont was inspired in his landscaping by the Claudian ideal. On his visits to Lord Bruce at Tottenham he would have met Henry Hoare, Bruce's neighbour and future father-in-law, and seen Stourhead. Hoare had in his collection a copy of Claude's *View of Delphi*; the picture with its version of the Pantheon was the source of Flitcroft's temple in its landscaped setting. It remains today the chief glory of Stourhead's gardens.

There was nothing particularly advanced in the Claudian concept.

* Dr Henry Quin, an eminent physician in Dublin.

Gentlemen, all over England, were out and about determining the Claudian potential of their demesnes, using that fashionable piece of equipment, a Claude glass which, silvered or blackened and slightly convex, reduced the most extensive scene to the dimensions of a small drawing.

Charlemont had in his possession, at least by 1761, a painting purported to be by Claude. This was probably the picture, 'Landscape with Cattle; signed,' which was in the Marino sale catalogue in 1875. However it is with a painting known as *The Marriage of Isaac and Rebecca*, with its columnar temple, that Roberts' view has most affinity; it would seem to have been the source of Charlemont's inspiration so far.[5] There were to be other buildings, including another temple, built in contrast to the Casino, and for which other influences will have to be considered. The improvements at Marino were a long drawn out, ever expanding, process.

We do not know how long it took to build the Casino – neither when building began nor when it was completed – but, at the most conservative estimate, it was no less than fifteen years. The leisurely pace is usually attributed to shortage of money, and it is assumed that all work ceased when money ran out and Chambers was no longer employed.

It is reasonable to assume, in spite of some evidence to the contrary, that building commenced in the summer of 1758. Charlemont had mortgaged his estates, therefore signifying his intention to commence operations. A receipt for a pear-wood model of the Casino by Bononi Thacker was, according to a nineteenth-century source, dated February 1758.[6] That receipt, and the model, have since disappeared, but there are no grounds for doubting their authenticity.[7] In 1759 the *Treatise* was published and the Casino entered as 'now erecting'.

In his *Views of the Seats of the Nobility and Gentry* 1783, Thomas Milton records (while admitting both the dates and the inscription were committed from memory, his notes having been mislaid or lost), that the foundation stone was laid in either 1761 or 1762 and that it carried a brass dedicatory plaque, that read, 'This Building was erected as a Testimony of Gratitude to Public and Private Virtue, during the Administration of William Pitt, when the glory of the British Empire arrived at its highest pitch'.[8]

Lord Bute replaced William Pitt in 1761. The inscription is in the past tense and, in view of Charlemont's British patriotic sentiments as expressed in his design for the Triumphal car in Rome, we cannot reasonably doubt Milton's accuracy. Yet again, we find Charlemont's Roman circle in accord: Thomas Scrope designed a small half-domed rotunda, which he erected at Coleby and dedicated to Pitt.

The explanation may be that the foundation stone was, in fact, laid in 1761 or 1762, work having started three or four years before. What is not apparent from Chambers' plans for 'the Cellary Storey' is the actual extent of the subterranean offices. Substantial vaults were constructed to circumvent the basement areas at the west, east and south sides. A tunnel was built that ran to a chamber some thirty yards to the west. It then continued on towards an unknown destination, perhaps turning south to Marino House to the south.

The major contribution to the first delay was the unexpected discovery of a copious spring in sinking the foundations. Perhaps taking heart from the classical aspect of this apparent misfortune, and his exploration of the fountain of the Acropolis at Corinth, Charlemont had the spring contained within excellent masonry; spacious steps were cut and laid down to the well.

In October 1761 we hear for the first time from an outside observer of the progress at Marino, and it is ironic that there was, at the time, some expectation of the building being completed within a year. George Montagu, the friend of Horace Walpole, came to Ireland in the train of his cousin, the new Viceroy, Lord Halifax. In a letter dated 1 October 1761, he first mentions Charlemont to Walpole, 'the paragon of this kingdom Lord Charlemont is making an Abs Court farm and Casino that promises to be very pretty'.[9]

In replying on 8 October, Walpole remarked, 'Lord Charlemont's villa is in Chambers' book'. Apparently Montagu did not give this his full attention because he wrote on 4 November, 'I have been to see Lord Charlemont's villa, the situation of the house beautiful and the whole edifice finished in about twelve months. The design, by what I can judge of it, will be vastly pretty; there is an old couchant lioness on one side of the landing-place, extremely well executed. The stone and artificers are from England and the work is well performed. Perhaps it is in Chambers' book.'[10]

There is a certain ambiguity in Montagu's account, and one has the impression Charlemont was not present to clarify. The presence of English artificers and the lioness on the terrace suggests that building had risen to ground level, but not necessarily that the dedication plaque had been set in. Pitt had only just been forced into resignation (to be replaced by Lord Bute), and the inscription was probably an outlet for

Charlemont's political and patriotic indignation. We may conclude that Milton was correct in the date between 1761 and 1762 for the plaque; the foundation stone itself must have been laid long before unless Milton confused it with the stereobate of the *piano nobile*.

Montagu's observance on the lioness has a particular interest. The lions, copies of the antique Egyptian lions of the Capitoline, are traditionally the work of Joseph Wilton. The presence of a single lion suggests either a model for Vierpyle or, more likely, the first of the four to be carved by him from a plaster cast of the original. The reliefs with which Charlemont replaced the fountains of the design in the *Treatise*, can reasonably be supposed to have been carved by Vierpyle, but the source of this variation to Chambers' design has not been identified.

Towards the end of December Montagu wrote again, 'I have been to see Lord Charlemont's collection. He has some charming things that would merit a show even at Strawberry. His medals are very fine, a charming Titian of Borgia, two Carlo Marats, a Claude, two fine vases, a Queen Elizabeth that he says was in Dr Meade's collection three quarters carved in onyx, a lion's skin of yellow that serves for a veil, a brave collection of books and an edition of a Voyage to Nubia printed in Copenhagen that on comparison with Backerville absolutely excels.'[11]

To which Walpole replied rather tartly, 'Lord Charlemont's Queen Elizabeth I know perfectly well, he outbid me for it. Is his villa finished? I am pleased with the design in Chambers.'

In February Walpole sent Montagu the first volumes of *Anecdotes of Painting in England* in which, under an entry for Valerio Belli (called Valerio Vicentino), the cameo was described: 'a fine bust of queen Elizabeth on onyx, *alto relievo* in profile and very large, by the hand of this master.'[12] A footnote recorded that Lord Charlemont bought it at Dr Meade's sale. When this cameo was exhibited by the 3rd Earl in 1872 at the Dublin Exhibition of Arts and Industries (Loan section), it was described as 'carved in full relief with large ruff and elaborately ornamented bodice, clothed in lion's skin and jewels'.

Evidently Montagu had seen the *Anecdotes* in manuscript, because he wrote on 27 February 1762, 'A thousand thanks to you for your books; though I had read them before. I shall show them to the Bishop of Derry [William Barnard] and Lord Charlemont, the only two people who understand any of the matter. It will not hinder the sale, but promote it.'[13]

Earlier, on 18 February, Montagu had warned Walpole, 'You may send your books in three parcels directed to Mr Secretary Hamilton ... No books, even yours, are never sent over here; they never read. Hamilton says he never found a book or a whore in any one's house since he came to Dublin.'[14]

Under the cover of waggery was Hamilton's and Montagu's discomfiture. These houses were where they dare not go for fear of Irish customs of hospitality, the same that Charlemont deplored. Rather than submit themselves to the drinking habits of Dublin society, they chose to be regarded as freakish and stayed in of an evening.[15]

NOTES

1. Registry of Deeds, Dublin, Memorial 2634.
2. Sir John Barrow, *Life of Richard, Earl Howe*, London 1838, pp. 45-51 Edward Augustus, Duke of York, midshipman, served with Commodore Howe in 1758, not 1757. Charlemont greatly admired Howe; Hardy, p.366.
3. Hardy, p.422
4. *A Philosophical Survey of the South of Ireland*, a series of letters to John Watkinson, M.D. (T. Campbell) London, 1777, p.24.
5. I am indebted to Patrick Bowe, who drew my attention to this. K. Lamb and P. Bowe, *A History of Gardening in Ireland*, 1995, p.35.
6. *The Irish Times*, 16 Sept. 1886 p.6. Proceedings of the Royal Dublin Society, 20 Jan. 1870.
7. Said to have been dated Feb. 1758 with a receipt for 50gns. Neither model or receipt have been traced.
8. T. Milton, *Views of Different Seats of the Nobility and Gentry*, London and Dublin 1783, pl.5.
9. W.S. Lewis and R.S. Brown ed. *Horace Walpole Correspondence,* Yale edition, Vol.9, p.391. Editor's note see E. Brayley, *Topographical History of Surrey*, 1850, vol.2 p.320.
10. Walpole Correspondence, Vol.9, p.400.
11. Ibid p.414.
12. Walpole, *Anecdotes of painting in England*, 3rd ed. London 1782, Vol. 1, p.276.
13. Walpole Correspondence, Vol.10, p.17.
14. Ibid p.11.
15. Ibid, Vol.9, pp.393, 399-400.

20

CHARLEMONT, HOGARTH AND WALPOLE

It is not clear from the correspondence of 1761 between Walpole and Montagu whether Walpole had by then met Charlemont. Walpole's interest could have arisen from seeing the designs for the Casino in the *Treatise* and some pique at having been out-bid for the cameo.

Charlemont, as we know, held Walpole in high regard and in the final years remembered him as an old and kind friend and 'undoubtedly the most pleasing Companion I ever knew'.[1]

Today the comparison is frequently made between the two masterpieces of architecture in miniature, Chiswick House and the Casino, and it is not so curious that all Walpole wrote of Chiswick should apply so aptly to the Casino. Both were beautiful buildings regarded by contemporaries as very ill-fitted for dwelling; 'His lordship's house at Chiswick ... is a model of taste, though not without faults, some of which are occasioned by too strict adherence to rules and symmetry ... Yet these blemishes, and Lord Hervey's wit, who said *the house was too small to inhabit, and too large to hang to one's watch*, cannot depreciate the taste that reigns in the whole.'[2]

Charlemont may have found some satisfaction in identifying, in spite of the disparate of styles, his aspirations for Marino with those of Walpole at Strawberry Hill. Strawberry, like Marino, was created, not from some grand and noble estate, but from comparatively humble material, a delightful site and a small, cramped and featureless house. On first seeing it, Walpole's friend, Etheldreda, Lady Townshend had exclaimed in profane dismay, 'Lord God! Jesus! What a house! It is just such a house as the parson's, where the children lie at the foot of the bed',[3] which was synonymous with Murphy's opinion that the money would be better spent elsewhere than at Marino.

The earliest meetings between Walpole and Charlemont, both patrons of Hogarth, may well have taken place in the artist's studio.

We know that Walpole was a spectator to, and had much to say about, the scandal that arose out of the terms under which Hogarth was persuaded by Charlemont and Sir Richard Grosvenor to reverse his decision in 1757 to abandon history painting. This was in effect a notice of Hogarth's intention to paint no more morality subjects or 'drolleries' in the manner of the *Rake's Progress* and *Marriage à la Mode*.

Hogarth wanted to devote his time and remaining energies to portraiture and engraving, more reliable and profitable sources of income, but he agreed to paint for each of them a subject picture. Because of the unusual circumstances, he was to choose his own subject, finish the work in his own time, and charge whatever he thought proper. It was, of course, a recipe for trouble.

Charlemont's picture was finished first; *The Lady's Last Stake* was all he could have desired.

Sir Richard, hoping for as much or more, had to wait. When at last he saw his painting, he was at first incredulous and then very angry. The money asked, four hundred guineas, meant little to Sir Richard, a very rich man, except as an insult in its topical allusion and as a sneer at a group of connoisseurs, among which Sir Richard accounted himself. A *Sigismunda*, for that was the subject Hogarth had chosen, had been sold in May 1758 from the collection of Sir Luke Schaub, who was rated by Vertue as a prime minister among connoisseurs and, as Sir Luke had pronounced it by Correggio himself, it had fetched four hundred guineas.[4]

Walpole's account of the affair does not excuse Hogarth and gives good reason for Sir Richard's complaint. 'From a contempt of the ignorant virtuosi of the age, and from indignation at the impudent tricks of picture-dealers, whom he [Hogarth] saw continually recommending and vending vile copies to bubble-collectors, and from having never studied, indeed having seen, few good pictures of the great Italian masters, he persuaded himself that the praises bestowed on those glorious works were nothing but the effects of prejudice. He talked this language till he believed it; and having heard it often asserted, as is true, that time gives a mellowness to colours and improves them, he not only denied the proposition, but maintained that pictures only grew black and worse by age, not distinguishing between the degrees in which the proposition might be true or false. He went farther: he determined to rival the ancients – and unfortunately chose one of the finest pictures in England as the object of his competition. This was the celebrated Sigismonda of Sir Luke Schaub

... said to be painted by Correggio, probably by Furino, but no matter by whom. It is impossible to see the picture or read Dryden's inimitable tale, and not feel that the same soul animated both. After many essays Hogarth at last produced *his* Sigismonda – but no more like Sigismonda than I to Hercules. Not to mention the wretchedness of the colouring, it was the representation of a maudlin strumpet just turned out of keeping, and with eyes red with rage and usquebaugh, tearing off the ornaments her keeper had given her. To add to the disgust raised by such vulgar expression, her fingers were bloodied by her lover's heart that lay before her like that of a sheep's for her dinner ...'[5]

In a later note Walpole adds that the fingers on inspection are unstained by blood and perhaps his memory is at fault, but that he had seen it when it was first painted, and 'bloody they were'.

Hearing that Henry Hoare was in the market for a Hogarth, Sir Richard seized upon the excuse. He wrote to Hogarth that he had no objection to Hoare having the picture since 'the performance was so striking and inimitable that the constantly having it before one's eyes would too often occasion melancholy thoughts to arise in one's mind, which a curtain being drawn before it would not diminish in the least'.[6]

This devastatingly rude letter put Charlemont in a quandary. Hogarth was furious and would not forgive the insult. Charlemont, ecstatically pleased with his picture, did not want to fall out with Hogarth or to take his side against Sir Richard. Moreover he did not want and he could not afford to pay what might then be presumed to be the exorbitant and going rate.

Without anything settled, Hogarth began a portrait of Charlemont. It was never finished. But in its incomplete state, Charlemont appears young, amiable, weak and foppish and with nothing of that expressive animation that his contemporaries found so agreeable. Perhaps it reflects the vacillation of the sitter in the affair of *Sigismunda* and the *Lady's Last Stake*.

Charlemont left for Ireland without settling for the picture, which was left in Hogarth's studio at the artist's request for engraving. Horace Walpole saw it there with the *Sigismunda*.

Before he left London Charlemont wrote Hogarth a note of fumbling apology. 'I am still your Debtor, more so indeed than I shall ever be able to pay, and did intend to have sent you before my Departure what trifling recompense my abilities permit me to make you. But the truth is, having wrongly calculated my expenses, I find myself unable for the present even to attempt paying you. However if you be in any present need of money, let me know it and as soon as I get to Ireland, I will send you, not the Price of the Picture, for that is inestimable, but as much as I can afford to give for it.'[7]

Back in Dublin on 29 January 1760 he resolved his difficulties by sending a sum which was on par with the usual rates rather than the terms of the agreement. He wrote to Hogarth, 'I send you a note upon Nesbitt for one hundred Pounds and considering the name of the author and the surpassing merit of your performance, I am really much ashamed to offer such a Trifle in recompense for the Pains you have taken and the Pleasure your Picture has afforded me. I beg you wou'd think that I by no means attempt to pay you according to your merrit, but according to my Abilities. Were I to pay your deserts I fear I should leave myself poor indeed. Imagine that you have made me a present of the picture, for literally as such I take it and that I have begged your Acceptance of the enclosed Trifle ...'[8]

Hogarth was not dissatisfied. According to Mrs Hogarth after her husband's death, he had always spoken of Charlemont with 'the greatest pleasure and gratitude'.

In 1763 Hogarth planned some breakfast lectures on his engravings for, among others, Charlemont, Walpole and Topham Beauclerk. (Topham Beauclerk was the only one of Dr Johnson's circle with whom Charlemont kept up a regular correspondence). Before the lectures, Hogarth selected some impressions to form a basis for Charlemont's collection of prints. It was a collection that Charlemont did not at first take very seriously; twenty years later he was looking for the *Cockpit*, the *Five Orders of the Periwig, Credulity, Superstition* and *Fanaticism* to fill the gaps. Such acquisitions as he had made in the meantime were not engravings but paintings and included the '*Gate of Calais*'.

Although there is no documentary evidence to pinpoint the date of Charlemont's first contact with Walpole, it is well-nigh impossible to think Charlemont's decision to build Gothick was not influenced by him. Since George Montagu could hardly have failed to mention to Walpole the beginning of such building at Marino in 1761, it would seem that the Gothic Room, a temple at the northern end of the lake was erected in unusual haste by Charlemont's standards, between 1762 and 1763. When in October 1763, Lady Northumberland visited Marino the painted windows were in situ.

The most complete description of the Gothic Room is that of

Caesar Otway, writing in 1835; by then the building was in a ruinous state. 'An erection in the enriched Gothic style; the front representing a highly ornamental screen, adorned with tracery and niches: a noble pointed doorway with receding columns, and fretted mouldings, opens in the centre, and a crocketed pinacle a little retired conveys the idea of a spire; the interior has been fitted up to imitate the nave, and side aisles of a cathedral, with clustered columns, deeply moulded arches, and groined ceiling; the hearth at the upper end, has been, when perfect, a beautiful composition of elaborate tracery; the light is admitted by four quaterfoil windows of stained glass, and the floor is constructed of marble in Mosaic; in its original perfect state, this edifice was supposed to present as pure a model of a Gothic, as the other did of a Grecian temple.'[9]

Leaving aside Otway's misconception about the style of the Casino, and that when he was writing the Gothic temple was a ruin, it is clear that he has taken the point that they were built for the effect of contrast.

Most visitors were struck by the windows but unfortunately made no reference to author or subject. They were of painted glass (not stained in the present meaning of the word) and the evidence suggests that Thomas Jervais had executed them.

Jervais is now best known for the great window of New College Chapel, Oxford which he painted to the designs of Reynolds, and the equally large Resurrection of St George's Chapel, Windsor. He was a native of Dublin, who was employed at Rathfarnham Castle and also by the Duke of Leinster on the bow windows of Leinster House before he left for England in 1770. Very little of his early work survives; in contrast to his later work, it seems to have been all on a very small scale. Some idea of the delicacy of his paintings on small panels of glass can be gauged from the sale catalogue of Cremorne Villa, Chelsea in 1827 when a window he had painted for Sir Thomas Dawson (Charlemont's compatriot Grand Tourist in Rome, afterwards Lord Dartrey and Viscount Cremorne) came under the hammer; it consisted of 'twenty eight compartments, containing copies from Italian and Flemish masters, beautifully finished' and was sold with 'a large magnifying glass on a tripod stand'.[10]

That Jervais was patronized by Charlemont is known since he recommended him to Horace Walpole when Jervais departed for London. A report in the *Gentleman's Magazine* of 27 February 1807 read: 'A fire broke out in the dwelling house of the beautiful demesne of Marino, the residence of the Dowager Countess of Charlemont, near Dublin. The Northern Wing of the building was destroyed, in which was a very beautiful drawing room, the windows of which were ornamented with some of the most masterly productions in stained glass, by the late celebreated Jervis.'

The drawing room was a part of the extension to Marino House undertaken by Charlemont around 1775, some five years after Jervais' departure and so one concludes that the painted glass that ornamented the windows had been acquired previously and, perhaps, at the same time as those of the Gothic Room.

There is an unexplained entry in the bill of a Dublin carver and gilder, Ignatius McDonagh, who is known to have been employed at Marino House and the Gothic Room between 1774 and 1776, which apparently refers to the windows: May 1776 'To a man sinking glass at the Gothic Room 0.5.0.'[11] Presumably this related to repairs, and not the removal of the glass panels from the Gothic Room to the drawing room of Marino House because, when T.K. Cromwell visited Marino in 1820, he saw Rosamund's Bower, as the Gothic Room came to be named, with stained glass Caesar Otway recorded, in 1835, four quatrefoil windows of stained glass.

Apparently it was Charlemont who named the building Rosamund's Bower. John O'Keefe, the dramatist, tells us in his *Memoirs* that in about 1776 he, with a friend, was walking through Donneycarny when Lord Charlemont, standing at the entrance to his splendid villa and grounds, invited them in and showed them the Casino and 'his Rosamund's Bower, which had a beautiful window of stained glass'.[12]

T.K. Cromwell described Rosamund's Bower as being at the upper extremity of the lake, 'in a dark sequestered retreat, embosomed with trees'[13] and from others we hear of the approach through winding paths in the thickest part of the shrubberies. There was no maze or labyrinth, but the place exemplified the legend of the bower of Henry II's mistress, Rosamund Clifford; the legend of which Walpole wrote in his *Essay on Modern Gardening*, that 'it was no doubt more difficult to find her in a park than in a palace, when the intricacy of the woods and various lodges buried in covert might conceal her actual habitation.'

Fair Rosamund's tombstone at Godstone Abbey church bears the whimsical couplet, of which Henry II is said to have been the author:

'This tomb does here enclose
The world's most beauteous rose,
Rose passing sweet erstwhile,
Now naught but odour vile.'[14]

On a rock close by the Gothic Room, where a fountain cascaded into the lake, Charlemont had carved by one of his masons this epitaph to a lost love:

'*Le penchant nous unite*
Le Destin nous separe.'

When Thomas Jervais decided to seek his fortune in England, he went with Charlemont's blessing. It is perhaps significant, in view of the particular work that he had done for Charlemont, that it was to Walpole that Charlemont recommended him. None other of Charlemont's circle, except Thomas Bagot, were building Gothick.

Walpole wrote on 17 October 1770 from Arlington Street, 'an artist that your Lordship patronizes will, I imagine, want little recommendation, besides his own talents … I am yet guessing only at Mr Jervais's merit; but though he has lodged himself within a few doors of me, I have not been able to get to him, having been confined near two months with the gout, and still keeping my house. My first visit shall be to gratify my duty and curiosity.'[15]

The remainder of Walpole's letter is concerned with Walpole's tragedy, *The Mysterious Mother*, an inscribed copy of which from the author, was to be one of the treasures of Charlemont's library. 'I am sorry to say, and beg your Lordship's pardon for the confession, that, however high an opinion I have of your taste, in the arts, I do not equally respect your judgement in books … After so saucy an attack, my Lord, it is time to produce my proof. It lays in your own postscript, where you express a curiosity to see a certain tragedy, with a hint that other works of the same author have found favour in your sight, and that the piece ought to be sent to you. But, my Lord, even your approbation has not made that author vain; and for the play in question it has so many perils to encounter that it never thinks of producing itself. It peeped out of its lurking corner once or twice, and one of those times, by the negligence of a friend, had like to have been, what is often pretended in prefaces, *stolen* and *consigned to the press*. When your Lordship comes to England, which, for every reason but that, I hope will be soon, you shall certainly see it; and will then allow, I am sure, how improper it would be for the author to risque its appearance in public.'[16]

Walpole's friends were greatly divided on the merits of the play. George Montagu was particularly appalled by the repugnant subject (incest), however movingly and with what a power and suspense, the plot was sustained; Charlemont was apparently unequivocal in his admiration.

Impressed as Charlemont undoubtedly was by Walpole, it is still difficult to assess the extent of Walpole's influence on Charlemont's only essay into Gothick architecture; more especially because the architect Charlemont chose to employ had been dismissed from Strawberry Hill in 1759.

Johann Heinrich Müntz's capability for architecture had not been explored at Strawberry, where he had been since 1755 employed as painter and decorator. It was after his dismissal by Walpole for gross impertinence that he had offered his *Proposals for Publishing by Subscription a Course of Gothic Architecture.*[17]

Müntz, was a man who could have appealed to Charlemont, and indeed Walpole had at first thought him humble, modest and reasonable; he 'has seen so much, and knows so much, of countries and languages that I am not likely to be soon tired of him' Walpole had written.[18] A Swiss of extraordinary versatility, he had been at one time an engineer in the French army; he had studied Moorish architecture in Spain, and he had been in Rome at the same time as Charlemont and Chambers. It was Chambers who, it is supposed, had brought his Moorish designs to the notice of the Royal patrons at Kew through Lord Bute, and it may have been Chambers who first introduced him to Charlemont. However while he was in Rome he had worked on a treatise on ancient vases, a subject close to Charlemont's heart. Müntz had made drawings from the collections of the Borghese, from those at the Villa Medici, from the excavations of the Baths of Diocletian and from the workshop of the sculptor-restorer, Cavaceppi, and, incidentally, from the collection of Patch's old enemy, the Bishop of Tivoli. From Rome he had gone to Paris and Nantes and then to Jersey. It was in Jersey that Richard Bentley had come across him and had sent him to Walpole.

Müntz in his *Proposals* of 1760 refers to drawings for 'a Temple in a garden, in the Moresque stile, of the Author's composition, and which is going to be executed at a Nobleman's Country Seat'. This could have been Marino, although two existing drawings 'Plan for the

Egyptian Room at Marino, Dublin' and 'Section of an Egyptian Room for Lord Charlemont' are dated 1762.[19]

Despite their captions the designs are Gothic and there is no very satisfactory explanation for the term Egyptian. Michael McCarthy in *The Origins of the Gothic Revival* suggests that it was for the antiquities the room was designed to house, that the room was named. We see from the section that Müntz is again on the old tack of vases. Eventually Charlemont's Egyptian collections were to be gathered in the corridor at Charlemont House, where they were seen by Pool and Cash in 1780. In 1762 work at Charlemont House could barely have begun and we cannot discount the idea that Charlemont intended there should be another reference at Marino to his Egyptian travels, in the Gothic Room as with the lions of the Casino.

The question is, of course, whether Müntz's designs were executed. No elevation of the Egyptian Room has been found and the unusual oval plan,[20] unpreceded in Gothic architecture, is, if it was carried out, not noticed by Caesar Otway in his description. A slight pencil sketch by Thomas Leeson Rowbotham, and another by Samuel Frederick Brocas, distant views of the building in the trees at the head of the lake, are inconclusive.[21]

Apart from the Gothic Room and the designs of 1762, there is indisputable evidence for Charlemont employing Müntz in 1768 when Chambers wrote 'I have seen Müntz & press'd him to finish your Lordship's design several times, he says now your Lordship shall have a sketch of it by the next post.'[22] This design was almost certainly for the Gothic seat, situated as we know from the Ordnance Survey of 1837, to the south west of the lake and the subject of one of Thomas Leeson Rowbotham's drawings.

If Charlemont had not been satisfied with the designs of 1762, it is unlikely he would again have employed Müntz. This gives some support to the supposition that Müntz was the architect of the Gothic Room even if it was built to designs of his other than the ones we know.

Müntz's section drawing could, at a stretch, be found to relate to Otway's side aisles (with clustered columns and deeply moulded arches with a groined ceiling), but it is the plan which holds the clue. A Pennsylvania stove is specified in Müntz's plan. This type of iron stove was still an innovation since it was only, as far as is known, in 1759 that it was first introduced into England and made at the Carron Works in Scotland.

The operation of this stove, in appearance like a protruding oven, raised on legs with closed front plates and with neither draft door nor smoke pipe, depended entirely upon the conveyance of heat through concealed flues from an adjoining fire or furnace in another room. Müntz's plan, although specifying the Pennsylvania stove, gives no indication of the source of heat. Traditionally the Gothic Room was said to be used for banqueting. This would suggest there might have been a kitchen and there is some evidence for this. Heat could have been conducted from cooking ranges or an oven for the Pennsylvania stove, depending on the kitchen's exact position.

Returning to Otway's description, we find at the upper end of the room in the position of Müntz's Pennsylvania stove, simply a *hearth* with elaborate tracery (the front plates of the stoves were often heavily ornamented). Little could be read into this had not J.D. Prendergast, the historian who edited the Charlemont papers for the 3rd Earl, writing some fifty years later, observed. 'There remained to the present Earl's time, a tall, ivy-covered chimney and the mullion windows of the ruined banquet hall as well as the *kitchen adjacent*. For amid ferns and ivy could be traced the oven and *hot-hearth*. The late Lady Charlemont made the ruin her fernery. In Sautelle Roberts' *View of Marino*, now at Roxborough, Rosamund's Bower forms a prominent object.'[23]

Thus, not so much as on a slender thread of evidence but upon the weight of a cast iron stove, hangs the case for Müntz as the architect of the Gothic Room![24]

If it was the same stove that Chambers referred to, without much enthusiasm, in a letter of circa 1769, Charlemont had long to wait. Chambers wrote, 'Jackson has finished the stove and it will be sent, price 26.5, hope your Lds will like it. No doubt it will answer.'[25]

NOTES

1. HMC Rept. 13, App. pt. VIII, p. 281.
2. Walpole, *Anecdotes*, Vol. 4, p. 233.
3. R.W. Ketton Cremer, *Horace Walpole*, London 1945, p. 134.
4. R. Poulson, *Hogarth*, Yale University Press, 1971 Vol. 2, pp. 275-6.
5. Walpole, Vol. 4, pp. 167-9.
6. Poulson, p. 275.
7. Poulson, p. 279.
8. Ibid.

9. R. Armstrong, 'Fingal', pamphlets, Dublin 1835, Chap. 2 by Caesar Otway, p. 26.
10. M. Wynne, 'Irish Stained and Painted Glass' in *Crown and Glory*, Norwich 1982, pp. 58-60.
11. RIA, 12.R.10, nos. 77, 78.
12. J. O'Keefe, *Recollections*, London 1826, p. 257.
13. T.K. Cromwell, *Excursions Through Ireland*, 1820, p. 193.
14. N. Williams, *Royal Homes of Great Britain*, London 1911, p. 28.
15. Hardy, p. 157.
16. Ibid.
17. M. McCarthy, *The Origins of the Gothic Revival*, Yale and London 1987, pp. 180-2.
18. Ketton Cremer, p. 149.
19. Lewis, Walpole Library, Farmington, Connecticut.
20. McCarthy, p. 112.
21. M. Wynne, 'The Charlemont Album', Irish Georgian Society Bulletin, Vol. XXI, Jan.-Jun. 1978.
    P. Butler, The Brocas Collection, National Library of Ireland, 1997 p. 108.
22. RIA, 12.R.12, no. 55.
23. *The Irish Times*, Sept. 9, 16, 17, 1886. The picture has not been traced.
24. Teresa S. Watts, 'The Life and Work of Johann Heinrich Müntz (1727-1798)'. Ph.D. thesis, University of Toronto, 1986. Her research continues into Müntz's role at Marino.
25. RIA 12.R.12, no. 63

21

THE TOWN HOUSE

We hear again of the Egyptian collections, although still with no detail, when Charlemont House was included, curiously but pertinently enough, in R. Pool and J. Cash's *Views of Public Buildings in the City of Dublin* in 1780. In the corridor connecting the main block with the celebrated Library wing at the rear, were handsome statues and Egyptian curiosities.

By 1780 Charlemont House was at its heyday, a centre of social and cultural activity where Charlemont received distinguished visitors to Dublin. The doors were ever open for literary and scientific discussion, and it was here that Charlemont appeared to the world, the most polite, the most agreeable and accomplished nobleman of his day. The town house did not make 'what Greece, what Rome, could boast of' theirs, but in fixing the Graces upon their native shore, it was with its urbane elegance eminently more successful in contributing to reform the taste of his countrymen than Charlemont's avant-garde ventures at Marino. Charlemont House was to become known as the Holland House of Dublin.

The earliest extant letter in the Charlemont-Chambers correspondence is concerned, appropriately enough in view of its future role, with the facade and the space for carriages drawing up at the street front. On 12 March 1763 Chambers has sent 'a design of the manner in which I think the sweep walls should be ornamented, if the upper part of the house be of brick then the space between the rustics of the Niches should likewise be of brick, but if of stone that should also be of stone. As you cannot have a Court deep enough to turn carriages in without throwing the house too far back ... as to receive any advantage from the fine prospect, I have designed two entrances with piers at the two extremities of the court and the space between them may be closed with an iron grille which will look well and show the house to advantage. I have made the piers plain as the rest of the design is so; the whole space occupied is 100 ft in front.'[1]

There is a lapse of five years before the correspondence is resumed. Apart from any missing letters, we have today to contend with alterations to the main block, the demolition of almost the entire library wing and the dispersal of the collections. Charlemont House, the most frequented and public of Charlemont's buildings, has acquired a cloak of mystery that was never intended.

Thus any visual reconstruction, even in the mind's eye, must depend upon the comments of passing visitors, not necessarily accurate in their accounts; on the correspondence between Chambers and Charlemont, which survives only intermittently and can therefore be misleading; on some old photographs taken of the interior before or at the time of demolition; on nineteenth- and twentieth-century sale and exhibition catalogues with imprecise, and often quaintly inaccurate, descriptions; and, on a rare occasion, as with the rediscovery of the Charlemont House medal cabinet in 1984 at Elvedon Hall, Suffolk, of the identification of a specific item from the dispersed collections.[2]

Let us begin with the prospect mentioned by Chambers in the first letter. This is described by the Rev. Thomas Campbell in 1778: 'Lord Charlemont's cannot be called a great house, but nothing could be more elegant ... it stands upon a little eminence, exactly fronting Mosse's Hospital and between them lie those beautiful gardens where the genteel company walk in summer evenings and have concerts of vocal and instrumental music thrice a week.'[3]

The house was much greater than it appeared from the street. The site was long and narrow and the main block was connected by the corridor, which ran over vaulted basement passages through the garden to the 'large, handsome and well-disposed' Library apartments at the rear, mentioned by Arthur Young in his *Tour of Ireland* published in 1780. Here was 'a pretty ante-room, with a fine copy of the Venus de Medicis' which led into the most elegant room, the principal library, 30 by 40 feet with 'the light well managed coming in from the cove in the ceiling' and beyond were two small rooms, 'one a cabinet for pictures and antiquities, the other medals'.

When in 1767 the correspondence is resumed, it is with the furnishing of Charlemont House that Chambers is concerned and particularly with the medal cases for the cabinet, which we now know to be 14 feet and 7 inches long and to have filled the east wall of the little room on the garden side adjoining the principal library. Not only has the medal cabinet itself been found but, with it Chambers' drawings and working instructions. Thus, it is with hindsight we review the letters relating to it.

On 25 August Chambers wrote, 'I have inclosed the designs for the medal drawers. The poor man [Diederich Nicholas Anderson] who had the bronzes in hand hath laid at the point of death for some time and there is no hope of his recovery, so that as soon as I can get the models I must employ some other person to do the work ... Alken [Sefferin Alken] has carved one of the little heads for the corners of the doors of the medal cases. It is very fine, but as he tells me he cannot do them under three and a half guineas a head, I have stopped his further progress until I hear from your lordship, and I think antique patterae or nails which will cost but a trifle will answer the purpose almost as well. Be pleased to send the inscriptions which are to be on the shields of the medal cases, for Mr Anderson has lost the former ones.'[4]

We hear again of the cabinet on 12 September. Chambers wrote, 'Alken I have set about a head of Plato to match that of Homer, and also about a pattera to supply the places of the heads. The Hercules Musarem is Bosted but the wood being damp he has been to dry kiln it; when that is done he will set about the finishing and do it with all possible care.'[5]

The sixteen little heads for the roundel angles of the doors were, as we can see, replaced by patterae. The Hercules Musarem identifies with the centre medallion, a carved figure with a lion's skin, lyre and club.

On 2 October Chambers wrote that Anderson was dead and Mrs Anderson out of town, 'so that I know not what was begun and what was not: but I find the ornaments for the medals cases are cast and his man will finish them as well as he could have done himself'. The matter was not so easily resolved. On 19 December Chambers reported, 'Mrs Anderson has sent me home the bas reliefs for the medal cases but they are ungilt and incompleat so that I must get some one to finish & Gild them and they have lost the drawings so that I am greatly at a loss to know how they are to be put together I will however endeavour to get over all these difficulties & send the things as soon as possible to Chester.'[6]

Mrs Anderson, being in 'great distress for money', had brought her bill and expected to be paid directly, which Chambers had not done. The bill was considerable and he had not Charlemont's approval of the charges and, besides, had no money to pay her 'for the devil had tempted me to build again, the consequences of which everybody that hath built knows very well.' Charlemont's draft of 2 January 1768 was not paid, because Chambers was away, until 9 February, when Chambers wrote that it was exceedingly acceptable to her and 'she begd I would offer her most hearty thanks to your Lordship'. Still on the subject of the ornaments for the medal cases, some figured sketches had been sent and 'there is no mistake about the Ebony Shields &c; the mahogany ones mentioned in the Lady's bill having only been turned for models to cast the borders upon.'[7]

By 12 March the ornaments for the medals cases were nearly finished and would soon be sent and there is no further mention of the cabinet in the correspondence, which as it now becomes clear related only to the ornamentation of the carcase or frame constructed by Charlemont's workmen on the spot. All the mouldings, carved wood, veneers and gilded bronze sent with the designs and working instructions by Chambers from England; not only for the medal cabinet itself, but for the room in which it was to be contained. The unknown quantity is the chimney piece, now missing, upon which the cabinet was to be centred; it is not clear whether it was to be executed in Dublin, presumably by Vierpyle, or sent thither. The evidence points to the same division of work as with the cabinet; on 16 November Chambers wrote, 'Your Lordship desires me to send you any bills I may have by me here. Inclosed are three

Viz Alkens		34. 1. 7
Haywards		6. 12. -
Evans		1. 1. -
	£s	41. 14. 7.'[8]

Alken's bill speaks for itself. George Evans, painter and gilder, was probably the man brought in to finish and gild the ornaments for the medal cases. The statuary, Richard Hayward, whose bill was too small for any but a part of the chimney piece, perhaps was the carver of the crossed branches, lyre and ewer of Chambers' design. This would explain Chambers' instructions for the Dublin end, that the chimney piece 'must all be of White marble'.

There are some small discrepancies between the executed cabinet and the section drawing with the instructions, which read, 'AB the walls of this room must be painted in Oyle upon the troweld Stucco, of a faint peagreen colour dead, the Cornice, Architraves of the Windows, and door, also the frieze and cornice of the door the Base & Surbase and dado of the room with the Bas relief and ornaments over the chimney and the frieze, cornice & pediment over them must all be painted dead white. The chimney piece must all be of White Marble.

'The medal cases entirely of mahogany [crossed out] from A quite up to B and from C to D.'

'Instead of mahogany are to be of yellow sandal wood fineer'd upon Mahogany – The Ornaments, Moldings and carved work are to be of Turkey Box – The Flat Parts only of Sanders wood, fineer'd as marked on the Drawing – These woods I shall send from hence.'[9]

'The depth of the break at G is marked on the full size drawing.'

The full size drawing is missing, but, as can be seen from the above, the only major alteration was that the centre medallion and the pediment over it, was not left free-standing against the white painted wall background, but enclosed with veneered wood.

Chambers designed other furniture for Charlemont House, the present whereabouts of which is unknown, if indeed any has survived. The few clues we have, open up vistas of speculation, which invite exploration in spite of the salutary lesson of the unpredictable medal cabinet. Although there is little evidence, some light is thrown on Charlemont's involvement as rather more than a sleeping patron, in the plans for the Town House, and the claims made by Thomas Campbell that Charlemont designed it himself.

The first clue is an inscription in pencil, unmistakably in Charlemont's hand along the left hand margin of Chambers' letter of 12 September 1767, which reads 'Chippendale'.[10] It seems to bear no relation to the subject in hand, Alken's work on the little heads and the Hercules medallion for the medal cabinet. This brings to mind an incident of some six years later, when Thomas Chippendale came to Chambers with designs for furniture for Melbourne House. Chambers wrote to Lord Melbourne that the drawings seemed on the whole very well, 'but I wish to be a little consulted about these matters as I am really a very pretty Connoisseur in furniture.'[11]

There is no evidence that Charlemont had any direct dealings with Chippendale, but there is every indication that he consulted *The Gentleman and Cabinet Maker's Director* (1754), at least in one instance for Charlemont House. In the sale of the contents of Marino in 1875 there was, among other items advertised as coming from Charlemont House, 'the old secretaire with alphabet and fittings (after Chippendale) made to the order of the first Earl of Charlemont'.[12]

The sale of 1875, running over a series of days between 22 October and 4 November, with no catalogue except of the pictures, was conducted by a Dublin Auctioneer, J.J. Byrne. He advertised rather haphazardly in the local papers the offerings each day. What appeared in one paper as, 'Hand gilt chairs, period of Louis Quatorze' was elsewhere 'Handsome gilt chairs'. The period mentioned was but a loose description of any gilt furniture of the rococo style – an anachronism we meet with frequently in catalogues compiled in Dublin at this time! However, once we have grasped the jargon, the advertisements for the Marino sale turn out to be a better source of information than they would at first appear.

Furniture known, or believed, to have been designed by Chambers specifically for Charlemont House, and mentioned in the medal cabinet letters, include the Triton candlesticks, the sideboards for the French room and the girandoles for the ante or Venus room of the principal library.

The Triton candlesticks are first mentioned in a letter of 15 September 1567 from Chambers. 'I wrote to your lordship two or three days ago, so that I have nothing now to say only to let you know that one of the Tritons for the candlesticks is cast; but as I find the pair will come to 36£ by the time they are finished, exclusive of the models, I have stopt farther proceedings till I hear from your lordship. For my part, as these things are rather for show than use, I should recommend wooden ones well bronzed, which, at the distance they are to stand will look full as well as real bronze.'[13]

On 2 October Chambers wrote that the bronze candlesticks would be finished with all possible expedition, but in March 'the Triton candle-branches are nearly finished' and 'The Tritons are finished all but the bronzing, and they are so finely executed that it would be a pity not to have them quite complete. I have therefore ordered them to be entirely gilded for I feared the bronzing would make them appear dull and partly gilding upon the bronze would look tawdry. This will increase the expense of them, but I think it will answer when done.'[14]

Also in Chambers' letter of 15 September is the first mention of sideboards, and here we are on surer ground than with the Triton candlesticks, because Chambers gives dimensions and the intended location. 'Inclosed I send the design for the foot of the side-boards for the French room, I have made them 7 foot long 2.9 wide and about 3 feet high, that they may range with the top of the surbase which I suppose to be about that height. It is difficult if not impossible to make out all the twists and turns of these sorts of works by a design, but if your lordship's carver is able and a little acquainted with French contours he will easily comprehend my drawing.'[15]

A photograph *c.* 1929, recently discovered, of the larger rear room in the main block of Charlemont House before demolition, discloses, surprisingly, the style of the decoration of this room to be at variance with the remainder of the building's classical symmetry and to be uncompromisingly rococo. It is just the setting that would be expected for furniture with the twists and turns and contours of contemporary Louis XV taste.

Charlemont's carver may have been the same Ignatius McDonagh, carver and gilder, already mentioned in connection with the Gothic Room, who was employed between 1774 and 1776 carving and gilding picture and table frames for Marino and for Charlemont House. If indeed it was McDonagh, hitherto known only for having carved the massive staircase in Powerscourt Town House, and he had achieved anything approaching the virtuosity of an *ébéniste*, he has to be considered, not only for the sideboards of the French room but the 'handsome gilt chairs in different styles, period of Louis Quatorze' with 'handsome console tables, same period' which appeared in the first advertisements of the Marino sale (1875). The same console tables may or may not be those again advertised for the sale on Saturday 20 October, when they were described in *Freeman's Journal* as 'two exquisite carved pier tables in white and gold [period of Louis XIV again] from Charlemont House', but the latter would seem to agree with the sideboards for the French room.

Although there is a passing reference to seat furniture in the Saloon of the Casino, nowhere in the correspondence is there any mention of designs for chairs by Chambers for Charlemont House or elsewhere. Yet in 1767 and 1768 Charlemont was busy with all the other furnishings, carpets, tables, girandoles, candlesticks, decorative paintings and even plaster vases for the tops of the bookcases in the library. The explanation can only be that they had been designed by Chambers before the correspondence begins, or that Charlemont went elsewhere and perhaps not much farther than Chippendale's *Director*, with its several very pleasing designs for chairs in the French style.

The correspondence has, so far, been one-sided; few of Charlemont's letters have survived, but one, undated, which is concerned with the furnishings of Charlemont House is a model of that easy manner, that unaffected and perfect politeness with which he insisted on Chambers attending to his requirements down to the smallest detail. It gives us a very clear idea of the extent of his participation and how he chose to direct Chambers, while at the same time in no way obstructing the genius that he recognized in him.

'My dear Chambers,

There is yet one thing remaining with regard to the Library apartment – I mean the best method of lighting it – the Great Room, will, I imagine, be sufficiently illuminated by the Lights which are to stand on the Chimneypiece and by candles placed on the Tables, but with regard to the Ante Chamber I think that nothing could be more proper than girandoles of two candles each fix'd in the center of the two long panels at each side of the room. A design, however, which corresponds with the other ornaments of this beautiful room, will be necessary and such a one I beg you wou'd immediately send me – I should imagine that an Amazonian shield, cross'd by branches of Laurel and Palm might make a pretty ornament and might serve for the basis from whence the branches for candles might spring. But this I only mean as a hint in case nothing better shou'd occur to you. The dimensions and situation of the panels are as follows. (See page VII of art section.)

Whenever it may best suit your convenience I shou'd be much obliged to you if you wou'd choose for me among the many vases of plaister, which are so common in the Statuary's shops such as you may think proper to be put up on the upper shelf in the Library. They must be bronzed and not exceed twenty eight inches in height. Then as soon as you can procure, be so kind as to send them well pack'd as usual to Chester directed for me to the care of Smyth at the White Lyon.

I heard the other day from Cipriani, who has not yet finished the Chiaroscuros; Be so kind, my dear Chambers, to call on him and to hasten him as much as possible. I should not desire this favour of you but that I know your reasons for not interfering are now at an end.'[16]

The letter ended with a plea: 'Hasten Moore with the purple carpetting for want of which I am much distressed.' The carpet or carpets had been already sent and, if we are to judge by the rare surviving examples of Thomas Moore's work at Moorfields in the City of London, would have been magnificent and probably made to the designs of Chambers.[17]

The plaster vases, twelve in all, were ordered, packed and despatched, and a bill for the packing came from Chambers in due course, but other delays continued to vex Charlemont. Chambers wrote that he would not fail 'to torment Cipriani' until he had finished the chiaroscuros, and Wilton was to be pressed for the tables, but without effect and Charlemont turned to Joseph Baretti to see what might be done.

Baretti wrote on 3 April 1768 that Wilson and Cipriani had read the postscripts to Charlemont's letter, and that Wilton says, 'your table has long been done, but the man who was to make the frame has died and another will have to be found to do the work. As for Cipriani he was 'almost desperate with too much business. The King has long employ'd him and made him neglect the works of other people by sending every day to see how he went on with a ceiling for one of the Queen's rooms.' However, of the five pictures, four were finished.[18]

Cipriani's letter, addressed to Baretti, was not very gracious, but Baretti took it upon himself to forward it to Charlemont. Cipriani assured his compatriot, writing in English, that he would attend to the many gentlemen that had honour'd him with their commands, all 'wishing to be served first' as soon as he had finished the Queen's ceiling. 'My case,' he wrote, 'is different of that of Mr Wilton, for I have not help nor health sufficient to satisfy all my engagements except a decent time is allowed to me. Ask what his Lordship pleases to call me tedious, you may assure him that the painting in chiarascuro which I have already forwarded for him are extremely more tedious than his Lordship can imagine, as I am forced to paint them over and over again to bring them to one even Colour and after they are finished the white turns so much as to want to be cover'd intirely. So much that these pictures shall be the last that I will undertake in this kind of painting. You may, sir, assure his Lordship that the four medallions for over the doors will be finished and ready in a fortnight's time, but I should choose to send them all together with the basso rèlievo for the chimney for the reason above mentioned of keeping them the same colour.'[19]

The pictures were duly finished and found their place in the principal room of the library and were still there when the photographs were taken prior to demolition in *c.* 1929. Cipriani's bill of 10 December 1768 itemises *Philosophy, Moral History, Natural History* and *Poetry* for the overdoors at forty guineas, and the large painting for the chimney, *Minerva in Parnassus,* thirty-five guineas.[20]

The matter of two pier tables made by Joseph Wilton is not so straightforward, but the evidence suggests the lesser table, in point of cost and as the one finished first, being for the French room at

Charlemont House and the second, a very magnificent table, for the Casino.

In his letter of 2 October 1767 Chambers first mentions the pier tables, 'I should think 6 ft quite sufficient for the length of the pier tables and therefore shall not say anything to Wilton about altering the dimensions and I believe it must be the same sort of foot with the sideboards which I am glad to hear your lordship approves of'. This, of course, is ambiguous. The tables, one of which was completed except for the frame in April 1768 as we know from Baretti's letter, were never to be a pair, albeit of the same length and perhaps, though this is unsure, with the same style of foot. Wilton's bill, presumably on completion of all work, was not sent until 3 May 1773. In it he accounts for 'a very rich pier table veneered with Lapis Lazuli' at a cost of a hundred and twenty-three pounds and another pier table of Sicilian green jasper, 'formerly sent to Ireland' at £13.13.4.[21]

The supposition is, although hypothetical, that wherever the lapis lazuli table was intended for, it was not Charlemont House. It was the green jasper table that Charlemont was impatient for as the interior furnishing of the ground floor there neared completion.

NOTES

1. HMC Report 12 App. Pt. X p. 273.
2. G. O'Connor, 'The Charlemont House Medal Cabinet' *Irish Arts Review* Vol. 1 No. 2, Summer 1984, pp. 23-27.
3. T. Campbell, op. cit., p. 24.
4. H.M.C. Rept. 12, App. pt. X, p. 283.
5. Ibid, p. 284.
6. R.I.A. 12. R. 10. no. 16.
7. Ibid., 12. R. 12. no. 52.
8. Ibid., no. 61.
9. C. O'Connor, p. 26.
10. RIA.
11. J. Harris, *Sir William Chambers* London 1970, pp. 197, 227.
12. *Dublin Evening Mail* Oct. 22 & 30, 1875.
13. H.M.C. Rept. 12, App. pt. X, p. 284.
14. Ibid.
15. Ibid.
16. R.I.A. 12. R. 30b.
17. H.M.C. Rept. 12, App. pt. X, p. 285.
18. Ibid.
19. Ibid, pp.314-5.
20. RIA, 12.R.12, no. 10.
21. HMC Rept. 12, App. pt. X, pp. 314-5.

22

THE CASINO

Work on the Casino had not kept pace with the building, decorating and furnishing of the Town House, which would appear to have been more or less completed by 1768. When, in 1761, George Montagu had visited Marino there had been expectation of the Casino's being finished by the following year, but when the correspondence relating to the Casino resumes in August 1767, it is evident that much remains to be done.

It is generally assumed that the leisurely pace was due to shortage of money.[1] We do not know how long the Casino took to build. There is no evidence of a date of completion and belated work seems to have been in progress in 1787, more than twelve years after the parting between Chambers and Charlemont. The length of time would seem to be mainly due to Charlemont's quest for perfection in putting before the world a work of art, which was to be a monument to his own connoisseurship and, at the same time, a compendium of his ideas and a model of Neo-Classical taste.

Inevitably, as with his *Essays*, edited and re-edited in the light of extended knowledge, some of the youthful vision was lost and the spirit, under the weight of practical difficulties, sometimes flagged. Of this Charlemont himself may have been sadly aware. In 1792 Edmund Malone was to plead with Edmund Burke to revive and enlarge *A Philosophical Enquiry into the Origins of Our Ideas of the Sublime and Beautiful.* Charlemont's comment to Malone was that if Burke had really given up politics, literature must be his only resource, but 'I cannot, with you, recommend a revival of the *Sublime and Beautiful*, since, notwithstanding the miraculous texture of the brain, thirty years I fear may have taken from him more in fire and fancy than they have given him in experience'.[2]

The fire and the fancy could still have been riding high when the Vicereine, the Duchess of Northumberland, visited Marino in 1763. By then Charlemont was in better health and had found there was after all some congenial company in Ireland.

The Vicereine's account of the visit in her journal for 27 October gives us some idea of how far the improvements had progressed and also of the itinerary of inspection. She wrote, 'I went in my post chaise with Mrs Graham to Ld. Charlemonts at Marino with whom we found Lord Drogheda. We walk'd thro' the Kitchen Garden wch. is 6 1/2 Irish Acres to his Hot House it is 170 Feet long; in the *Anti Room* of which we breakfasted. The Walls were all Tapstried with Myrtle and an innumerable quantity of flowering Plants perfumed it on every side by their Fragrance. The rest of our Company were Lord and Ly. Stopford, Lord Tyrone and Lord Powerscourt. We then visited the Stables which are grand and handsome, the Farm Yard Barns &c. Then we walk'd thro' a very pretty Shrubbery to a very handsome *Gothic Room* (the Windows of painted Glass). We then went to the *Temple*. The stonework is admirably well executed all of Portland Stone, it is a beautiful Building but very ill qualified to be a Dwelling House.'[3]

Apparently it was still Charlemont's intention that the Casino should be his *palazetto abitabile*.

Almost four years elapse between the Duchess' visit and Chambers' next extant letter relating to the Casino and we are left without any record of progress. When the correspondence resumes on 25 August 1767, the iron gates for the entrance to Marino are under consideration. Chambers has sent a sketch in which his clerk has made some errors, but he thinks the smith will understand it sufficiently, if not he can send a more correct drawing.

Charlemont is evidently impatient, but perhaps not only with his Dublin work force. Chambers writes, 'I am sorry to find your lordship so much distressed with your workmen. Give me leave to offer a piece of Italian advice; *bisogna aver phlegma* I am not sure the spelling is right, but I am sure the prescription is the only efficacious one yet discovered.'[4] At the same time Chambers is protesting that he has already sent the pattern head and also the pattern for the cove cornice of the mezzanine and that he has sent to George Barret to tell him to despatch at the first opportunity a sample of the 'Sky-blew'. 'I am sorry there is no person in Ireland to rely on for fixing the tints of the painting as there is no probability of sending patterns over unaltered, the want of air always making a very considerable alteration in the colours before they arrive in Dublin.'[5] One is given the impression that at some inconvenience to Chambers, Charlemont is insisting that Barret, (whose early paintings of Powerscourt and the Dargle not being as well received as they deserved, had gone to England in 1762)[6] must be employed.

The next mention of the Casino is in the letter dated 12 September 1767. Chambers wrote, 'I have sent here inclosed a border for the flat of the Casino ceiling, but can send no design for the centre till I have the dimensions for the flat exactly, and if I could have a tracing on this paper of the whole ceiling it would be better still.' Chambers is clearly referring to the ceiling of the Saloon because on 2 October he sent 'a design for the Apollo's head and also one for a new Galloss as the one before sent cannot be reduced to 4¾ ins without being too trifling'. Possibly the design for the head had also been revised.[7]

We hear no more of the Casino until the following year when in two undated letters, a new project is introduced and Charlemont is considering designs for a Lodge, (of which more hereafter), and adds, 'Now with regard to the Casino I must ask you some questions which I beg you wou'd answer as soon as possible. How is the Freeze of the Door Head to be ornamented? With oak leaves as in the engraved elevation, or as the Freezes of the window Frames, with Fasces or Reeds bound together? For my part I shou'd prefer the Oak leaves, as richer and more varied from the rest. How are the angular Recesses to be paved, with plain white Portland, or chequer'd black and white, or with Marble?'[8]

These questions are of course about the exterior, the door head of the entrance and the paving of the angled recesses of the platform. Some seven or eight years after building has commenced the Casino is still a shell. Charlemont, in the same letter, is putting forward alterations to the Saloon – the same room about whose ceiling, Chambers had, months before, been consulted.

'In the Section of the Saloon there is one thing that I wish could with any Propriety be alter'd. I mean the two false Doors, which not only crowd a small Room with five Doors, but take up the place of necessary Furniture, chairs or sophas. This is a nice Point and I shou'd be glad you wou'd consider it. I have not yet received your sketch for the parketted Floors; nor the Design for the ornamenting the Boudoir with Flowers &c, nor Munt's Gothick Design [probably for the Gothic seat] – All of which I beg you wou'd expedite for me.' There is a postscript to this letter. 'Pray be as good as to let me hear from you as soon as possible.'[9]

Chambers' answer, also undated, is primarily concerned with the designs for the Lodge, but he touches briefly on the queries about the Casino. Oak leaves would do best for the frieze of the door. The false doors in the Saloon could be safely left out, 'it would be even best to leave them out'. He wrote, 'I have sent a drawing for the Plafond of the angular recesses & another for the Pavement composed of Portland and black marble, which I think will do better than [dove]. Some of the octagons are larger in my drawings than others, which I did to make them range with the Bases of the Columns, but it will be better to make them all of a size. The top of the Casino may be flat it will make a pleasant gazebo. Lead will be best covering at least 7 lb to the foot superficial, copper is more expensive than lead, poisons the rain water & cannot easily be made tight.'[10]

For the first time Chambers mentions Vierpyle, the modest self-effacing character, whose part, except as a surpassing stonemason, in the building of the Casino has until recently been overlooked. 'Your Lordship's letter & another received the same post from Verpyle makes mention of some designs for parquetted floors for the Casine, it is the first newse I heard of them.'[11] The designs were going to require some thought but he would send them in a post or two, also drawings for the Boudoir.

Charlemont had already enquired about designs for the parquetted floors, which Chambers for his own reasons chose to ignore. The bold patterns suggesting Masonic symbols, of the floor in the Saloon are evidence of Charlemont's at times independent way of thinking, and his predilection for iconography. This begs the question as to whether Charlemont was a Freemason. There is no evidence of him belonging to an Irish lodge, but a letter from a Turkish member of the brotherhood claimed him as such.[12] Incidentally, the same question is now being asked about Lord Burlington and whether or not Chiswick House was a Masonic temple.

The drawings for the Boudoir, designs for 'ornamenting it with flowers etc' have, as we now know, been mistakenly connected with Chambers' selection of a Chinese wallpaper for another, unspecified room. On 22 March 1769 Chambers wrote, 'I went to Starks where there is a great choice of India paper & chose one which I think remarkably handsome, the ground is a fine blew and the flowers are very well painted and of a small pattern as your Lordship desired'. There were grumbles about Vierpyle's confused dimensions which neither Stark nor he could understand, but enough, even some to spare, was being sent and the price very reasonable. 'Stark says the silver grounds are apt to turn black and therefore I would not take one'.[13]

There are no clues for what room the paper was intended, but certainly not the Boudoir. A fire destroyed the little room in the early nineteenth century, but two sources provide accounts of its original decoration. J. D'Alton in 1838, remembered 'a most exquisite chimney-piece, small but highly sculptured with fruit, flowers and shells'.[14] Recently, Rolf Loeber and Magda Stouthamer-Loeber discovered a more detailed account of 1797. '... the boidore is decorated with some compartments of looking-glass placed in the wall, round which is some light and elegant stucco work of various fruits and flowers, branching a little upon the surface of the glass, and all, as I was informed were to be intended to be painted so as to represent nature; there is in this room a most exquisite marble chimney-piece, of small size, but highly sculptured with corresponding fruits, flowers, and shells.'[15]

So much for the Boudoir still unpainted in 1797, two years before Charlemont's death. In 1764 the colours for the Saloon were under discussion.

The painstaking investigation of the colours undertaken by Ian Bristow during the restoration of the Casino showed that in principle and in certain of the details, Chambers' scheme was adopted.[16] The touches of blue, discovered under layers of later paint, were revealed as a very delicate pricking out of blue upon the white of the architraves of the doors and the enrichments of the cornice.

The overall effect we have today is not entirely satisfactory. This is not due to a misreading of the evidence or any historical defect, but for two obvious reasons. There is too great an expanse of unrelieved blue wall hanging, which originally would have been broken up by pictures and perhaps a pier glass over the table facing the chimney piece. The floors, without the corresponding magnificence of the original chimney piece and the furniture, have taken on a predominance which was never intended, and indeed, their impact throws out the balance and proportions of a room which is only 19 feet 4 inches by 15 feet 1 inch, and a total of 17 feet 6 inches high.

Not only has the original furniture with the chimneypiece, which would have restored the proper proportions, disappeared without trace, but the evidence for what it consisted of is extremely hazy. In the light of the unexpected proportions of the rediscoved Charlemont House medal cabinet, that evidence has to be treated with rather more than usual caution.

Charlemont's pictures are well documented, but there is no evidence of any of the listed works hanging in the Casino. A Titian (spurious) and doubtful Rembrandt (perhaps school of) were seen at Charlemont House, where the collection of Hogarths were also hung and, perhaps, Reynolds' *Venus Chiding Cupid.* None of these would have been appropriate to a classical temple set in a *ferme orné.* One turns more hopefully to pastoral subjects and considers some of those pictures which might have strayed from the Casino to the nearby Marino House, where the sale of 1875 was conducted. These included the Claude, and also a set of four upright decorative landscapes by George Mullins (now in the Irish National collections), works by Caspard Dughet, Richard Wilson and Orizonte, all Italianate and pastoral in subject.

In speculating along these lines, we come across the pair of Zuccarellis which Charlemont commissioned from the artist in London. These paintings are mentioned on 22 March 1769 in the correspondence between Charlemont and Chambers dealing with the Chinese wallpaper and the colours for the Saloon. Chambers then wrote, 'Zucharelli's pictures are now finished'[17] and would be sent the following week. They are now in a private collection in Ireland.

With the chimney piece and the table we are on surer ground, but there is nothing conclusive since the only known contemporary description of the interior of the Casino does not refer to either. The furniture had to be sparse, as dictated by the size of the room and the pattern of the floors, but that it had to be magnificent in order to counteract their otherwise overpowering brilliance. Bearing this in mind, we examine the clues.

In a letter of 1769, undated, in which Chambers writes, 'I have sent to Wilton about the table' (in the singular, and certainly not the green jasper table, which according to Wilton's bill was sent first), Chambers advises about a table in relation to the chimney piece and the floors of the Saloon. He writes, 'Think any border the shape of the table before the Chimney of the Saloon will have a bad effect & therefore should advise to keep the slab as at first intended and make nothing under the table but let the floor be continued there as it is elsewhere.'[18]

Common to Wilton's second and much richer table, and a chimney piece ordered by Charlemont from Francis Harwood in Florence, was the use of lapis lazuli in combination with statuary marble and, in the case of the chimney piece, gilt bronze and in the table, gilt metal. It is well within the bounds of probability that the chimney piece and the table were *en suite*. That the chimney piece was ordered specifically for the Saloon is supported by the article in the *Irish Builder* of 1894 which tells of a slab or plaque, 5 inches by 12, of lapis lazuli, which had formerly been part of the chimney piece in the Saloon, but had disappeared, as had more recently the chimney piece itself.

The *Treatise* contains the designs for the chimney pieces for the Casino; the principal presumably for the Saloon. But neither that nor the others fitted the fireplaces, and when drawn out the templates showed them as too large for the other rooms and too small for the Saloon. The present chimney piece came originally from Marino House and though neither of the quality, nor imposing enough, to be anything more than a makeshift, happily the motif of a ram's head makes it more appropriate than it first appears.

The bills from Florence, and Francis Harwood's letter of 9 February 1768,[19] are informative and detailed and in some particulars would seem to conform to the principal engraving in the *Treatise*. Without drawings and dimensions a proper reconstruction cannot be carried out, even though a picture begins to emerge from the white statuary marble terms by Francis Harwood, from the blue of lapis lazuli worked by Cosimo Siries of the *Opificio delle Pietre Dure* (the tablet mentioned in the *Irish Builder*?) and the gold of the gilt bronze of a life size ram's head and festoons of laurel leaves.

The richness of the effect can be appreciated even if the details are not sharp and, according to Harwood's letter to Charlemont, 'among the many, Sir Horace [Mann] did me the pleasure and highly approved of its elegance and execution', which may have appeased any misgivings Charlemont had about the cost, which amounted, with carriage only as far as Leghorn, to nearly a hundred and thirty pounds sterling.[20]

The curiosity is that Charlemont should send to Florence when he had Vierpyle at hand to sculpt the marble, and Wilton to call on for the lapis lazuli. The answer must be that it was for the sculptural bronze work, unheard of, at this time, as a component of English chimney pieces. Only in Florence could he find the practical collaboration of founder with sculptor and lapidary.

The lapis lazuli, at fifty pounds, was the single most expensive component (although there was no itemised bill, Harwood having paid Siries and entered the payment in his own account), but the emphasis was on the bronze, the gilt head and the festoons of laurel leaves. The gilt bronze head, '*una testa di Bronzo rappresentante di un*

Caprone di grandezza al naturale, cesellate con due Caschate di nastri', was mistaken by the founders for a goat's head, but Harwood who made the model for casting and was of, course, directly accountable to Charlemont, refers to it as a Ram's head.[21]

Rams' heads are to be seen at the angles of the cornice of the Saloon, and the motif is repeated, with the additional festoons of laurel leaves, on the podium urn outside and beneath the window of the room. The flocks on the lawns surrounding the Casino spoke also for Charlemont's penchant for sheep, but it is the ram's head of the chimney piece with the ribbons, 'due *caschate di nastri*,' which would seem to be an echo from December 1749 of Charlemont's delight in the flocks at the approach to Athens, each 'preceded by its *vir gregis* with his horns richly gilded and adorned with ribands.'[22]

It is difficult to reconcile Charlemont's sending to Florence with Chambers' view that neither the Italian nor French excelled greatly in the composition of chimney pieces and that, in this particular, England surpassed all other nations, 'not only in point of expense, but likewise in taste of design and goodness of Workmanship'. We do not know whether this was one of Charlemont's independent moves or whether he had persuaded Chambers to make a fresh drawing based on the one in the *Treatise* (which was now ill-fitted to the room because of the alteration to the number of the doors), and to waive the objection to foreign workmanship on the grounds that Francis Harwood was an Englishman and almost certainly well-known to them both.

The lapis lazuli table, which had been so long in Wilton's hand, had been designed, as we believe, by Chambers for the Saloon prior to the introduction of the parquetted floors and before contours of the table fame were found (in 1768) to be inconsistent with their pattern. Chambers, as we have seen, recommended making no alteration either to the slab of the facing chimney piece or to the floors beneath the table.

The table had probably not by then been delivered. It was not until 17 May 1773 that Wilton wrote to Charlemont and enclosed his bill dated February of the same year. Wilton was in no immediate need of money since his father had died and left him a very good estate (as Chambers had informed Charlemont previously) and Wilton was renowned for the high style of his living and the hospitality of his board. It is possible that the bill may have been sent long after delivery, as was the case with the Sicilian green jasper table, known to have been finished in 1768 and now accounted for as previously sent. The cost of that table was in the region of £12, but for the lapis lazuli it was almost the price of the Harwood chimney piece, at around £124. It is not possible to be precise as allowance has to be made for the carriage and packing of several items, not only the tables but emery and other materials used in the work.

That part of Wilton's bill which relates to the 'very rich pier Table veneer'd with Lapis Lazuli' is extremely detailed, but for all that, uninformative. However, several points emerge clearly: the so-called table was the top of a table only and no frame or support was supplied by Wilton; that a length of 9ft 8ins of 2ins deep of 'chosen Statuary' was used; Panzetta, Wilton's assistant and incidentally also his godson, put in one hundred and fifty days of work 'on joining, inlaying and polishing'; and that apart from a scalloped border, seemingly in white marble, of 7ft 6 ins, there was the same length of a gadroom of husks and a 7ft. run of 'galoss inlaid *Giallo Anticio*', both water-gilt.[23]

The use and quantity of the statuary marble would seem to suggest a white ground upon which the lapis lazuli was inlaid, possibly in a pattern and with the *giallo antico*, to form a mosaic rather than an unrelieved field of blue stone, which one would associate with a later period and that found in Russian furniture of the early nineteenth century. The lapis lazuli used in the eighteenth century is more usually of a delicate shade of smokey blue, sponged or faintly mottled. This is to be seen in the tablets of the Croome Court Tapestry chimney piece*, supplied by Wilton, and in the chimney piece made for Leinster House, now at Carton, Co. Kildare, possibly also supplied by him.

If we are correct in our assumption that the Casino and particularly the Saloon, was furnished sparsely but magnificently, there remains only, the chairs and lights to consider. In the correspondence there is nothing to suggest that Chambers designed the chairs for the Saloon, and no mention is made of lighting. In the matter of the offending doors, which were removed to give space for the necessary seat furniture, we find that in the letter of 25 August 1767 that Mr Moor had just been with Chambers and that the chairs would be ready very soon, but he 'must have the dimensions of the Setee before he can send the stuff for it'.[24] There is nothing here to suggest that

* Metropolitan Museum, New York. I am indebted to James Parker for permitting my close inspection of this item some years ago.

the chairs or the settee were destined for the Saloon, but it is evidence for Charlemont having the upholstery, or at least the covering for the seat-furniture, done in England.

The remaining correspondence about the Casino is concerned chiefly with the roof, the chimney vases and the positioning of the statues. As late as 30 January 1771 Chambers was sending drawings for vases which would, he thought, look well and 'leave room for the smoke to pass as the funnels may be reduced to 9" diameter without making them too narrow, these vases will do best of lead or some sort of mettal painted & sanded to look like stone'. He added 'I am not sure of the measure as I cannot find any figured copys of the Casino they must therefore be drawn on a board to the full size then cut out and put in the place by which means you will be able to judge of the proportions.'

'With regard to the statues* they are proportioned to the Columns & cannot be made less their heads now reach to the under side of the Attick Cornice and they will when seen from below particularly if the spectator be near appear higher than the Attick but that will have no bad Effect however the plinths on which they stand may be made a little lower making its top to level with the plain part of the Case of the Attick instead of levelling with the top of its mouldings as it does in the design.'[25]

Thereafter all reference to the Casino ceases except for an entry in Chambers' bill of 1773. 'May 14th drawings & directions for painting the Vestibule of the Casine ... 2.2.'[26]

If, as might be supposed with the painting of the Vestibule, that the Casino, by the end of 1773 or 1774 was completed, it had taken at least fifteen years to build and to decorate. But if, on the basis of the evidence of two witnesses, we believe the interior unfinished, first in 1778, and then in 1787, we are forced to think in terms of thirty years. For this reason the visit of the Vicereine, Lady Shelburne, to Marino on 11 September 1769 as recorded in her journal, although hardly the last word, is, nevertheless, the best since it is the only description of the interior of the Casino we have.

Marino House she regarded as 'indifferent ... the curiosity of the place consists of a very fine Temple, Lord Charlemont is building at very great expense. The Architecture is v. correct and the stonework well executed. In the inside is a room for dining in & over looking the fine prospect, which may contain the company of 12 or 14 people.

* Apollo, Venus, Bacchus, Ceres.

On one side of it is a closet which is to hold books, the ceiling is a dome on which is to be painted the northern hemisphere and round ye frieze, ye signs of the Zodiac. On ye other side is a little drawing room of the same size. Over these are 2 tolerable bedchambers and two smaller ones for servants. The floors are parquetted in the most sumptious wood, painted satin furniture, gilding & every other expense is lavish'd on ye decration of it – a less sum might have built a v.g. dwelling house. This can never answer that purpose and is at the same time too large for a garden building.'[27]

NOTES

1. J. Gough, *A Tour in Ireland in 1813 and 1814*, by an Englishman 1817 p. 176, estimating the cost at £30,000.
2. RIA 12.R.17, no. 33.
3. E. Malins and the Knight of Glin, *Lost Demesnes*, London 1976, pp. 138-9.
4. HMC, Rept. 12, App. pt. X, p. 203.
5. Ibid.
6. Strickland re Barret p. 30.
7. HMC, Rept. 12, App. pt. X, p. 284.
8. Ibid, Rept. 13, App. pt. VIII, p. 372.
9. RIA, 12.R.21, no. 135
10. Ibid, 12.R.12, no. 55
11. Ibid.
12. RIA, 12.R.14, no. 13 from A Raish of Constantinople, member of the Order of Freemasonry claiming Charlemont as a brother.
13. HMC, Rept. 12, App. pt. X, p. 291.
14. D'Alton, *History of Co. Dublin*, 1838, p. 64.
15. Written communication R. Loeber and M. Stouthamer-Loeber.
16. I.C. Bristow and J. Redmill, 'The Casino at Marino' *Association for Studies in the Conservation of Historic Buildings*, Vol. 9 (1984).
17. HMC, Rept. 12, App. pt. X, p. 291.
18. HMC, Rept. 12, App. pt. X, p. 292.
19. RIA, 12.R.10, no. 17.
20. Ibid.
21. Ibid.
22. Stanford and Finopoulos, p. 119.
23. HMC, Rept. 12, App. pt. X, pp. 314-5.
24. Ibid, p. 304. I am indebted to Cliodna Devitt for drawing attention to upholstery by Moore at Audley End. Wendy Hefford 'Thomas Moore of Moorfields', *Burlington Magazine*, Vol. 119, Sept.-Dec. 1977.
25. RIA, 12.R. 30th Jan. 1771.
26. RIA, 12.R.10, no. 79.
27. Communicated to me by the Knight of Glin.

23

RETRENCHMENT

The Vicereine's views on the indifference of Marino House and the impractibility of the Casino, recall Lord Chesterfield's well-known quip about General Wade's house in Cork Street. The house was ill contrived and inconvenient, but with so beautiful a front designed by Lord Burlington, that Chesterfield could only advise 'as the General could not live in it to his ease, he had better take a house over against it and look at it.' This is more or less what Charlemont came to do: he made alterations and additions to Marino House and lived there instead.

He might still have persisted in his intention to make the Casino a dwelling, had he not, to the astonishment of society, married at the age of forty a penniless young woman of minor gentry origin.

The apocryphal story of how Charlemont overcame his deep aversion to the married state,[1] is that walking one day at Marino with Francis, who by this time was married and had a son, his brother was so tactless as to admit his lack of interest in the demesne and his intention, on inheriting, of sweeping the improvements away.

Charlemont, greatly distressed at this prospect, allegedly ran to Dr Lucas to know what should be done. The physician prescribed and recommended Mary Hickman, 'the daughter of a decayed gentleman of his acquaintance',[2] a country girl from Co. Clare, whom, one supposes that in his professional capacity, he regarded as young, strong and healthy enough to fulfil the purpose for which she was required.

Charlemont fell in love with her to judge from the drafts of letters he wrote her (which may or may not have been sent). He admitted it was to his self-confessed shame, for the first time he felt 'a passion whose purpose and designs were perfectly virtuous'.[3]

His sudden marriage on 2 July 1768 completely surprised society. Francis wrote on 12 July that he had heard of it and offered the conventional congratulations. So surprising was it that Charlemont should marry a penniless provincial girl, who apparently had not even great beauty to recommend her, that even to this day there persists among Dubliners a sort of King Cophetua and the beggar maid tradition that she was the daughter of a common sea-captain and that all her poor relations came to live with him and so bothered him with their idle and vulgar chatter that he built the Casino as a refuge!

Nearer the truth was that the new Countess was a gentlewoman and connected with the O'Briens of the ancient royal line of Thomond; that Mary brought her sister, Miss Hickman, to live with them, and that Charlemont regarded her with the same sort of affection he felt for his half-sister. (She was now Mrs Ross, he was very fond of her and continued to be after his bitter and final quarrel with her father, Thomas Adderley.)

Dr Leland,* the historian (who had been Francis' tutor) wrote Lady Charlemont a delightful letter with just a bare hint of advice that she would have to reconcile herself to the width of her husband's outside interests and perhaps suffer a little neglect on their account. Charlemont had already forestalled him by warning her of the disadvantages for her in their marriage, first that he had got into a long and inveterate habit of living for himself; that his fortune was not what it might have been and that due to his chronic ill health she might begin her married life by becoming a nurse.[4]

The marriage, undoubtedly a happy one, provided Charlemont with that quiet, stable domestic background which at the age of forty he needed and for so long, had avoided. There had been many affairs, and even the birth of an illegitimate child about which we have no information except that of a letter from Robert Wood (once more the go-between), asking on the mother's behalf for some regularized provision, not for herself but for the child.[5]

What we suspect was at the root of Charlemont's distaste and fear of marriage was, happily, never realised: Mary survived safely the birth of five children. Nevertheless, there was sadness and, from another quarter, shocking tragedy. Charlemont was greatly afflicted by the death of their second child in 1773 and, the first-born being a daughter (Lady Elizabeth Caulfeild) it was not until the birth of Francis William on 3 January 1775 that the original purpose of the marriage was substantiated. At the end of the same year, by some dreadful irony, Francis, on his way back from London where he had been greatly exercised in trying to find some relief for Charlemont's nearly desperate financial situation, was lost in a violent storm at sea

* Dr Thomas Leland 1722-1785 wrote a *History of Ireland*, *Life of Philip of Macedon* and translated *The Orations of Demosthenes*.

with his wife (Lord Eyre's only daughter Mary), their infant child and their coachman. To add to the tragedy there were two other children of the marriage to provide for, but for them after some discussion, Lord Eyre agreed to take responsibility.

After his marriage Charlemont went to London less often. At first his Countess accompanied him on his visits, but it tells something of her unsureness in fashionable London society that, according to Hardy, the politeness and 'affectionate courtesies' she received from Lady Northumberland, were for ever 'cherished in her grateful remembrance'. One fears that the little provincial wife was snubbed by others when Charlemont was not present to protect her.

With a wife and children, the wife of a retiring and home-loving disposition, all thoughts of the Casino as a dwelling had to be abandoned and Marino House began to come into its own through the need for family accommodation. But by the time Charlemont undertook the alterations and an extension to the House, money was short and, for the first time, Charlemont realised that he could not any more be a chooser and that the richer effect which he had formerly preferred had to be sacrificed to economy.

The fire at Marino House in 1807 destroyed the greater part of his work there and with it much of the evidence which would perhaps have shown whether extensions and alterations bore any resemblance to the designs for a Hunting Lodge,[6] which Charlemont commissioned from Chambers in 1767. These were presumed to have been abandoned, but which may perhaps have been re-hashed into plans for the extension to the House.

In 1767 Charlemont was not yet married and his money difficulties had taken on no serious proportions. With Charlemont House not finished and the completion of the Casino not even in sight, that he should commission an entirely new building at this stage, seems symptomatic of building-mania. There was no question then of the designs being for Marino House; Chambers' undated letter of *c.* April 1768 is clearly about an unattached building, whose foundations had yet to be laid, with a front and a garden front for which plans and elevations exist.

That this building was intended for Roxborough, Charlemont's estate at Moy, Co. Tyrone seemed questionable. Charlemont, having made some improvements for the benefit of his tenants in the village there in 1763, thereafter took very little interest in his northern properties, other than for the mortgages to subsidise his building programme in the south. He states clearly in his political memoirs, 'My health to which sea-bathing, and the social nei'bourhood of a Metropolis were absolutely necessary, would not allow me to settle on my estate in the North ...' When he was courting Mary Hickman he explained to her he could not follow her into the country because 'my health will not permit me in its present state to venture an intermission of sea-bathing'.[7] It is difficult to think then the letters exchanged between Charlemont and Chambers in 1768 were about a building as far from the sea as Roxborough, and yet the least likely place for a Hunting Lodge was as close to the city as Marino.

Nevertheless we have to think of Charlemont as a builder of beautiful buildings for which usage was of secondary importance. Chambers' designs are for a 'hunting Lodge', all Charlemont's references to it are simply as 'the Lodge'.

Charlemont's routine, according to Hardy, included every day a morning ride (such as Lady Sandwich had recommended him so many years before) but one never hears of any hunting; that was left to Lord Bruce for whom Chambers designed the Hunting Casino for Tanfield Hall in Yorkshire. It was about Lord Bruce that Richard Phelps had once written to Charlemont: 'He is fit to be Huntsman Royal to Diana. He is out every morning an hour & a half before day & sometimes brings night home with him; he has lowere'd the price of Dust brooms by the infinite quantity of Fox's brushes that his Huntsman & Grooms distribute about and his Stable Doors look like an Indian habitation cover'd over with Scalps.'[8]

Charlemont's use of the word 'Lodge' in connection with the new building adds a fresh complication to the puzzle. J.P. Prendergast, (entering once more into the lists), in *The Irish Times* of 16 September 1886, wrote, 'Marino was an appropriate name as the waters of Dublin Bay wash its verge. It was once called the Lodge.' In editing Charlemont's correspondence for Charlemont's grandson, the 3rd Earl, Prendergast tabulated the letters of 1768 as 'about plans for a Lodge at Marino; – for additions to the house.'[9]

Although by April 1768 he was beginning to have reservations about the stabling, Charlemont intended a hunting Lodge as we learn from the following letter: 'Dear Chambers, I have received and thoroughly considered your Designs for the Lodge, of which in general I approve exceedingly. The Front is just as I cou'd wish it, but I shou'd be glad to have a Design for the Garden-Front also, which by the present Disposition of the Plan, if rightly comprehended, would not I believe look so well, on account of the too great Projection of the Break and the Return of the cornish of the Wings, which I fear wou'd not have a good effect. I would also have some changes in the Plan – viz – What is intended for a stable B, I would have changed into a dining Parlour and wou'd have it enlarged by making the Breadth what is now the Length. That is to say I wou'd have it made proportionally long to its Breadth of two and twenty feet, by which means it will make an excellent eating Room, and the Break in the Garden Front will be so much lessen'd, which I think will be an Advantage. I wou'd also have a Door of communication between it and the Drawing room A and another from the Study C. It will I believe be best lighted from the Side and the Chimney may be opposite the Windows, but this I leave entirely to you. The Kitchen wing must be enlarged in the same proportions, as an eating room shou'd always be very lofty. I believe there can be no Room over it, but I wou'd have it coved, and shou'd desire a Section with the cove mark'd. The Stables I intend to build in a cover'd situation at some distance from the House. So much for the Lodge ...'[10] and Charlemont went on to ask the questions about the Casino, the false doors, etc., by which we can more or less date the letter.

The above and Chambers' reply, also undated, cannot be related to Chambers' known designs for Lord Charlemont's Hunting Lodge and perhaps preceded these. Chambers sent on drawings for the garden front, which he hoped would please, 'and the plan of the ground floor is now much more convenient, the dining room is of a fine size but I have not drawn a Cove for I think it will be better without ... the little apartment in the Wing opposite the dining room will I think answer your Lordship's purpose for a private Study & bedroom – the offices are underground, they are not numerous though sufficient I apprehend for a building of this kind. The stair A is necessary to serve the table without passing through the drawing room or Study, the Kitchen's and Butler's pantry are lighted by an Area which I suppose may be easily made & the Servant's hall, stair and pantry must be lighted by openings in the ground covered with grates. All the flues of the Chimneys must be brought into Wall C and terminate in Stack D. As I am unacquainted with the Exposition of the Building I may perhaps have placed some of the rooms improperly. The dining room should not have its principal light to the West or the private Study to the East; the Larder & pantry should look North, a south or East light will be rather inconvenient for the Kitchen. These things I mention that they may be attended to in planting the building.'[11]

It is clear from the above that Prendergast is mistaken; this is no plan for an extension to an existing building, but for a small house to be built upon a vacant site. Thereafter there is no specific mention of the Lodge as such in the correspondence, and the idea seems to have been abandoned.

There has been some speculation, since a hunting lodge at Roxborough seemed so unlikely, as to whether the plan was intended for Hollybrook on the Marino estate on the other side of the Dublin-Malahide road. Hollybrook, with a house and a parcel of land, was sold by Charlemont's son, Francis, 2nd Earl of Charlemont, in 1861 to his niece, Margaret Zoë Caulfeild and her husband, John Calvery Stronge. The Stronges demolished the original house, known as Mount Temple and built the present Victorian mansion. Could Mount Temple have been built by Charlemont?

In the light of a letter written by Charlemont's brother Francis, who up until his death was member for Charlemont's Borough in Armagh, credence must be given to the Roxborough supposition. Francis wrote, 'I have seen a farm of yours near Moy which tho' small I think will do tolerably well for me to build on'.[12] Francis was in straitened circumstances and had neither the wherewithall nor Charlemont's experience in building and one may suppose this was the propitiatory sop for the loss of his expected inheritance through Charlemont's marriage. At all events, with Francis' death, all mention of the Hunting Lodge ceases.

In reviewing the correspondence relating to the Hunting Lodge, we find for the first time, evidence of Charlemont and Chambers not being in complete agreement. Charlemont had asked for a coved ceiling for the diningroom, but Chambers thought it would be better without. Charlemont's request for a kitchen wing had been brushed aside for offices underground.

However some months before Francis' death in November 1775 there was a change of direction and plans for a hitherto unmentioned Gallery and a Drawing room are under discussion, which can have nothing to do with the Lodge.

On 19 April Chambers sent designs for 'a Cornice, Frieze and necking for the Drawing room with a door, Entablature, Base & surbase for the same room all drawn of the full size'. He also sent a design for a chimney-piece and a cornice for the Gallery, a fret for its ceiling with sketches of the form of the room figured. 'A design of the Niches in my dining room, I have also sent according to yr. Lds. desire.'[13]

Without any of that urgency which had formerly characterised his letters, Charlemont replied on 9 July, three months later, 'The Designs which you sent me, like everything that comes from you are perfectly pretty. Indeed the entablatures and other ornaments for the drawing room are so very pretty that I am to ornament the ceiling also; since, if it were left quite plain, it wou'd I fear ill correspond with the other parts, all of which are enrich'd. I must therefore trouble you to send me a Design for the ceiling, which however I would wish Light, plain and not expensive – a *light architrave* ceiling if I may so call it, divided into compartments would, I fancy be the cheapest, and the dossils of the Joysts might be ornamented with Vitruvian Fret. But this I leave entirely to you as you are the best Judge of what will look best and lightest. The Dimensions of the Room, which you may have forgotten, are 30 feet 6 inc. long by 22 feet broad and 16 high. Be as exact as possible in marking and figuring the Projections as I would leave as little as possible to our Workmen. The opening of the Chimney Piece, which you sent me is no more than three feet eight inches and I should conceive that for a Room of the above Dimensions less than four feet would not answer. The aperture may, however, I suppose, be increased, without alterating the Proportions of the other parts. You forgot to figure the Design of your Nitch. Be so good as to send me its Dimensions.'[14]

In his reply of 2 August, Chambers wrote, 'I do not in the least recollect the Nitch which your Lordship mentions, but as it was not figured, it has probably a scale which may be attended to.' Do we begin to detect a little tetchiness in these exchanges over dimensions and a niche, which had certainly been mentioned by Chambers in his letter of 19 April and which appears in Chambers' final account (the fatal bill that Charlemont left unpaid).

However the rest of the letter is perfectly equable. Chambers was glad to hear that the designs sent gave satisfaction and hopes that the one for the ceiling enclosed will do the same: 'the ornament must have very little relief, from 1/4 to half an Inch & as the design is large they cannot go wrong provided the workmen be good. I have coloured a part to show how it might be done; but it will look very well all white.'

'I know not how the chimney came to be sent only 3 ft. 8 ins. it will do better four feet but the ornaments which surround it need not be altered they will do equally well.'[15]

The ceiling, which we take to be for the said drawing-room, is mentioned once again in Chambers' letter of 7 September:'I am glad the ceiling pleased your Lordship with regard to the projection; the ornaments as I have said before should not project above half an inch in the highest parts, but some of the mouldings may project more, else they would have no effect, the common rule is to make their projection about 3/4 of their width, excepting in astagals which need not project above a third.' Chambers added, with a rough sketch of a cornice, 'there will be no difficulty in the Junction of the Cornice & ceiling as to the best of my recollection there is a plain space all round this'.[16]

With that letter ended the correspondence in so far as it related to Charlemont's building, and without any evidence for the exact location of the drawing room and gallery under discussion. Chambers' final bill, which included the account for 1773, is no more informative, although in its detail the latter part fits neatly enough with the letters of 1775.

'Dr the Rt. Honr. Lord Charlemont in acc. wh. W. Chambers.

				L	s	d
	1773					
Jan. 30th	Various designs for flower stands with a pavillion in the center			8.	8.	-
	Two sections of the Library coloured being patterns for the painter			4.	4.	-
May 14th	Drawings & directions for painting the Vestibule of the Casine			2.	2.	-
	Ditto for the antiroom of the library			2.	2.	-
	Design of a pedestal for an Antique bas-relief				10.	6
	A new design for a flower stand			3.	3.	-
15th	A design of a Therm chimneypiece sent by letter to Mr Verpyle			3.	3.	-
				Ls:23.	12.	6
	1775 [*this part of the bill in guineas*]					
Apr. 19th	Designs for finishing a drawing room Cornice frize & Door & window architrave frize and cornice Case surbase and chimney piece	6.	6.			
	Cornice galoss &c for a gallery Sketches of the room Designs for a Therm & other ornamts of a Nich	2.	2.	13-	13-	0

Aug. 2	A design for a Ceiling for a Drawing room partly coloured	5. 5	
			Ls:37. 5. 6

This bill[17] and Charlemont's reasons for not paying, apart from the most obvious one, we shall come back to later. It would appear from the entry for 15 May 1773 that Vierpyle was still in Charlemont's employment and was to make a chimney piece with terms, and that, therefore, building at this indeterminate site was either contemplated, or in progress, between 1773 and 1775.

Prendergast, in editing the correspondence, believed that the letters referred to alterations and extensions to Marino House, 'once called the Lodge'. Certainly there was a drawing room there, because in February 1807 a fire broke out destroying the northern wing with 'the very beautiful drawing room, the windows of which were ornamented with some of the most masterly productions in stained glass, by the late celebrated Jervis'.[18]

The term 'Lodge' appears in the memorial of Charlemont's will and is taken to refer to Marino House, left to Lady Charlemont for her life. The Lodge is also mentioned by Ignatius McDonagh, the Dublin gilder and carver, employed by Charlemont between 1775 and 1776 in making picture and table frames, and in repairs to the Gothic Room. Among the entries in his bill for 1776 we find the following:

To two pieces of Ornamt. to each side the tablet to Ram's Head chimney piece	1.	7.	0.
To an ornamental frieze and two Capitals for the Boe Parlour at the Lodge	2.	5.	6.[19]

Since McDonagh was a wood carver, the ram's head chimney piece cannot be Harwood's chimney piece of statuary marble, bronze and lapis lazuli. There is no reason to doubt that this was the 'original mantel' of the report and plans of Marino House, published by the *Irish Georgian Society* in 1913, when it was recorded as being in the drawing room.[20] The Marino House chimney piece is, as already mentioned, now in the Saloon of the Casino.

With no mention of a gallery in the 1913 report, we are left to doubt Prendergast's assumption that the 1775 correspondence referred to Marino House; there remains only Charlemont House to consider. Chambers' bill for 14 May 1773 accounts for drawings, and directions for painting the Vestibule of the Casino, 'Ditto for the antiroom of the libary'; but before that, on 30 January, there is 'two sections of the Library coloured being patterns for the painter'. It was supposed that these entries referred to minor redecoration of Charlemont House library, and there seemed to be no connection with the designs of 1775 for a drawing room and a gallery. But in his letter of 9 July 1775, Charlemont gives the dimensions of the drawing room, which he thinks Chambers may have forgotten; a strong indication that Chambers had already provided designs for this particular location sometime before.

Descriptions of Charlemont House in its heyday agree in general, as to the appearance of the library wing and to the collection of paintings and sculpture displayed in the house, giving an impression of consummate elegance throughout.

It is then with astonishment that we learn from the Loeber discovery of a Tour of Dublin in 1797, the principal floor of Charlemont House was unfinished and the walls and ceilings not even plastered.'[21]

While this makes a good case for relating the correspondence of 1775 to the first floor of Charlemont House, the implications are not without pathos. Charlemont's financial situation did not allow him to carry out plans, but he continued to indulge himself in ordering designs.

NOTES

1. Irish Political Characters, 1799, p. 84.
2. Craig, p. 151.
3. HMC Rept. 12, App. pt. X, pp. 286-289.
4. Ibid, p. 290.
5. RIA, 12.R.12, no. 26.
6. J. Harris, *Sir William Chambers*, London 1970, pp. 52,174, 245, pl. 69 (V & A.).
7. HMC, Rept. 12, App. pt. X, p.
8. RIA, 12.R.21, no. 157.
9. Ibid, 12.R.12, see index, no. 55.
10. HMC Rept. 13, App. pt. VIII, pp. 272-3.
11. RIA, 12.R.12, no. 55.
12. RIA, 12.R.10, no. 4.
13. RIA, 12.R.12. no. 4.
14. Ibid, 12.R.30a.

15. Ibid, 12.R.12, no. 3.
16. Ibid, no. 5.
17. Ibid, 12.R.10, no. 79. HMC Rept. 12, App. pt. X, p. 338.
18. Gentleman's Magazine, 1807, Pt. 1, p. 269.
19. RIA, 12.R.10, nos. 77, 78.
20. Irish Georgian Society, Vol. 5 (1913), p. 86.
21. Communicated by Rolf Loeber and Magda Stouthamer-Loeber.

24

THE PARTING WITH CHAMBERS

In 1774 Charlemont's heir was born, Francis William, the future 2nd Earl of Charlemont; the future of Marino too, it was hoped, was made secure against Charlemont's brother Francis's threatened devastation. Francis' death, by a terrible irony, followed in 1775. At the same time money ran out and all building ceased.

Chambers, on 25 July 1774, had written Charlemont his congratulations on the birth of his son, and recommended to him a Piedmontese custom told him by Baretti. A thousand poplars should be planted, which by the time the young gentleman came of age, would be worth a thousand pounds and serve for his portion. This would ensure an easy way to provide for posterity, 'which might with great success be introduced into Ireland; where waste lands are frequent, and well prepared for the growth of poplars. 'By the help of this secret', Chambers wrote, 'your Lordship may have as many sons as King Priam and make for them any provision you think proper; you may then, as now, build temples upon every occasion without fear on the consequences; and I shall be your Lordship's Architect with infinitely more pleasure, when I know your fund is inexhaustible; fifty good poplars will produce a tolerable sized column; five hundred, a pretty temple; five thousand a villa, a Bridge, a triumphal arch; a Casino; a paralaia; a Boudoir; or anything that five thousand pounds can purchase; *a viva il Baretti.*'[1]

A delightful letter, but under the circumstances of Charlemont's pecuniary affairs, not very tactful. There was no secret about Charlemont being in bad financial straits, being dunned even for the ground rents of Marino and, at the same time, trying to raise money to buy out his landlord, Sir Francis Lumm. He was protesting he would pay when he could and in the meantime his creditors could try Sir Annesley Stewart or wait.[2]

It was to Sir Annesley, a cousin of Charlemont's, also his banker and adviser, that Francis, who was then in London trying to help sort out Charlemont's affairs, had written on 16 September 1775: 'I am excessively glad to hear my brother intends to borrow money instead of selling so much of his estate. You and he may depend on it I shall expedite matters as much as possible. I mention'd it to Wm. Chambers by mistake, the money shall be paid on Monday to Sr Jos. Reynolds ... I will come over as soon as I hear from you unless this offer of 50,000£ should require my attendance.'[3]

He added that he intended to sell his annuity as surely any brother would be more pleased at getting £450 by the death of a stranger than his own brother. On 4 October he wrote again to Sir Annesley that the matter of the annuity had been agreed and he hoped to set out in a day or two.

In a fearful storm in the third week in November, Major Francis Caulfeild, returning to Ireland to take up his duties as M.P. for Armagh was, with his lady and an infant and their coachman, lost at sea.

It may have been out of delicacy or perhaps only the customary delay, but Chambers did not present his final bill until January 1777, nearly a year and a half after the last entry of 2 August 1775 for a ceiling design for a drawing room, partly coloured. The total was, as we may recall, the comparatively small sum £37.5.6.

Until recently a note on the reverse of the account in faint pencil, but unmistakably in Charlemont's hand, had escaped notice. His comment refers to the entry for 30 January 1773, 'various designs for flower stands with a pavilion in the center' at a cost of £8.8.0. and for another of 14 May 1773, 'A new design for a flower stand' £3.3.0. Charlemont wrote, 'There is, I believe, a Mistake in the charge of £8.8.- for *Various Designs for Flower Stands*. There were but two such Designs exclusive of that which is afterwards charged £3.3.-, and which alone answered my purpose, the others being only unsuccessful attempts, which if it were intended that they should be charged, as I rather suppose it was not, ought not certainly to be set at a higher price than that Design which alone was of any sort of use to me.'[4]

A fragmentary letter of Chambers' of which only half survives, and which if it had been complete would still seem to be unusually short and abrupt, throws no light on the subject of the design for the offending flower stands. It reads, 'My Lord, I have sent another d.......... pavillion which I th.......... first I have drawn the f.........., if it were made Octagon .... in the side views and a .... flowers would l..... Honour to be, My Lord, Yours ....'[5]

In his letter of 18 January, when Chambers first took the liberty of enclosing a small bill (the first presentation as far as we know of the fatal account) Chambers wrote that it had been a great while since he had had the honour of hearing from his Lordship and he concludes that 'you have done little of late in the building ... I have done nothing for these fifteen months past but labour at the works of Somerset House, so extensive and complicated that they require all my attention and have reduced me to the necessity of declining all private employment ... if your lordship should be in want of any designs, Mr Gandon of Broad Street, an old pupil of mine & very ingenious would I daresay do them to your Lordship's satisfaction, he knows nothing of this recommendation nor have I seen him these seven years but in the street, yet from various designs of his which have appeared in the exhibitions, think he merits encouragement and wonder he has been so little employed. Your Lordship's protection would probably make him more known than he now is and more valued according to his desserts.'[6]

Chambers did not write again until 20 May 1779 and this time with a little more emotion: '... if anything could make me regret the having quitted a troublesome business it would, among a very few other things, be the loss of your Lordship's correspondence; the letters with which you honoured me on many occasions formerly, are preserved very carefully; I frequently read them over with much pleasure and a great deal of pride; as testimony of your Lordship's former kindness to me, but with a mixture of mortification at receiving no more such marks of distinction. I have not I flatter myself forfeited your Lordship's favour, yet cannot help having some apprehension which nothing but seeing or hearing from your Lordship can effectively remove. I wish it were in my power to pay you a visit at Dublin.'[7]

The letter could not have failed to soften the hardest heart had it not ended, 'Some time ago I sent over a bill for some designs done for your Lordship from Ja. '73 to August '75 amounting to 37.5.6 which I apprehend has been forgotten.'

Between the parting with Chambers and the employment of James Gandon on the Rockingham Room in the mid 1780s (Rockingham died in 1782), Charlemont was apparently without an architect and one might have concluded that the Casino was finished and work had come to a halt. The loan of £50,000 had not materialised and Charlemont was still looking for that sum at the end of the 1780s, but his situation had been eased in the meantime by a legacy from his maternal uncle.[8]

In 1778 John Wesley visited Marino and recorded in his journal for Thursday 16 July, 'Went with a few friends to Lord Charlemont's two or three miles from Dublin. It is one of the pleasantest places I have ever seen, the water, trees and lawns so elegantly intermixed with each other, having a serpentine walk running through a thick wood on one side, and an open prospect both of land and sea on the other. In the thickest part of the wood is the Hermitage, a small room, dark and gloomy enough. The Gothic temple, at the head of a fine piece of water, which is encompassed by stately trees, is delightful indeed. But the most elegant of all the buildings is not finished; the shell of it is surprisingly beautiful and the rooms well contained both for use and ornament. But what is all this unless God is here? Unless life is known, loved and enjoyed? Not only vanity unable to give happiness but vexation of spirit.'[9]

Vanity of vanities saith the Preacher. Wesley is not speaking figuratively of an empty shell when he states it is unfinished. Ten years later, an anonymous commentator[10] writing about the Casino, declared the same but specifically mentioning the interior. We have to conclude that the Casino was not nearly as advanced as the documents indicate when Chambers and Charlemont parted, or that there was some alteration, not necessarily of a structural nature, made to the interior.

As the Casino is presented today there are very obvious stylistic discrepancies, the plaster work in the boudoir and the crimson flock wallpaper in the little room for books, are clear indications of nineteenth-century renovation after the Casino had fallen into disrepair following Charlemont's death. The attic storey is not so easy to explain. The King's bedroom suggests some interference with the original at the time of George IV's visit in 1821 but, on stylistic grounds alone, the State bedroom looks to have nothing to do with Chambers, and yet is of late eighteenth-century design.

There are no known designs by Chambers for the attic storey. Lady Shelburne had mentioned in 1769, 'two tolerable bed chambers and two smaller ones for servants'. This description cannot be related in any way to the almost ostentatious decoration of the so-called State bedroom, so much in contrast with the simplicity of the three other rooms.

Until fresh documentation comes to light, we can only speculate about what happened at the Casino after the parting with Chambers. Did Charlemont with the assistance of Vierpyle, struggle on, adhering to the working designs of Chambers? Or did he, free from Chambers' restraining hand, take it upon himself, or another architect, to design what we suspect are the innovations of the attic storey?

In the 1791 edition of the *Treatise*, Chambers was to allow that the Casino 'was built by Mr Verpyl with great neatness and taste after models made here and instructions sent from hence'. It was a tribute, but one that ensured Vierpyle was kept in his place as Clerk of the Works and stonemason of the Casino.

The modest Vierpyle was content to have himself listed in the Dublin directories as a stonemason or, alternatively, a stonecutter and yet it was as a sculptor that Charlemont had brought him from Rome. Very little sculpture had come from his hand after his arrival in Dublin; two portrait busts in 1758 and a 'Meleager' and a portrait bust in 1765 are known. But when Murphy was writing to Vierpyle about the value of the series of the Emperors' heads, which he was thinking of presenting to Charlemont, he addressed his letter to him as Simon Vierpyle, *Statuary* and *Architect*.[11]

After his work for Charlemont was done, Vierpyle was employed as a stonemason in the building of the 'Blew Coat Hospital'; but it was as all three – statuary, architect and mason – that Ralph Howard in 1785, commissioned him to design and build the Wicklow family mausoleum at Kilbride, Arklow. It still survives, although the ornamental carving has been desecrated, commanding as it was originally intended 'a good prospect all round'.[12] In the form of a pyramid, its design perhaps owed something to Vierpyle's former patron.

Murphy's addressing Vierpyle as Architect draws attention to an otherwise almost imperceptible undertone of antagonism or rivalry between Chambers and Vierpyle. There was the incident of Vierpyle's confused dimensions for the Indian wallpaper, which neither Chambers nor Stark could make out; the letter from Vierpyle about the parquetted floors, the first news Chambers had heard of them, and the matter of a pedestal for the Fighting Gladiator made by Vierpyle for Charlemont in Rome, for which Chambers could not send a design since there were 'no dimensions nor any cast of it in London'. It appears Charlemont wanted to put the Gladiator up at the centre of the radiating paths in the walled-in garden, the spot from which it was removed by the 3rd Earl at the time of the sale of Marino. It only required that Chambers consult Vierpyle about the dimensions and not make an issue of it with Charlemont.

If, in fact, Charlemont was in want, at this late stage, of working designs for the so-called State bedroom, or any other innovation that occurred to him, and was not confident about Vierpyle's capacities, he might have preferred that the employment of another architect, other than Gandon whom Chambers himself had recommended, was kept as much as possible a secret.

With little or no documentation to guide us, it is tempting to take a hint from Hardy that Charlemont was ever on intimate terms with James Stuart. Stuart was employed around 1780 by Robert Stewart, the future Lord Londonderry at Mount Stewart, where Charlemont was a frequent visitor. For Robert Stewart, 'Athenian' Stuart built the Tower of the Winds.[13] He had also been employed at Wentworth Woodhouse and had worked for Lord Bagot at Blithfield.

NOTES

1. RIA, 12.R.13, no. 1.
2. Ibid, 12.R.10, nos. 84, 85. Christine Casey's discovery of Sir Annesly Stewart's accounts and payments made on Charlemont's behalf, clarifies this.
3. Ibid, 12.R.10, no. 60.
4. Ibid, no. 79. I indebted to John Redmill for drawing my attention to Charlemont's notes.
5. Ibid, loose page, unlisted fragment with no. 38.
6. Ibid, no. 79.
7. Ibid, no. 93.
8. Ibid, 12.R.26, no. 6.
9. N. Curnoch ed. *The Journal of the Rev. John Wesley* Vol. 6, p. 204.10.
10. Trinity College Dublin Library, MS 891.
11. H. Byrne 'The Speculative Building Activities of Simon Vierpyl', *Irish Georgian Society Bulletin*, Vol. XXXVI, 1995, pp. 31-40.
12. Wicklow papers. Remains of the pyramidal vault in Kilbride churchyard still survive. Another pyramid, erected as a garden building at The Neale, Co. Mayo by Charlemont's brother-in-law, Sir John Browne was said to have been built to a plan and drawing supplied by Charlemont. E. Malins and the Knight of Glin, pp. 141-2.
13. Ibid, pp. 110-111.

25

ARBITER ELEGANTIARUM

It was for Reynolds' *Venus chiding Cupid* that Francis, shortly before his death, had arranged payment in London. Charlemont, on taking delivery the following year, wrote to Sir Joshua, 'I have pleasure in thinking that by this importation I shall in a great measure contribute to reform the taste of my country.'[1]

He appears to write with all the confidence of the unchallenged *arbiter elegantiarum* of Ireland, and figuratively at least he could be said, as with his self-appointed role of Minerva on the triumphal car in Rome, to preside over the Arts and Sciences. There were to be no more such importations. His money was spent; he had parted with his architect; the Casino was apparently unfinished; and yet there was some room for complacency. Noblemen and gentlemen all over the country were building or rebuilding their houses and improving their estates.

It was twenty years since Charlemont had returned to Ireland and begun the landscaping of Marino. Although he would have been too modest and too moderate in his opinions to think that he alone had promoted the fashion, he knew that in the improvements and through the building of the Casino and Charlemont House, he had set an unrivalled standard and had eventually attracted the attention of his countrymen towards the Arts.

There is little evidence for Charlemont, at the beginning, having encouraged native artists or talent. He had relied almost exclusively on the importation of ideas, Vierpyle and works of art. He employed Matthew Peters, but only after first sending him to England to study up-to-date methods. He had patronised Jervais, having presumably seen his work for the Marquis of Kildare at Kildare (Leinster) House. And there had been Ignatius McDonagh. Recent research has revealed that the stuccodores of the Casino's superb plasterwork were Irish, but here, at least, native skill had triumphantly developed from the introduction of Italian artists such as the brothers Lafrancini in the 1730s.

Nevertheless his interest in the activities of the Dublin Society, which had been founded in 1731 primarily for the improvement of husbandry, but also other 'useful arts', was the basis upon which the school of eighteenth-century Irish landscape painting was founded. Premiums were awarded for draining, levelling and fencing, and for the planting of thousands upon thousands of acres of trees. This was an incentive to the laying out of parklands, gardens and lawns of demesnes as building became fashionable. When the Dublin Society extended beyond agriculture to the fine arts and opened its drawing schools, Charlemont was said to have been involved in superintending classes.

Premiums were again paid to the most promising pupils. By 1765 the Society of Artists in Ireland had been founded and the first exhibition was held.[2]

Painters of portraits in oil and chalk, miniature painters, architectural and topographical draughtsmen, glass painters, sculptors, carvers, engravers, still-life and landscape painters exhibited their works. The portrait painters almost invariably did not name their sitters, but the patrons of the landscape painters put no such condition of anonymity upon the views they had commissioned. These view-painters of gentlemen's seats, because that was how they were employed rather than as landscapists, were in demand; gentlemen who were building and improving all over the country were ready with their patronage.

Not surprisingly, Marino demesne was featured prominently and there may have been other paintings and drawings since the extant catalogues are incomplete.

In 1767 *A View of the Casino at Marino* was exhibited by Jonathan Fisher. In 1770, James Coy's *View of Marino* was exhibited. The brilliant, but short-lived, Thomas Roberts showed, in 1772, *A View of the right Hon. the Earl of Charlemont's domain, taken from the Gothic Room*, and in the following year *A View of the Earl of Charlemont's Casine at Marino.* Also in 1772 there was a drawing by the architect and draughtsman, Thomas Ivory, *A View of the Right Hon. the Earl of Charlemont's Casine at Marino*; the drawing was afterwards engraved. Although George Mullins was known to have been patronised by Charlemont, it is not possible to identify him from the catalogue descriptions, as the painter of the four large decorative paintings which were sold from Marino in 1875. After he left Ireland, he exhibited at the Royal Academy in London *A View from the Gothic temple at Morina the seat of the Earl of Charlemont in Ireland in which is introduced the story of Diana & Acteon.* There is also, although it was not exhibited at the Society, the drawing by Francis Wheatley, which was engraved for Thomas Milton's *Views* in 1780.

Before the Society's exhibitions ceased in 1780, some fifty views of noblemen and gentlemen's seats, many duplicating the subject but by different artists, were exhibited. In almost every instance they were painted for known associates of Charlemont. These included the Lords Tyrone, Drogheda and the 3rd Viscount Powerscourt, (brother of Charlemont's friend), all of whom were of the company at Marino when, in 1763, Lady Northumberland visited there. Agmondisham Vesey was his own architect at Lucan, but in consultation with William Chambers and James Wyatt. Thomas Dawson was now Lord Dartrey of Dawson's Grove. As Slane Castle was included, with the improvements by Lord Conyngham, Frank Burton's uncle, and also views of the Boyne from nearby Beau Parc, (believed to have been designed by Burton's father-in-law, Nathaniel Clements), Burton himself was not so far away.

Nathaniel Clements, of the Treasury, was the amateur architect responsible for Viceregal Lodge (Aras An Uachtaráin); he had built Lodge Park for Joseph Henry's father at Straffan. Neither Lodge Park nor Russborough were, as far as we know, subjects for the early view painters. Lady Kildare, who visited Russborough in May 1759 commented, 'The house is really fine and the furniture magnificent; but a frightful place.'[3]

Lady Kildare was qualified to judge: she had changed the course of the Ryewater and built the bridge at Carton to the designs of Thomas Ivory. Views of the transformed landscape were painted by Thomas Roberts and George Barret.

Barret, the protégé of Lord Powerscourt, painted for Joseph Leeson a series of Italianate decorative landscapes for Russborough, which were far removed in subject and style from the views he painted of the hilly, wooded demesne of Powerscourt with its spectacular waterfall; so far removed and so effective that Lady Kildare feared when he came to paint Carton and Castletown for her sister, Lady Louisa Conolly, that Castletown was too flat ever to make a pretty picture.

When Barret was brought by Lord Powerscourt to Carton, Richard Marlay visited with them. The man, who had once seemed to Charlemont to be his only friend in a strange country, was still very much of Charlemont's circle in Ireland. In London, Marlay, known as the witty, worldly Dean of Waterford, was one of the Johnsonian set. He was also, as it happened, the uncle of Henry Grattan, whose association with Charlemont was to have such far-reaching political effect.

The intimacy between Charlemont and the Kildares dated from at least 1761 when the *Beggar's Opera* was performed at Carton with Charlemont in the part of Peachum. In August of the same year, Joseph Henry returned from eleven years abroad and Charlemont begged leave to present him to Lady Kildare. After Lord Kildare's elevation to the Dukedom of Leinster in 1766, Chambers wrote to Charlemont,'I shall with great pleasure obey her Grace's commands on this and all other occasions',[4] which might suggest some obligation to Charlemont for her patronage.

The fashionable circle of those engaged in building and improving have already been shown to have bestowed much of their patronage on the same view painters. As time went on they inclined, more and more, to employ resident and native artists, craftsmen and artisans, particularly those who had received instruction in the Dublin Society's schools. At these schools, plaster casts, after the Antique, and prints, after the Old Masters, were readily available for study. Many of the casts and prints had been presented by the Grand Tourists in their efforts to promote the highest standards. Joseph Henry, continuing in this tradition, presented a Venus di Medici and a Dancing Faun, both in marble, in 1786.

The concerted movement of fashionable society towards the ornamentation of Ireland was conducted at speed, as if to make up for lost time. The dearth of the arts in the country had caused an earlier commentator from England to remark, 'To expect many works of the fine arts in a country, but just recovering from an almost uninterrupted warfare of near six hundred years, would be to look for the ripe fruits of autumn in the spring.'[5] By the 1770s the movement was hastening towards summer.

During the 1770s the state of the country, with many references to the fine arts, came under the review of two English tourists, one the eccentric Dr Twiss, the other the distinguished agriculturist, Arthur Young.

Dr Twiss made himself very unpopular in Dublin with offensive remarks about the ignorance and eating habits of the Irish and he was more than unchivalrous about the thick legs of Irish women. A Dublin earthenware manufacturer contributed, very profitably, to avenging his country's honour with some chamber pots printed inside with a portrait and a motto playing on the rhyme of Dr T— with P—. Nevertheless his *Tour in Ireland* was a best seller and, like Arthur Young's, ran to several editions.

Twiss gives us a detailed, although not necessarily accurate account, of collections of paintings in Dublin at the time. Mr Stewart had a hundred pictures, including a large nativity by Rubens; Lady St George's house, and the Earl of Ely's Rathfarnham Castle, a good number. Lord Moira's collection included a Murillo, a Correggio and portraits by Rosalba, a warrior's head by Rembrandt and pictures by Salvator Rosa. Of Joseph Henry, he wrote that he had a few pictures, among the best a madonna as large as life by Carlo Dolci 'estimated to be a chef d'oeuvre'. Henry had also two pictures by Batoni (presumably one was his own portrait, now in the Walters Art Gallery, Baltimore), four by Vernet, a nearly life size St Peter and St Paul by Andrea del Sarto, and several views of Naples and its surrounds, Aranjuez, Madrid etc., by Antonio Joli painted in 1750. Among these was a bullfight and Joli had engraved a plate of it for Mr Henry.[6]

Twiss formed the opinion that there were no other collections, apart from a few pictures by Mrs Angelica Kauffman, in the whole island, and chose to ignore Ralph Howard's collection at Shelton and that of Joseph Henry's uncle Joseph Leeson, now the Earl of Milltown, at Russborough.

However, he did visit Charlemont House and Marino, both of which he contrived to dismiss fairly briefly. At Charlemont House he saw 'one of the finest pieces Rembrandt ever painted' and Hogarth's *The Lady's Last Stake*. 'It represents a lady sitting in a desponding air, and an officer offering her his hat full of money and jewels which he has just won of her: eager desire is expressed in his countenance and in her repentance and hesitation'. At Marino he saw 'an elegant Casino of which it is sufficient to say that Messrs Adam were the architects and that a very fine print is engraved of it, by Mr Rooker from a drawing by Thomas Ivory. The building is a square of sixty feet to each side and from the top is a view of Dublin, the bay, the sea &c. The gardens (termed improvements in Ireland ...) are not extensive but are created with taste.'[7]

Arthur Young's report was of a very different calibre. He had arrived in Dublin with a letter of recommendation from Edmund Burke to Charlemont. His prime interest was agriculture and at Marino he noted the new lawns of white clover, trefoil and rib-grass, and also the well-planted thriving shrubbery. He described the Casino: 'on a rising ground a banqueting room, which ranks very high among the most beautiful edifices I have anywhere seen; it has much elegance, light and effect, and commands a fine prospect',[8] which he thought might have been more perfect if the city had been planted out.

In Young's conclusion on the general state of Ireland, he wrote: 'Ireland has been absolutely new built within these twenty years, and in a manner far superior to anything that was seen in it before. It is a fact universal over the whole kingdom; cities, towns, and country seats; but the present is the era for this improvement, there being now far more elegant seats rising than ever were known before.'[9]

Arthur Young's mention of the cities and towns gives some indication that this flurry of architectural and artistic activity was not entirely elitist or confined to the country seats of the aristocracy and their Dublin houses. By the simple economics of upper class prosperity and the provision of new opportunities for industry and employment, the movement based upon something so nebulous as Taste, began to take root and spread throughout the country.

In 1768, it was not members of the aristocracy, but the merchants of Dublin who offered a premium for a design for the Royal Exchange (the first Neo-Classical public building to be erected in Dublin). Charlemont took pains to try to procure the job for Chambers, but after some delay the prize was awarded to Thomas Cooley, a Londoner who had worked in association with Robert Milne, of Blackfriars Bridge fame. Chambers did not hesitate to suggest to Charlemont that to a mercantile soul, it was a matter of money and there is even a hint that a bribe would bring about the desired result.[10]

To judge from newspapers of the period, politics rather than money, influenced and shaped the course of the movement and generated a new interest among the rising classes.

Twice weekly the *Public Monitor*[11] gave vent to its opinions in a column entitled 'View of Stephen's Green', purported to be written by Amos Griffith, although he denied the charge. The paper justified its most virulent attacks by proclaiming that for the blackening of one character, fifty were favourably reviewed. The greatest abuse was reserved for those whose honours were seen as bribes to buy their allegiance to the Castle and Viceroy, Lord Townshend's unpopular administration. On the other hand, those whose sympathies were with the Opposition, the national or 'patrotic party' were eulogised, and these included notably the artists whom they employed. Members of the Society of the Artists of Ireland were given a tremendous puff. Articles and letters from the *Public Monitor* were reprinted as *Baratariana*,[12] edited and written by Henry Flood and Henry Grattan in 1773.

Of all the characters seen perambulating the Beau Walk of Stephen's Green, none was more vilified than Joseph Leeson senior, now the Earl of Milltown. 'There goes Joe Taplash, the Right Hon. Earl of M——n, who was the son of a Brewer, who was the son of a Butcher, who was the son of a Huxter, who was the son of a Shoeboy, who was the son of a W——.'[13]

When Simon Vierpyle was seen approaching he was 'one of the greatest Artists in the World, and the best statuary on Earth. Lord Charlemont brought him from England merely for his amazing Excellence, he is now the Chief undertaker of the Royal Exchange.'[14]

There were compliments for Henry Tresham, 'that genteel young man in brown ... a celebrated limner and an honest, worthy soul'; for the Roberts brothers, Thomas and Thomas Sautelle, both promising to become ornaments of their country. And most especially for the Healys.

'Healy is the greatest Mechanical Genius that now exists ... he is sent for to the most remote Parts of the Kingdom by the first Nobility to erect Chinese turrets, superintend Grottoes and to ornament Entertainments ... his abilities are superlative, as may be seen by his decoration of Lady Mo-ra's Room ...' The commentator also mentions Healy's son Robert, who, as we know, made drawings at Castletown of Tom Conolly's horses and hounds;[15] he had died two years before.

Healy's decorations at Moira House were described by John Wesley when he waited on Lady Moira in 1775. He was surprised 'to observe, though not a more grand, yet a far more elegant room than any I ever saw in England. It was an octagon, about 20 feet square and 15 or 16 high having one window, the sides of it inlaid throughout with mother-of-pearl reaching from the top to the bottom; the ceiling, sides and furniture of the room were equally elegant'.[16]

The Earl of Moira, a member of the Society of Dilettanti, had a scholarly taste in literature and a very fine library. In politics, Lord Moira was, like Charlemont – his coadjutor in the Irish House of Lords – a Whig; that is to say, a member of the more liberal of the two political parties. He and Charlemont had much in common and they were friends. A further connection was the marriage of Lord Bruce (Ailesbury), after the death of his first wife, to a daughter of Lord Moira's. Joseph Henry married another.

One venture of Charlemont's, Moira's, and others of the former Grand Tourist circle including the 2nd Duke of Leinster, was a failure. Arthur Young wrote 'An ill-judged and unsuccessful attempt was made to establish the Italian opera ... *La Buona Figliuola, La Frascatana,* and *Il Geloso in Cimento* were repeatedly performed, or rather murdered, except the parts of Sestini. The house was generally empty, and miserably cold'.[17] *The Dublin Evening Journal,* in a scathing attack by *Anti-Castrato,* went further, straight to the very roots of the fine art movement and burlesqued the building activities of the aristocracy.

'My Lords and Gentlemen, You have imported a company of itinerant vagrants; you have turned yourself into a committee for conducting their theatrical movements and are therefore ostensible to the public for their conduct; since the first night of performances the town has been insulted by the impudence and caprice of YOUR company – If the Sestini imagined an indisposition, the opera is postponed, "Good Heavens, your grace! I can't sing tomorrow; the straps of my cork-rump are loosened – I'm dead with hoarseness." His Grace flies to the Committee – the physician-in-waiting is dispatched to examine the premises – reports the complaint to be fundamental! There's no opera ...'[18]

For the last performance of the 1778 season, a Benefit for the distressed Manufacturers of the city, the ladies Antrim, Moira, Bective, Charlemont, Ely, de Vesey and Kingsborough with mesdames Pery, Gardiner and Adderley were distributors of tickets. It was to the ladies that *Anti-Castrato* addressed himself.

'Castle building has been a favourite amusement with the nobility of this country. I don't mean the aerial castles which are constructed in the imagination, those baseless fabricks of a vision which leave not a wrack behind nor do I mean the fortified edifices of hair which your Ladyships erect upon your heads, tier after tier ... but permanent substantial castles, founded upon the principles of masonic stability, as the castle of Marino, without a room in which a large man could turn – the Castle of Leinster, not quarter, furnished – the castle of Powerscourt, without courtyard or area – and the castle of Clare, like a broken-down barrack or hospital. Now, ladies, I am informed your lords and husbands are determined to build one castle more before they finish or furnish those already on hand, they intend to erect an Italian opera house by subscription. Pray, ladies, how is this to be done? Will it not rouse, at this era of calamity, the inpineness of judgement, creditors and mortgages? ANTI-CASTRATO.'[19]

The attempt to establish Italian opera came to an end.[20]

The castle builders are of course Charlemont (the Casino), the Duke of Leinster (Leinster House), Lord Powerscourt (Powerscourt Town House), and Robert, Viscount Clare, Earl Nugent (Cabinteely House). The Duke of Leinster was Grand Master of the Grand Lodge of Ireland and Earl Nugent, the Junior Grand Warden. The implication is that Charlemont and Powerscourt were also Freemasons.[21]

NOTES

1. HMC Rept. 13, App. pt. VIII, pp. 382-3.
2. G. Breeze compiled, *Society of Artists in Ireland*, 1765-1780, lacking 1774, 1775, 1777, National Gallery of Ireland 1985.
3. B. Fitzgerald, ed. *Correspondence* Duchess of Leinster, Vol. 1, p. 70.
4. HMC, Rept. 12, App. pt. X, p. 203.
5. 'A Philosophical Survey of the South of Ireland', *Dublin Evening Journal* 9, May 1778.
6. R. Twiss, *Tour in Ireland in 1775*, London 1776, p. 24.
7. Ibid.
8. A. Young, *A Tour of Ireland 1776*, Dublin 1780, Vol. 1, p. 3.
9. Ibid, Vol. 2, p. 195.
10. HMC, Rept. 12, App. pt. X, p. 290.
11. *The Public Monitor or New Freeman's Journal*, Dublin 1772-3.
12. *Baratariana*, Dublin 1773.
13. *Public Monitor*, p. 205. (Dec. 19-21 1772).
14. Ibid, p. 249.
15. Ibid, (27 Mar. 1773), p. 282.
16. Maxwell, *Dublin under the Georges*, p. 80.
17. Young, p. 5.
18. *Dublin Evening Journal*, April 23 1778.
19. Ibid, 7 May 1778. 'Clare' refers to Robert, Earl Nugent 1776, Viscount Clare 1766.
20. T.J. Walsh, *Opera in Dublin*, 1973, pp. 184-199.
21. Indebted to the Archivist of the Grand Lodge of Ireland for this information.

26

PATRIOTS, POLITICIANS AND PEOPLE

The 'pleasing hours', much as Charlemont was enamoured of the Arts, could never, perforce as much as by inclination, be totally separated from politics. To fix the Graces upon his native shore demanded more than the building of an architectural masterpiece on Irish soil, or the making of Charlemont House a centre of learning and culture in Dublin. It was not enough to forego the pleasures of life in London and become resident in a country where, at first, he had no friends. His compatriots, unless shaken out of the state of their semi-barbarism, and abjection, and brought to a sense of national pride, would continue as before, the gentlemen only interested in 'claret, horses and dogs' and the ladies in 'dress and scandal'.[1]

Conscious from the first of those responsibilities attached to his inheritance, he had taken his seat in the Irish House of Lords on 7 October 1755, three months after his return to Ireland. While he kept a house in London for the next fifteen years, his visits there were strictly between sittings; when duty called he was to be found in Dublin or Armagh, the county to which he had been appointed Lord Lieutenant in 1748. As time went on he came to accept that mere duty was not enough, and only by a total and full involvement in Irish affairs, could he hope to serve his country.

It is perhaps difficult, in the light of Ireland's subsequent history and contemporary thought, to accredit to a nobleman of planter stock, whose loyalty was to the Crown, the most sincere patriotism and disinterested statesmanship. More particularly since he was a Northern Protestant and, while sympathetic to the miserable lot of his Catholic countrymen, his politics stopped short of Catholic emancipation.

Charlemont's effectiveness as a politician owed nothing to rhetoric. In the days of the great orators, he was incapable of any public speech, but his integrity and high-mindedness was never in doubt. His object was an Irish Parliament constitutionally free to govern

Ireland for the Irish, without pressure through fear and favour from England; and unlike so many of his peers, whose grovelling self-interest disgusted him, he could not be bought.

So tainted with corruption were the conferments, the honours and the sinecures by which England wielded power in Ireland that Charlemont was constantly at loggerheads with his Sovereign's Viceroy. When offered the Earldom for what he considered minor services, he hesitated and accepted only on the condition that he remained free to oppose the Government, and that it be understood that it was not for his own services, but for those of his ancestor, the first Lord Charlemont, for whom an earldom had been intended during the reign of James I.

Charlemont was never accused of running with the hare and hunting with the hounds, but through the friendships and connections formed on the Grand Tour, he was in a unique position to carry his views into the English camp. The story is told of Charlemont dining with Lord Rockingham and one of the company expressing his surprise that Charlemont, Lord Rockingham's friend, should oppose his Viceroy in Ireland. Whereupon, the noble Rockingham exclaimed, 'Lord Charlemont is perfectly right. He may approve of us here and, therefore, I presume, he would support us here; but we may be erroneous in some part of our conduct towards Ireland, and, if he thinks so, as the Irish Parliament is the more immediate sphere of his public duty, no doubt he should oppose us there.'[2]

Charlemont, for whom Adderley, with Francis as the unsuccessful candidate, had contested the Armagh election of 1753 on the side of the Opposition, had long since declared himself an independent. He had cut himself off, not only from the 'undertakers' of English interests, and the hated and wily Primate Stone (who acted during the Viceroy's absence), but from the Opposition party itself.

The small services, for which indirectly Charlemont received his Earldom, were (although Charlemont had chosen to live in and near Dublin), in the North, and among his own people and tenantry. When in February 1760, news had come of a French squadron having appeared in Belfast Lough and having taken Carrickfergus Castle, Charlemont, as Lord lieutenant of Armagh, hastened northwards. By the time he had reached Carrickfergus, the French, without moving on Belfast, had departed leaving behind only the wounded General de Flobert and a small party of men. The prisoner was brought back to Dublin, and all but fêted, before being released on parole to return to France. Charlemont was going to London and, at de Flobert's request, he accompanied him; de Flobert entrusting Charlemont with his money, for fear of brigands along the way.

Charlemont had seen how 'singular and formidable' had been the peasantry, many of them his own tenants, who with astonishing regularity and rapidity, had rallied in martial array to the defence of Belfast.[3] It was these men in their thousands who would later form the strength of the Irish Volunteers with Charlemont as their Commander.

In 1763 the Oak-Boy disturbances took him again to the North. Headed by farmers of respectable acreage, bands of four and five hundred men, wearing oak branches in their hats, were rampaging the country. They erected gallows and threatened 'ineffable perdition to all their enemies' in protest against the exactions of the clergy in their collection of tithes, and the heavy taxes laid on the country for the making and repairing of roads. Charlemont believed that, as usual, the people had in the beginning good reason for ill-temper, but would soon put themselves in the wrong by some outrageous excess, and he felt it his duty to intervene. He signified his intention to Primate Stone (acting for the Viceroy), who promised military backing. Charlemont considered it undesirable, and he rode north to see what he could do.

Reaching Newry, he was met by local gentlemen, who were much alarmed by the situation and advised he proceed no farther without a guard. Charlemont would not think of going into his own country with a military force. But after the gentlemen still urged the dangers, he consented to stay the night if scouts were sent out to test the mood of the insurgents. If the reports were unfavourable, he would set out in the morning, not with a guard, but with the gentlemen themselves, should they think it proper to accompany him. To this they agreed. The scouts returned with assurances from the leaders that they had no thought of molesting his Lordship and, accordingly, he rode on with the two gentlemen who had come with him from Dublin, and two servants, all of them armed.

They met with no resistance, but near to Armagh they came to a newly constructed gallows astride the road. This they were obliged to pass under, which Charlemont did with cool self-possession, commenting only on the excellence of the cord.

There was no violent cruelty and not a single life was lost. The insurgents, with the propensity of the 'the lower Irish' for jibes and jokes, obliged all who fell into their hands to swear they would not levy more than a proportion of the tithe or the tax. One Dr Clarke, 'a respectable clergyman', whom they alleged was the first to exact more than he was entitled to in tithes, they forced to go on the top of his own coach and dragged him through the country. It was a species of conduct, as Charlemont observed, that was in total contrast to the Catholic insurrections of the South, not because of the diversity of religion, but because of the greater oppression under which these unfortunate people laboured. 'A rebellion of slaves is always more bloody than an insurrection of freemen.'[4]

Charlemont remained in the North until order was restored; and although troops were brought in, it would seem that through his intervention, the gaols were not, as he feared, filled to unwieldy proportions and only the leaders were apprehended.

These small incidents, long lost in the shadow of subsequent and greater events, mark the beginning of Charlemont's political awakening through personal and practical involvement with the problems which confronted the country. An earlier assay would appear, at least on the surface, even more trivial since it was concerned primarily with ladies and their dresses. In fact it was the first, however puny a blow, struck by him in the cause of national identity.

For the marriage of the as yet uncrowned George III to Charlotte of Mecklenburgh-Strelitz on 8 September 1761, and the coronation on 22 of the same month, the Irish peeresses had bought expensive dresses only to be informed by the Vicereine, the very formidable Duchess of Bedford, that there would be no place for them in the procession. Charlemont, appealed to, took up the cause of the disappointed ladies in London to find no support from the Irish peers there; 'the honour of their country was an idea totally foreign to their thoughts'. Single-handed, he battled on alone, applying first to Lord Middleton, his former associate in the patriotic prank of the Carnival car in Rome, when national honour had also been at stake (albeit of a different nation.) Middleton accompanied him to Lord Halifax, the succeeding Viceroy to the Duke of Bedford, and the matter was brought to the King's attention, who ordered a council for the following day at which Charlemont was, to his astonishment and some distress, required to furnish precedents. Remembering at last Lord Egmont, an authority on heraldry and all such matters, and with only a few hours left, he appeared early in the morning with a thousand apologies, in that nobleman's bedchamber before he had risen and came away furnished with hastily written notes on precedents with which to strengthen his petition. His claim was violently opposed by Lord Delawar, but Lord Halifax was for him. No decision being arrived at, the matter was left to the King, and it was through Lady Hervey, having the ear of the influential Lord Bute, that it was settled that at the Coronation the entire Irish peerage would appear as a separate body.[5]

During Lord Halifax's Viceroyalty, the so-called Catholic question was brought to the fore. Charlemont, while advocating amelioration of 'the truly deplorable' situation of the Catholic gentry, stopped short of emancipation and, in this respect, his reputation as a totally disinterested patriot has suffered. But his own statement should dispel any notion of his Protestant bigotry or hatred of Catholics, of which even during his life time, he was unjustly accused.

'One measure, proposed by the Earl of Halifax's administration, was not, I confess, so disagreeable to me as it certainly was to the majority of Irish Protestants. The situation of the Catholic gentry of Ireland was, at this time, truly deplorable. The hostile statutes enacted against them, however their necessity may have ceased, were still unrepealed; and, respecting devise and inheritance, they laboured under the greatest hardships. In time, however, it might be hoped that these difficulties would be palliated, or perhaps removed; but they were subjected to one inconvenience, which was so interwoven with the existence of a Protestant interest and government, that sound policy, and, indeed, necessity, must for ever prevent its being remedied. Their sons were destitute of profession; the only occupation left them was foreign service, and of this they availed themselves; but as the French service, in which a national brigade had been formed for their reception, was that to which they most frequently resorted, they often found themselves compelled to fight against their king and their country ...'[6]

The measure, prompted by England's war with Spain, was to allow the Portuguese, Great Britain's allies, to raise among the Catholics of Ireland six regiments, to be officered by Irish gentlemen of the same persuasion and taken into the pay of Portugal. This measure was warmly opposed on the grounds of the danger of having so great a number of Catholics arrayed, armed and disciplined, who might at some unforeseen, but possible crisis, return to their native land and rise against a Protestant church and state. It was also said that Ireland could not spare so many of her inhabitants, particularly from the Catholic areas of the south and west, which were thinly peopled.

Charlemont wrote, 'Though I felt the weight of these arguments, the liberality of the plan was so pleasing to a youthful heart, free from prejudice, and deeply impressed with the wretched situation of my Catholic countrymen, that I could not help wishing its success; and the bigotted zeal, which evidently appeared to be the real basis of the opposition, undoubtedly added strength to my wishes.'[7]

But the very arguments that Charlemont at that time disputed, with reference to the many of his countrymen he had met abroad in foreign service, became the basis of his later opposition to franchise for Irish Catholics. Against the background of the revolution in France, a growing Catholic representation in Parliament would, in the end, he feared, break the connection with England, and then Ireland, not big enough or strong enough to stand on her own, would inevitably fall a victim to England's enemies.

At the very end of his life, he changed his opinion, but by then his dream of a separate kingdom was shattered. Though he did not live to see the Act of Union, he died knowing that it was inevitable and that Catholic emancipation, although in different circumstances than he would have wished, would eventually follow. Had not he been one of the first to try to alleviate the misfortunes of his Catholic countrymen by introducing the abortive Catholic Relief Bill of 1770, which being defeated at the third reading in 'the House crowded with zealous supporters of orthodoxy and oppression', (his own words), had left him, 'not wholely unsuspected of being little better than a Papist'.[8]

At this time Flood was the very able leader of the Opposition. He was successful in 1771 in having a money bill sent over by the Privy Council in London rejected, and for the second time, on the grounds that the bill had not originated in the Irish House. Charlemont and Flood, united in the cause of an independent Irish parliament, were close friends, and exchanged verse, criticism and gossip.

In 1775, Charlemont wrote, 'my friend Flood – the dear partner of my heart and of all its councils – anchor of my hope and pillar of my trust – Flood gave way, and deserted the glorious cause in which he had been triumphantly engaged', which is to say Flood accepted a seat in the Privy Council and the office of vice-treasurer at three and a half thousand pounds a year.[9]

But in 1775, 'By the vacancy which Mr Caulfeild's death occasioned in Parliament, the Electors of Charlemont were enabled, under the auspices of his Lordship, to return a man to the House of Commons, who was destined to act a more conspicuous part than any one who had been deputed to serve there'.[10] That man, of course, was Henry Grattan, who took his seat in the same session in which Flood became a minister.

The members for the Borough had been Francis and a Mr Moore. Adderley had been dismissed by Charlemont, in 1760, from all involvement in family, business and political affairs.

The exact causes of the quarrel are not easy to fathom, but from the copy Charlemont made of his letter to Adderley, 'the most disagreeable I ever wrote', it seems the bones of contention were 'the Affair of my Brother's marriage', Adderley's conduct in Parliament the previous winter and 'the Transaction with Miss Ward'.[11] Charlemont had considered Francis's marriage improvident. If he had doubts about Adderley's political and moral rectitude, these were later justified when, in 1783, Adderley as Treasurer of the Barrack Board was found, in an enquiry conducted by the Viceroy, Lord Temple, to be 'deficient in a very large sum'. Charlemont refused to use his influence to stay the action against him. As to Miss Ward, although a very different construction has been placed on this affair to the effect that Charlemont and Adderley were rivals for her hand,[12] according to Mrs Delany, Miss Ward, her neighbour at Mount Panther, Co. Down, was the daughter of a clergyman and 'with no great fortune'. She was to have been married to Mr Adderley.[13] But instead he had married Miss Margaretta Bourke, a co-heiress. Afterwards he became the member for Bandon and, in his favour, did much to establish linen and cotton industries around Innishannon.

Grattan, the new member for the Borough of Charlemont, the friend of Flood, who with him in *Baratariana* had written 'And Charlemont firm, may the Heavens reward him! Whose heart is still to us open, like his garden',[14] was now to supersede Flood in Parliament and in Charlemont's heart. Grattan's powers of oratory were surpassed only by Burke's. Both men had been educated at Trinity College, Dublin, and had been inspired by their studies of the orators of antiquity. The 'patriot party' could scarcely have dreamt of a more persuasive leader.

At the same time England's quarrel with her American colonies came to a head and in 1775 Washington was appointed Commander-in-Chief of the American army. Following the withdrawal of British troops from Ireland for America, fears of a French invasion began to outweigh Irish sympathy with the colonists. In 1778, eighteen years after Charlemont had seen the Belfast Protestants rally to the defence of their town, the whole of Ulster, with the same astonishing rapidity was ready to rally to the defence of the country and to place itself in arms under the leadership of the local gentry and nobility. Charlemont found himself commanding the first Company of the Armagh Volunteers.

By the following year the Volunteers of the City and County of Dublin, with Grattan their Colonel, and the Duke of Leinster in command, were parading in College Green before William III's statue, with brass cannon bearing the placard, 'Free Trade – or this'. The Volunteers were testing their political strength, much to the disquiet of Dublin Castle.

The movement gathering rapid momentum, there were soon 40,000, then 80,000 Protestant merchants, tradesmen and farmers in uniforms of Irish cloth, drilled and armed and officered by gentlemen, throughout the country conducting themselves with a business-like air and with a polish that was surprising in an irregular army. They brooked no authority but their own conventions and in 1780 they elected Charlemont to their head as Commander-in-Chief.

The danger of a French invasion receded, but the Volunteers continued to drill and their Commander to ride continuously from manoeuvres to reviews in all weathers, often under the strain of recurring ill-health, but untiringly devoted to the causes of free trade and a free constitution. A great spirit pervaded the land and the nation found its self-respect and confidence and, with the removal of trade restrictions, industry and agriculture moved into an area of prosperity.[15]

But as quickly had come those glorious days, so was their passing. Their effects would linger on until the infamous Act of Union, which Charlemont without living to see, would die knowing it to be inevitable. At the finest hour of the second Dungannon Convention of February 1782, presided over by Charlemont and Grattan with Flood, who had returned to the fold, all had agreed on the resolution that 'the claim of any other than the King, Lords and Commons of Ireland to make laws to bind this kingdom is unconstitutional, illegal and a grievance', and, equally so the powers exercised by the Privy Councils of both kingdoms under Poynings' law.*

Grattan's motion that 'as Irishmen, Christians and Protestants, we

* The repeal of Poynings' Law (1782) ended the right of the English parliament to legislate for Ireland.

rejoice at the relaxation of the penal laws against our Roman Catholic fellow-subjects', was carried. The relaxations were no more than Charlemont had always advocated. But when, in the Irish Commons, Grattan urged full civil liberties for the Catholics, neither Flood nor Charlemont were behind him. Further, while Grattan was content with the Constitution and the recognition of Irish parliamentary independence in the British and Irish Houses (May 1782), Flood wanted a formal Renunciation as a guard for the future, and on this point hostility flared into open and vindictive oratory between them.

At the third Dungannon Convention, 3 September 1782, in the absence of Charlemont and Flood, it was decided to hold a National Convention in Dublin in November. Charlemont regarded this with foreboding. It was apparent from the presence of the Earl-Bishop at Dungannon, that he intended to enter the arena as the newly appointed Colonel of the Londonderry Corps in an endeavour to promote his own reforming schemes for Catholic emancipation through the Volunteer movement. In this matter, if no other, Frederick Augustus Hervey, Lord Bristol, was consistent and sincere, but as Charlemont had anticipated, the Earl-Bishop, never content with the side lines, was dead-set on leadership and was preparing his move to oust Charlemont. His entry into the city was triumphal. Drawn in an open coach by six horses bedecked with purple ribbons, and attended by servants in magnificent livery, the Earl-Bishop sat making 'dignified obeisances'[16] to the gathered crowd. He was dressed in purple, his knee and shoe buckles were of diamonds, his gloves hung with gold fringes and tassels, and he wore the hat of a colonel of the Volunteers. A troop of Derry cavalry formed a guard of honour and behind came the carriages of his supporters.

Charlemont, who admitted he was often puzzled by the 'astonishing contradictions'[17] in the behaviour of this most eccentric man, was on this occasion ready for him. Anticipating a courtesy call at Charlemont House, he issued orders that a guard of infantry and a squadron of horse should be drawn up at the door to salute, as was fitting, the Derry troop on arrival. But he ordered that the Earl-Bishop's coach should be prevented from coming too close to the door, so that he should receive him at some distance from the house. This would ensure that the salute, as they walked together, should appear to be made to himself as General, and not to the Earl-Bishop. The ruse worked, and the Earl-Bishop, who understood perfectly, had difficulty in concealing his displeasure.

Out-witted by tactics that perhaps owed more to Charlemont's observation in Constantinople of the haughty Turk's reception of foreign ambassadors, than to his own inventiveness, the Earl-Bishop continued on his way, making a great display as he was driven through the city, only to be again thwarted at the Convention. It was Charlemont who was elected President of the Assembly.

Charlemont, who would not have thanked them for it had he known, had on his side the Castle, where he was regarded as manageable or at least predictable, which the Earl-Bishop was not. And the Castle faction, then in the person of the Earl of Northington, was doing all it could, through agents, to contribute to the general confusion of ideas and plans with which to harass the committees. Everybody was agreed on reform, but to what extent and how, could not be decided, and some of the schemes put forward were of the 'wildest and most ridiculous nature'.[18]

'The Bishop, disappointed of the chair, lost no time in rendering it a 'seat of thorns', and heckled the President at every opportunity. He taunted Charlemont with being timid or lukewarm on the issues of reform, and even with a change of heart. Charlemont was driven to defend his position. He would do everything to promote their object; except endanger the public peace and throw the country into civil war. And this was not without its point, as the Earl-Bishop in an earlier exchange had cried out, 'We shall have blood, my Lord, we shall have blood'.[19]

The Castle could hardly have dreamed of the level of their success in discrediting the Convention. Flood, forming an alliance with the Bishop, hastily drafted a reform bill in the face of Charlemont's opposition, and carried it straight from the Convention to the House. The bill, because of the manner in which it was presented, was immediately thrown out. Charlemont, before any more damage could be done, adjourned the Convention and, with that, virtually ended his political life, and any further close association with either Grattan or Flood, whose mutual jealousy and rivalry had, in any case, parted them.

As for his own arch-enemy and rival, Charlemont, who had in common with the Earl-Bishop, a love of Italy, travel, patronage and collecting, besides their inveterate building schemes, would describe him as an 'eccentric and baleful comet, whose short perihelium of unnatural heat is contrasted by ages of torpid frigidity'.[20]

NOTES

1. C. Maxwell, *Dublin under the Georges*, London 1946, p. 201.
2. Hardy, p. 116.
3. Ibid, pp. 57-9.
4. Ibid, p. 95.
5. Ibid, pp. 61-4.
6. Ibid, pp. 65-6.
7. Ibid, p. 67.
8. Ibid, pp. 190-1.
9. RIA, 12.R.7, p. 97.
10. Hardy, p. 184.
11. RIA, 12.R.9, no. 81.
12. Craig, p. 114.
13. Lady Llanover ed. Delany *Correspondence*, Vol. 3, p. 511.
14. *Baratariana*, Dublin 1773, p. 295.
15. Grattan on 16 April 1782 made the famous declaration, 'I found Ireland on her knees. I watched over her with paternal solicitude: I have traced her progress from injuries to arms, and from arms to liberty. Spirit of Swift, spirit of Molyneux, your genius has prevailed! Ireland is now a nation.'
16. HMC Rept. 12, App. pt. X, p. 121.
17. Ibid, p. 124.
18. Ibid, p. 124.
19. J.A. Froude, *The English in Ireland in the 18th Century*, London 1874, Vol. 2, p. 420.
20. RIA, 12.R.7, p. 550.

27

THE FRUITS OF AUTUMN

On 3 June 1782 Charlemont reviewed the Leinster Volunteers in Phoenix Park. To mark the occasion a linen printer of Leixlip, Co. Kildare manufactured a printed fabric, which he advertised as 'on cotton from copper plate a Volunteer furniture in chintz colours, which is an exact representation of the last Provincial Review in Phoenix Park'. The busy spectacle is presented with great attention to detail and some robust humour. Banners display the motto LOYAL AND DETERMINED. Red-coated and bayonetted soldiers stand to attention. Mounted officers on prancing dock-tailed horses accompany the General, as he reviews the troops, bareheaded with his tricorne hat in his hand, riding a splendid charger. Diminutive drummer boys beat their drums. Lady Charlemont watches from a carriage displaying the Charlemont cipher, with a wide-eyed child beside her, presumably her eldest son. Under the surrounding trees, picnickers gather and deer abound. One tree-climbing lad is tumbling towards a picnicker below. The flaps of the Volunteer tents are open to give a glimpse of the prepared victuals laid out on linen-covered trestle-tables within. Elsewhere, a small family group, presumably having overstepped the spectator's bounds, is seen off at the point of a volunteer's bayonet, a rent in the back of the lady's overskirt suggesting that he has been rather too rough. Over all Lord Chesterfield's Phoenix monument rears its august head.[1]

Meanwhile below in the city, in the Dublin Society's schools, cannon volley from the Park shook the foundations and sent Ajax and Apollo, the plaster casts in the figure room, reeling. Hercules stood firm. Instruction had to be abandoned, but Francis Robert West got the undivided attention of his pupils with a discourse upon Charlemont, Grattan and Flood. Using his brother as a foil, West played out the scene of Grattan's attack on Flood. While Grattan was undoubtedly the hero of the hour (a grateful nation had voted him £50,000), it was obvious to West's pupils that West's heart was with

Lord 'Charleymount' because he was the greater lover of the arts.[2] Charlemont had presented a number of casts to the schools, including the Laocoon.

On 12 June, Edmund Burke in a letter to Charlemont wrote, 'I find that Ireland among her other marks of her just gratitude to Mr Grattan (on which your Lordship will present my congratulations) intends to erect a monument to his honour, which is to be decorated with sculpture', and Burke went on to put forward the name of a young Irishman, John Hickey, whom he thought, as far as his judgement went, was 'fully equal to our best statuaries, both in taste and execution'. His employment would encourage 'the rising arts in the decoration of the rising virtue of Ireland ... I am sure there has ever been a close connection between them in your mind.'[3]

In 1782, four months after the Phoenix Park Review, Lord Temple (future Marquis of Buckingham) the newly appointed Viceroy, arrived in Ireland and intimated his Majesty's intention of creating an Irish Order of Knighthood.[4] Temple asked Charlemont if he might put his name on the list for the King's approval. Charlemont hesitated because, although the conception of an Order of the Knights of St Patrick was extremely gratifying, coming so soon after the establishment of an independent parliament, there was the consideration that, apart from the Duke of Leinster, the majority of the proposed Knights differed from him in 'every political principle'.

Temple was married to the daughter of Robert, Earl Nugent, and that may have contributed to Temple's better understanding of Charlemont's predicament. Earl Nugent, as Viscount Clare, had been one of those builders of castles 'founded upon the principles of masonic stability' so decried by *Anti-Castrato* in the *Dublin Evening Journal* four years before. At all events, Temple agreed to the Volunteers, in conjunction with the King's troops, manning the streets at the approach of St Patrick's Cathedral on the day of the Installation. Thus the Volunteers, with cheering crowds behind them, could salute their General, a distinction not accorded to the other knights.

John Keyes Sherwin painted the scene in St Patrick's Hall at the Castle that night, when the Knights rose to drink the King's health. Charlemont subscribed for three of Sherwin's engravings of the picture. They were never delivered. Three years later Horace Walpole, having seen in Paris the long run of portraits of the Knights of the St Esprit in the convent of Les Grand Augustins, wrote to Charlemont from Strawberry Hill to suggest something similar for the Knights of

St Patrick. He added, 'But it is unnecessary to dilate on the subject to your Lordship, who, as patron of the arts, as well as patriot, will improve on my imperfect thoughts'. Charlemont must have given the idea some thought because he wrote to ask if the Knights of the St Esprit were drawn in their robes of ceremony.[5]

But as patron of the arts, Charlemont's course was nearly run. His pecuniary affairs were in a very bad state. An ugly rumour circulated in Dublin that on Grattan's receiving his award from a grateful nation, Charlemont had asked him for a loan of £5,000 and been refused.

Yet it was Grattan who pointed out that 'without pay or reward' Charlemont had for years presided over a large army and 'helped to accomplish a great revolution without a drop of blood' and had 'cast on the crowd that followed him, the gracious light of his own accomplishments; so that the very rabble grew civilized as it approached his person'.[6]

That army whose presence – and flexing of muscle – had brought free trade, had indeed promoted industry and all the minor arts and crafts for the demands of the newly-opened market with the British colonies. The glass industry flourished, and not only commercial glass, but glass of the highest standard engraved with the mottoes and symbols of the Volunteers;[7] the uniforms, saddlery, swords and tents were all of Irish manufacture, besides the damask woven with Volunteer emblems for their banqueting tables. Fashionable ladies also proclaimed their patriotism by wearing cambric and poplin at assemblies and balls until, with such encouragement, the manufacturers came to produce silks, satins and velvets.

It was now more than twenty years since Secretary Hamilton had put books and whores on the same par, neither being acceptable socially, and it became the fashion to read. Hardy put this down to those officers, gentlemen of liberal education, whose association in the field with those less informed, made them so ashamed of their own ignorance that they were induced to study, if at first only military manuals, until reading became the vogue and then a habit.[8]

It gave Charlemont great satisfaction when English and Scottish booksellers came to Dublin to attend the sale of the Rt. Hon. Denis Daly's library, 'in the expectation of finding Ireland, a land of ignorance, where the best books might be purchased for a trible', he wrote to Edmund Malone.* 'During the week of the auction the Dublin

* Edmund Malone, 1741-1812, Irish lawyer, devoted his life to literature. Authority on Shakespeare, but best known now for his *Life and Works of Reynolds.*

world was book mad. All men bought, they who could and they who could not read, and the prices were more than London could have afforded.'[9]

Charlemont himself admitted to collector's mania and now, with money so short, occasional book-buying was all he could afford. Malone kept a list of his desiderata, mostly Restoration plays, and acted for him at London book sales. One remarkable purchase stands out. Malone acquired for him the series of drawings by Governor John White of the early State of Virginia.[10] The drawings are now in the British Museum.

Less than three weeks after Burke had written of the rising virtues and arts of Ireland, the Marquis of Rockingham, to whom Burke had been secretary, died.

It was not until the following year, May 1783, that Charlemont wrote to Dr Halliday of his expectations from his uncle's will – expectations which were sufficient at least for him to contemplate building again, this time the Rockingham Room, an extension to the west side of the garden corridor at Charlemont House, to be dedicated to the memory of his friend.

Gandon, who was to be the architect of the Rockingham shrine, had, as already mentioned, been recommended by Chambers in such way as almost to bequeath him to Charlemont. Gandon, however, was the protégé of Viscount Carlow, later Lord Portarlington (for whom he had designed Emo Court) and had already been brought to Ireland, through Carlow's good offices. He was to undertake the new Customs House for John Beresford, the Chief Commissioner for the Irish Revenue and the most powerful man in Ireland. Gandon was under enormous pressure of work as, at every stage of the building, there was trouble. The vast proportions, the impractibility of the design for its purpose, and the enormous public cost outraged the merchants. Their resentment was communicated to the masons, who made every difficulty another excuse to down tools. Dr Halliday, following a visit to Dublin, referred to the Customs House as 'the Seraglio of the Commissioner'. Nevertheless, Gandon felt he could not refuse Charlemont, his 'earliest patron and friend', with regard to the Rockingham Room. Gandon's lodging in Mecklenburgh Street, close by the Customs House and the nearby Turkish baths to which Charlemont went every Saturday, afforded opportunities for the two men to get together for gossip about the fine arts.[11]

Dr McParland has pointed out the similarities between the

Rockingham Room and the vestibule of Gandon's other major public building, the Four Courts.[12] A photograph taken in 1865, before the library wing of Charlemont House was demolished, shows the ghosts of the past foregathered in the Rockingham Room; the Emperors' busts recalling the faithful Murphy and the labours of Vierpyle in Rome, joining that of the man Charlemont had first known there as Lord Malton some forty years before.

Much time and trouble was taken over the Rockingham monument and it fell upon Burke to deal with Nollekens, the sculptor of the bust, in London. Burke wrote to Charlemont on 18 July 1787, 'When I go to town I shall see Mr Nollekens and hasten him as much as I can [how familiar we are with that phrase]; there was no bust taken from Lord Rockingham during his life time. This is made from a masque taken from his face after his death, and of course must want that animation which I am afraid can never be given it, without hazarding the ground work of the features. Tassie has made a profile in his glass, which is I think the best likeness, which exists. I will recommend it to Nollekens; perhaps he may make some advantage of it though I have observed that artists seldom endeavour to profit of each other's works ...'[13]

Part of the delay was caused by Lady Rockingham insisting upon supervising the work. On 21 October she wrote to Charlemont. '... I must now speak a word upon its Merits; the marble is as beautifully perfect as anything can be & I really am as contented with the Resemblance as it is possible to be about that sort of thing. I hope you will think it has greatly profited from the pains I took and the patience that the artist exerted in following my directions. Be so good as to place it for the right side of the bust to strike the eye first, the front and left side having not to my eye so strong a resemblance, but on the whole I hope it is worthy of the place your Lord has kindly destined for it; and your accepting it as a mark of my gratitude for so flattering a testimony of your Regard to the Original will be the highest satisfaction you can confer on me'.[14]

Lady Rockingham's gift of the bust was tactful and generous. In the words of a contemporary, Charlemont's 'very enlightened and pure taste in virtu' had made him 'poor as a rat'.[15]

Charlemont composed so lengthy an inscription for the front of the monument that even Hardy thought it would have been better had it been 'more compressed'. However the part in which Charlemont pays tribute to Rockingham's patronage of the arts is interesting because it reflects the standard to which Charlemont himself aspired.

> A Patron of all the Arts, useful and ornamental,
> His Perspicuity discovered,
> His Influence protected, his Liberality encouraged,
> His Courtesy distinguished, and animated
> Innumerable Votaries to true Genius,
> Whose Modest Merit might otherwise have been concealed
> And lost to their Country.[16]

Through lack of funds and the cessation of building, Charlemont's inspirational promotion of the fine arts in Ireland might have ground to a miserable halt. Yet there remained a project which was to absorb his energies and, still more to his satisfaction, open up new vistas of interest to which he could bring an almost youthful enthusiasm. It began with the deliberations of a few scholarly men, among them John Hely-Hutchinson, Provost of Trinity College; the Rt. Hon. Denis Daly; Lord Moira and Col. Henry Burton Conyngham. They were soon joined by Richard Lovell Edgeworth; General Charles Vallancey; a number of Fellows of Trinity and some distinguished churchmen; the Primate of Ireland, Richard Robinson; Lord Rokeby; and the Bishops of Clonfert, Dromore, Killaloe and Waterford. At a meeting of the 'Neosophical Society' on 29 March 1785, the members were informed of Charlemont's approval of the founding of an academy for the promotion of study in 'science, polite literature and antiquities', and the first meeting of the Irish Academy took place at Charlemont House three weeks later.[17] Charlemont was elected President shortly afterwards and, through his good offices with the Viceroy, the Duke of Rutland, the Academy received the Royal Charter.

Dr Thomas Leland died the year the Academy was founded, but it was his *History of Ireland*, and Vallancey's Irish Grammar, which gave impetus to the growing interest in Irish antiquity. Leland had been absorbed by his studies in this field and had found some response with Edmund Burke, who on discovering two volumes of ancient Irish laws in manuscript on a London bookstall, had presented them to him. A search for Irish manuscripts was instituted all over Europe, and rewarded by presents from Rome of manuscripts, prints and inscriptions through the interest of the titular Archbishop of Dublin, Dr Troy, and another Catholic, Chevalier O'Gorman, in

Paris. Lord Kenmare, one of the few Catholic peers, presented a gold gorget which, with manuscripts and some objects excavated by Sylvester O'Halloran from a tumulus in Co. Limerick, combined to form the nucleus of the Academy's collections.[18]

At the first session Charlemont delivered what he described as 'a trifling essay' on the 'Antiquity of Wollen Manufacture in Ireland'; his source the work of Fazio delli Uberti, which made for an agreeable fusion of his old studies with the new. Thereafter he was to read three more papers, including 'An Account of a Singular Custom at Metelin', which recalled his visit to Lesbos.

Grattan and Gandon were made members, and Sir Joseph Banks a corresponding member, as the Royal Irish Academy gained in strength and reputation. By modern standards the work was not systematic, but it opened up new avenues of learning and created intense interest in Ireland's prehistoric past. It helped to soften the prejudices against the more recent Gaelic traditions which the country people still treasured in their hearts. It paved the way towards the later Celtic revival.

Nobody attended the meetings more assiduously than Charlemont. All his remaining energy and talents were expended upon the Presidency, his last and crowning effort to fix the Fine Arts or, rather, the Liberal Arts upon his native shore. His patriotism assumed the colour of extreme nationalistic pride. One of the members complained to Edmund Malone, 'Our amiable friend the President is more wild and postures on the subject of Ireland more than you can conceive ... There has arisen in Ireland within a few years such a spirit of extravagant, fulsome self-adulation that it exceeds everything human vanity has hereto made pretensions to ...'[19]

Charlemont's swansong is fittingly commemorated in the finest handiwork of William Mossop, the Dublin medallist, who in 1786, struck the Cunningham medal for the Royal Irish Academy. Charlemont's portrait as a Knight of St Patrick in the uniform of the Irish Volunteers is on the obverse and on the verso a figure of Hibernia with emblems of Astronomy, Chemistry, Poetry and Antiquity. So pleased was Charlemont with Mossop's artistry that he invited him to visit Charlemont House whenever he liked to study his cabinet of medals. Charlemont remained President until the year of his death. He read two more papers, 'Some considerations on a controverted Passage of Herodotus' and 'Some Hints concerning the State of Science at the Revival of Letters, grounded on a Passage of Dante in his Inferno, Canto IV v. 130'.

While it can hardly be claimed that the name of the Academy is synonymous with that of its first president, there are grounds for remembering that Dr Johnson is said to have chosen not to have Charlemont as a founder member of the Literary Club because he feared 'We shall be called Charlemont's Club; let him come in afterwards'.[20] But undoubtedly Charlemont brought to the Royal Irish Academy the imprint of his experience of Scipione Maffei's assemblies of the literati at Verona; we see the shades of Maffei's methods in his invitation to Mossop for the study of the medal collection at Charlemont House.

NOTES

1. Pieces of the 'Volunteer Furniture' survive at Castletown, Co. Kildare, at the Masonic Hall in Dublin and the Museum of Fine Arts, Boston, USA.
2. J.D. Herbert, *Irish Varieties*, London 1836, pp. 54, 70.
3. RIA, 12.R.16, no. 87.
4. P. Galloway, The Most Illustrious Order of St Patrick, 1983, pp. 1-10.
5. Hardy, pp. 247-8.
6. Craig, p. 266.
7. C. MacLeod, *Irish Volunteer Glass*, National Museum, pp. 1-4.
8. Hardy, p. 208.
9. Maxwell, pp. 201-2.
10. L. Binyon, 'The Drawings of John White, Governor of Raleigh's Virginia Colony', *Walpole Society*, XIII, pp. 21-4.
11. J. Gandon and J. Mulvany, *The Life of James Gandon*, p. 80.
12. E. McParland, *James Gandon*, London 1981, p. 119.
13. RIA 12.R.16, no. 97.
14. Ibid, 12.R.15, no. 20.
15. McParland, p. 120.
16. Hardy, pp. 432-3.
17. T. O'Raifeartaigh, ed. *The Royal Irish Academy* 1788-1983, R.B. McDowell, 'The Main Narrative', pp. 9-12.
18. Ibid, pp. 19-20 and E.G. Quin 'Irish Studies' p. 176.
19. Sir J. Prior, *Life of Edmund Malone*, London 1860, p. 138.
20. Ibid, p. 88.

28

DECLINE AND DEATH

Charlemont died before the Act of Union, but he lived long enough to perceive that all he had worked for politically would, in the end, be of little avail. In spite of that era of real prosperity which parliamentary reform and the Volunteer movement had procured for the nation in the 1780s, no stable remedy for Ireland's ills had been found; when the United Irishmen, with revolutionary France at their back, uncovered the weak point in England's defences in the Rebellion of 1798, England had then the justification they needed to enact the degrading solution.

By the 1790s Charlemont had become that kind of venerable nobleman that he in his youth had admired. But unlike the Baron de Lastio de Vigouroux, Maffei and Montesquieu, who had each enjoyed (or at least it had so appeared to Charlemont), the well-being of fulfilment in their old age, Charlemont's final years were darkened by Ireland's tragedy, by the death of his second son James in 1793 at the age of seventeen, his own increasing ill-health, and his poverty.

He disdained any retreat from his misfortunes and continued as actively as his health allowed, but he took refuge in a life of almost military precision. Like his Sardinian majesty so many years before, he moved by the clock and was always to be found at the precise hour at the same place and, also like King Charles Emmanuel, he became absorbed with economy. Bent and decrepit and burdened by care and failing eyesight, he, not unnaturally, became prone to irritation and prejudice.

When Parliament was sitting he was unfailingly to be found in the House of Lords and, just as surely, in the Commons later and 'those who have sat next to him, during a debate, cannot forget the vivacity and justness of his remarks, on the different speakers.'[1] It was here that his irritability showed the most, but any rebuke that he delivered to a recalcitrant in the lobby afterwards, was couched with the suavity of manner for which he was famous.

When Parliament was in recess, he would ride out every morning until one o'clock, when he went to his library and remained there until dinner time. Still adding to and re-editing his *Traveller's Essays*, his history and translations of Italian poetry, and Latin, Greek and French epigrams, he also kept up a copious correspondence. The wonder was that with so many visitors and interruptions he found time to write at all. There were letters to Burke, to Baretti and Edmund Malone, but his most regular correspondent of the later years was Dr Alexander Halliday of Belfast.

One memorable visit to Charlemont House is mentioned in a letter from Robert Jephson to Malone. 'I was fortunate enough to get a sight of the famous Pamela,[2] as I happened to be sitting with Lord Charlemont when they both came to see his library. She is elegant and engaging, I think, in the highest degree, and showed the most judicious taste in her remarks upon the library and its curiosities ... She promised Lord Charlemont with great good humour, to assist him in keeping her husband in order.'[3]

But to keep Lord Edward in order was beyond the power of Charlemont, his brother the Duke of Leinster, or his mother the Duchess for, according to Jephson, 'He is turned a complete Frenchman, crops his hair, despises his title, walks the streets instead of riding, and thence says he feels more pride in being on level with his fellow citizens.' When the ill-fated Lord Edward died from wounds following his arrest on the eve of the 1798 Rebellion, Charlemont, appealed to by his family, was too ill and too near death himself, to do anything to protect Pamela and her children from the attainder of her husband's estate.

One suspects that, even in retreat at Marino, an orderly routine was maintained. He was aware of having become a habitudinarian and admitted as much to Dr Halliday when physicians prescribed the waters of Bath for his ailing daughter, and it fell upon him to accompany her and Lady Charlemont there. It was not pleasant for him to give up Marino, still less his library; but to absent himself from public life, where his endeavours might possibly be of some small use to his country, was the least pleasant of all.[4]

On the day of his departure many friends came to wish him farewell, and the streets were thronged with people expressing their good will with prayers for his safe return. His political influence had waned but his popularity was as great as ever.

While he was in Bath (he stayed there six months) there was a move among his friends and admirers in the North to set up a public monument to him with his statue. He was averse to the idea, but gave way to the extent that it should conjointly honour the Volunteers. The project came to nothing and, indeed as we see now, there was no need. Charlemont had erected his own monument at Marino. Dedicated to the principles of Whiggism and Neo-Classicism, the Casino and its setting were an expression of his concept of both.

As to the first, the historian W.E.H. Lecky wrote of him, '… he had personal qualities of a kind which often go further in politics than great brilliancy of intellect, and he was one of the few prominent Irish politicians who had never stooped to any corrupt traffic with the Government … He was a Whig of Whigs – with all that love of compromise; that cautious though genuine liberality; that combination of aristocratic tastes and popular principles; that dislike to violence, exaggeration, and vulgarity; that profound veneration for the British Constitution, and that firm conviction that every desirable change could be effected within its limits, which characterised the best Whig thought of the time.'[5]

The dedication of the Casino to William Pitt the Elder is a manifestation of his Whiggism, and there can be no doubt about his abhorence of violence. His arch-rival, the Earl-Bishop, might cry for blood, but Charlemont once commenting on the terrible hunting down of the White Boys when it became 'the fashionable chase' recorded, 'I have heard the Earl of Carrick, speaking of a successful Hunt, with his son a very young boy participating, pronounce the horrible words, "I have blooded my young Dog, I have fleshed my Blood Hound"'.[6]

As to the ideology of his Neo-Classicism, it is expressed in the epitaph he wrote for Chambers on the architect of the Casino's death in 1796. 'The Best of Men, and the First of English Architects Whose Buildings, Modelled from his Own Mind, Elegant, Pure and Solid, Will Long Remain the Lasting Monuments of that Taste Whose Chastity Could Only Be Equalled By the Immaculate Purity of the Author's Heart …'[7]

Far more than a new and fashionable form of art and a reaction against the frivolity and floridity of Rococo, Neo-Classicism was as much a moral as an aesthetic reformation. The Neo-Classicists turned to the virtue and excellence of the Ancients and found in antiquity a source of purity, precision, stability and elegance, and as this first generation of Neo-Classicists believed, the way to enlightenment and triumph over ignorance, superstition and injustice.

At the time of its conception and when building began on the Casino, say in 1759, the design would have been avant garde in England and much more so in Ireland. This might explain the lack of contemporary comment from Irish observers who, perhaps abashed by its extraneousness and sophistication, had remained silent, not knowing what to say. Foreign visitors were more voluble but even Dr Twiss, usually very ready to give his opinion, had found his way out in a superficial reference to a print and an inaccuracy as to its architect.

Charlemont had intended an ornament to his country upon which he could expend his passion for the arts and indulge his own artistry. 'I speak as an artist,'[8] he once wrote, and the phrase has been construed figuratively or as a reference to his literary endeavours. But there can be little doubt that the claim was based upon his creation of the templescape at Marino. It was Pope who said, 'All gardening is landscape painting ... just like a landscape hung up,'[9] and Marino with all its contrivances of perspective and contrasting light and shade was his chef d'oeuvre.

In 1790 Charles T. Bowden visited Marino and wrote, 'This is one of the most beautiful and elegant seats in the world, happily situated and in a demesne improved in the highest taste ... laid out in plantations, sheep-walks, lawns and a delightful park. There are sheep here with four, six and eight horns – the temple is situated in the park – a monument of his Lordship's refined taste. The Gothic room is a very curious and beautiful structure. The hermitage is nature itself. There is also a cane-house constructed after the Eastern model ... What obligations are not the citizens of Dublin under to his Lordship for having the gates of this terrestrial paradise opened to them whenever they chuse to walk through it!'[10]

Bowden was shown round the gardens, 'very civilly' by one Mr Adams, who had a neat house on the estate. The mention of Adams gives us an approximate date for some notes in Charlemont's hand under the heading 'Regulation of future Expenses at Marino'.[11] The notes are sad evidence of Charlemont's worries and impatience with the management of his costly paradise.

For all the world Marino was an idyllic retreat but while his friend Dr Halliday could imagine a pretty pastoral scene with Charlemont sitting among his haymakers, the master of Marino was testily noting 'this article has hitherto been extravagantly done, but for the future I shall expect to make Hay nearly as cheap as my neighbours'.[11]

While another friend, Sir Edward Newenham could write delightfully of a lamb given him by Charlemont (perhaps from the flock of Barbary or Jacob's sheep seen by Bowden), 'Your lamb has been all the evening in the library and made the Lap dogs give way by butting them',[12] Charlemont was trying to balance the costs between 'Sheep bought in to stock the farm' and 'Sheep sold with their prices and mutton consumed in the Family at the Current market price'.

As for the cultivation of pineapples (which once he had presented to Mrs Delany with pride), he wrote, 'I will believe they can never be had in Quantity or Perfection 'till a proper Stove is built for them; but with regard to Melons they can, I am sure, as no Convenience or expense has been wanting. I shall therefore for the future expect a Quantity of this fruit far greater than I have yet had, care must be taken to have them early, which has never yet been the case, and to have them only the best kinds, as the Cultivation of the inferior kinds is no sort of use, and is in fact so much Room, Culture and Expense totally thrown away.' He added, 'This Adams must attend to or expect the consequences. Early garden stuff will also be expected: fruit and flowers.'

His letters to Dr Halliday, began to reflect the same sort of tetchiness, the complaints of an ailing old man, preoccupied by failing health and eyesight and above all his own helplessness as the darkening clouds, which presaged the Union, gathered with increasing menace. Armagh was agitated by sectarian warfare and he was powerless to do anything about it. His efforts, by now feeble, to rally the old spirit of the Volunteers, had met with little response and the Opposition party had dwindled away to almost nothing. Having believed the dispersal of the French fleet and the gallantry and loyalty of the South, would unite the country in its gratitude for a providential escape, disillusionment brought despair. Again his spirits revived when his son, Francis William, was elected member for Co. Armagh and made a creditable maiden speech on 5 March 1798; but almost immediately came the Rising. Rumours of the Union put him into further misery and when the motion was rejected on 25 January 1799, for a moment he was jubilant. The temporary stay gave him a fresh burst of strength, but by April it was evident the time had come for him to die. His friends came in numbers to Charlemont House until he could no longer receive them.

As he lay on his death bed, he went through his papers, and Lady Charlemont, under his instructions, burnt piles of letters, poems, ballads and rhymes. The letters were, it was said, the volumes of correspondence with the Contessa at Turin and the Marchesa in Rome. Near the lake at Marino was a stone bearing the inscription, '*Le penchant nous unite Le destin nous separe*', but perhaps, the much quoted passage he had written to Baretti many years before was more apt. 'I may love Italy as a mistress, while my Native Country claims from me the proper and just regard due to a wedded wife.'[13]

He died on 4 August 1799. It was intended the funeral should be private, but a great procession of carriages and horsemen trooped along the road from Dublin to Armagh, where he was buried in the family vault in the Cathedral.

NOTES

1. Hardy, pp. 425-6.
2. Lady Edward Fitzgerald. She was French, beautiful and reputed to be the daughter of the Duc d'Orleans.
3. Prior, *Life of Malone*, p. 198.
4. Hardy, p. 320.
5. Craig, p. 268.
6. RIA, 12.R.7, p. 50.
7. Harris, p. 17.
8. HMC, Report 12, App.pt X p. 269.
9. J. Harris, *Lord Burlington, His Villa and Garden at Chiswick*, p. 198.
10. C.T. Bowden, *A Tour through Ireland*, Dublin 1791, pp. 78-9.
11. RIA, 12.R.21, no. 84.
12. RIA, 12.R.14, no. 65.
13. RIA 12.R.12 undated. 'Italy must with justice allways claim a great share in my Regard and Affection. Many of the best years of my Life most agreeably spent in that delicious Country renders it by one Degree only less dear to me than my native soil, Nay perhaps my affection to it may be even warmer. I may love Italy as a mistress, while my Native Country claims from me the proper & just regard due to a wedded wife.'

EPILOGUE

In the early hours of the morning of 26 December 1863, Francis William, 2nd Earl of Charlemont, at the age of eighty-eight, died at Marino House of bronchitis, following an attack of influenza. His four children had long predeceased him and the title devolved upon his nephew, Charlemont's grandson, James Molyneux Caulfeild.

Francis William had complied as faithfully as was within his power with the wishes of his father's will, that whatever had to be sold to meet his debts, Charlemont House and the Lodge of Marino, 'with 30 Acres of land adjoining same and the edifice erected on another part of ye lands of Marino known by the name of Casino with 30 acres of land about sd. Casino, which were granted to him in perpetuation by the Corporation of the City of Dublin … and all other edifices erected on same …' should be spared, together with his collections. On 8 March 1834, while all his children were still alive, Francis William drafted a will declaring the Pictures, Busts, Statues, Medals, Prints and Books left him by his father to be in the nature of heirlooms, and he directed that upon his decease proper inventories should be taken of the contents 'in and about my said Houses in Rutland Square and Marino respectively for the better information of such of my family as shall from time to time succeed thereto.' That inventory, if it was ever made, has never been found.

Faced with the task of raising money without disposing of the buildings or the collections, Francis William almost at once gained, by the revocation, at the Act of Union, of James I's Charter granting the right of the Borough of Charlemont to return two members to Parliament, the sum of £15,000. In 1802 he married Anne Bermingham, who was beautiful and also an heiress. In the same year he leased the lands of Marino around the Casino to William and Elizabeth Sophia Jolly for 90 years, 'provided the said William and Elizabeth Sophia and the survivor of them should so long live', for which he received £3000 and an annual rent of £300 until the lease lapsed at the death of William Jolly in 1833.

During the Jollys' tenancy the Casino and the Gothic Room fell into disrepair and by 1833 the Gothic Room was a ruin. Francis William set about restoring the Casino and redecorating it, and again the gardens and grounds were open to the public. Marino House acquired a parterre and other manifestations of Victorian taste in the garden around the house.

At the succession of the 3rd Earl in 1863, the dispersal of the collections and the dismantlement of Charlemont House began. In 1865 he sent the coins, medals and books to Sotheby, Wilkinson and Hodges for sale. A fire in the auction rooms destroyed the major part of the library. The doors and some of the chimney pieces from the house were removed to Russborough, Co. Tyrone, to be installed in the grandiose Gothicized chateau there, a massive extension of a neat house built by Francis William, the 2nd Earl in the 1840s. The sale of Charlemont House to the Government followed in 1870. In 1875 the contents of Marino House were put up for auction, and in 1876 Marino estate was sold. The house was demolished in 1921.

BIBLIOGRAPHY

F. Hardy, *Memoirs of the Political and Private Life of James Caulfield, Earl of Charlemont,* 1810

M.J. Craig, *The Volunteer Earl,* 1948

Edited W.B. Stanford and E.J. Finopoulos, *The Travels of Lord Charlemont in Greece & Turkey 1749,* A.G. Leventis Foundation 1984

Historical Manuscripts Commission, Twelfth Report, Appendix Part X, 1891; Thirteenth Report, Appendix Part VIII, 1894

Dictionary of British and Irish Travellers in Italy 1701-1800 compiled from the Brinsley Ford Archive by John Ingamells, 1997

Arthur Young, *A Tour in Ireland* 1776, 1777 and 1778, 1780

Constantia Maxwell, *Dublin under the Georges*, 1957

Edward Malins & the Knight of Glin, *Lost Demesnes*, 1976

John Harris, *Sir William Chambers, Knight of the Polar Star* 1970

INDEX